NAPLEX®

Prep

2019–2020

NAPLEX®
Prep
2019–2020

Cynthia Sanoski, BS, PharmD, FCCP, BCPS
Amie D. Brooks, PharmD, FCCP, BCACP
Emily R. Hajjar, PharmD, BCPS, BCACP, BCGP
Brian R. Overholser, PharmD, FCCP

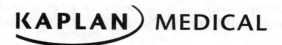

© 2019 Kaplan

Published by Kaplan Publishing, a division of Kaplan, Inc.
750 Third Avenue
New York, NY 10017

Printed in the United States of America

Retail ISBN: 978-1-5062-3596-7
10 9 8 7 6 5 4 3 2 1

Course ISBN: 978-1-5062-4559-1
10 9 8 7 6 5 4 3 2 1

Kaplan Publishing books are available at special quantity discounts to use for sales promotions, employee premiums, or educational purposes. For more information or to purchase books, please call the Simon & Schuster special sales department at 866-506-1949.

About the Authors

Cynthia Sanoski, BS, PharmD, FCCP, BCPS, is the chair of the department of pharmacy practice at the Jefferson College of Pharmacy at Thomas Jefferson University. Dr. Sanoski received her Doctor of Pharmacy degree from Ohio State University, and subsequently completed a 2-year fellowship in cardiovascular pharmacotherapy at the University of Illinois at Chicago. She is also a board-certified pharmacotherapy specialist and a fellow of the American College of Clinical Pharmacy. Dr. Sanoski serves as an instructor with Kaplan Medical, teaching NAPLEX review courses for graduating pharmacy students across the country.

Amie D. Brooks, PharmD, FCCP, BCACP, is a professor of pharmacy practice, director for the division of ambulatory care at the St. Louis College of Pharmacy, and a clinical pharmacy specialist in ambulatory care at St. Louis County Department of Health. Dr. Brooks is a fellow of the American College of Clinical Pharmacy. She received her Doctor of Pharmacy degree from the St. Louis College of Pharmacy and completed her pharmacy residency training at the Jefferson Barracks VA Medical Center in St. Louis, Missouri. Her research interests include clinical pharmacy services, diabetes, resistant hypertension, and collaborative practice.

Emily R. Hajjar, PharmD, BCPS, BCACP, BCGP, is associate professor in the Jefferson College of Pharmacy at Thomas Jefferson University in Philadelphia, Pennsylvania. Dr. Hajjar earned her PharmD at Duquesne University. She completed a pharmacy practice residency at the University of Rochester Medical Center in Rochester, New York, a geriatric pharmacy specialty residency at the Minneapolis Veteran's Affairs Medical Center, and a geriatric pharmacotherapy-epidemiology fellowship at the University of Minnesota, College of Pharmacy. Dr. Hajjar provides clinical services to the Jefferson Family and Community Medicine Senior Center Practice and the Kimmel Cancer Center Senior Adult Oncology and Outpatient Palliative Care clinics. Her research interests include geriatric pharmacotherapy and polypharmacy.

Brian R. Overholser, PharmD, FCCP, is associate professor of pharmacy practice in the College of Pharmacy at Purdue University and Adjunct Associate Professor in the Division of Clinical Pharmacology at the Indiana University School of Medicine in Indianapolis, Indiana. Dr. Overholser earned his PharmD and conducted his postdoctoral research in pharmacokinetics and pharmacodynamics at Purdue University. His primary teaching responsibilities include courses in pharmacokinetics, pharmacodynamics, and pharmacogenetics at both Purdue and Indiana University. Dr. Overholser's research program is focused on elucidating the pathological regulation that increases the susceptibility of arrhythmias in patients with heart failure.

The authors wish to thank the following expert reviewers:

Lauren Biehle, PharmD, BCPS
Clinical Assistant Professor of Pharmacy Practice
University of Wyoming School of Pharmacy
Denver, Colorado

Sarah Fowler Braga, PharmD, RPh
Associate Professor Pharmacy Practice and Director of
  Drug Information
South University School of Pharmacy
Columbia, South Carolina

Ashley Castleberry, PharmD, MAEd
Assistant Professor
University of Arkansas for Medical Sciences College of
  Pharmacy
Little Rock, Arkansas

Jamie Cavanaugh, PharmD, CPP, BCPS
Assistant Professor of Medicine
University of North Carolina
Chapel Hill, NC

Jill Chao, PharmD
Class of 2017
University of Houston College of Pharmacy
Houston, Texas

Kelly Clark, PharmD
Assistant Professor Pharmacy Practice
Coordinator—Integrated Pharmacy Skills Lab
South University School of Pharmacy
Columbia, South Carolina

Robert Clegg, PhD, MPH, MCHES
Associate Professor of Administrative Sciences
California Health Sciences University, College of Pharmacy
Clovis, California

Kimberly Ference, PharmD
Associate Professor
Wilkes University School of Pharmacy
Wilkes-Barre, Pennsylvania

Patrick R. Finley, PharmD, BCPP
Professor of Clinical Pharmacy
University of California San Francisco
San Francisco, California

Eric Z. Kao, PharmD
Class of 2017
University of Houston College of Pharmacy
Houston, Texas

Sonia Kothari, PharmD
PGY-2 Cardiology Pharmacy Resident
UMass Memorial Medical Center
Worcester, Massachusetts

Kelly C. Lee, PharmD, MAS, BCPP, FCCP
Professor of Clinical Pharmacy
UCSD Skaggs School of Pharmacy and Pharmaceutical
  Sciences
La Jolla, California

Megan Maroney, PharmD, BCPP
Clinical Associate Professor
Ernest Mario School of Pharmacy
Rutgers, The State University of New Jersey
Psychiatric Clinical Pharmacist
Monmouth Medical Center
Long Branch, New Jersey

Santhi Masilamani, PharmD, CDE, MBA
Director, Ambulatory APPE
University of Houston College of Pharmacy
Houston, Texas

Quamrun N. Masuda, PhD, RPh
Associate Professor (Pharmaceutics) & Assistant
  Director of the Center for Compounding Practice &
  Research
Virginia Commonwealth University, School of
  Pharmacy
Richmond, Virginia

Rebecca Stauffer, PharmD, BCPS
Assistant Professor
St. Louis College of Pharmacy
St. Louis, Missouri

James A. Trovato, PharmD, MBA, BCOP, FASHP
Associate Professor and Vice Chair for Academic
  Affairs
Department of Pharmacy Practice and Science
University of Maryland School of Pharmacy
Baltimore, Maryland

Ashley H. Vincent, PharmD, BCACP, BCPS
Clinical Assistant Professor, Purdue University College
  of Pharmacy
Indiana University School of Medicine
Indianapolis, Indiana

The authors also wish to thank the following test item writers: LeAnn C. Boyd, PharmD, BCPS, CDE; Elizabeth Langan, MD; Amy Egras, PharmD, BCPS; Stacey Thacker, PharmD; and Arneka Tillman, PharmD candidate, Xavier College of Pharmacy; and test item reviewers: Brittany Hoffmann-Eubanks, PharmD, MBA; and Michelle A. Vermeulen, PharmD.

The authors would also like to acknowledge the contributions of Karen Nagel, BS Pharm, PhD, and Steven T. Boyd, PharmD, PCPS, CDE.

Table of Contents

NOTE: Sections in gray appear in the digital version of this book only. See the "How to Use This Book" section for more details.

PART THREE: Pharmaceutical Sciences, Calculations, Biostatistics, and Clinical Trial Design

PART FOUR: Resources and Policy

Part One

Overview

How to Use This Book

Congratulations! You've taken the first step to prepare yourself for the NAPLEX®. The content of this book is designed to provide a concentrated and concise review of the competency areas tested on the NAPLEX. This book is not intended to replace standard textbooks in pharmacy. Rather, it should serve as a primary tool in the weeks and months prior to taking the exam. Our intention—and our hope—is that this book will be an integral part of your preparation for the NAPLEX.

Step 1: Access Your Online Center

The 2019–2020 edition of this NAPLEX review is delivered both in print and online. Log on to *kaptest.com/NAPLEX2019* to access your online center. You will be asked for a password derived from the text to access the online center, so have your book handy when you log on.

Your online center resources include the following:

- The **digital version** of the book, including all 31 content review chapters *plus* an exam overview and Kaplan's exclusive test-taking strategies.
- Chapter **quizzes** to assess your strengths and weaknesses as you complete each content area.
- **Two full-length practice tests**, each with 250 unique questions.

Step 2: Familiarize Yourself with the Digital Book

The digital version of *NAPLEX Prep 2019–2020* covers all of the areas tested on the NAPLEX in 31 chapters, arranged by disease state (such as pulmonary disorders) or concept discipline (such as pharmaceutics or biostatistics). The digital book is the master version of *NAPLEX Prep 2019–2020*.

Each disease-state chapter focuses on the following:

- Definitions of the disease
- Diagnosis
- Signs and symptoms
- Guidelines
- Guidelines summary
- Drug tables (*author-determined "Top 200" drugs are indicated with a star*)
- Storage and administration pearls
- Patient education pearls

Step 3: Familiarize Yourself with the Print Book

The printed version of *NAPLEX Prep 2019–2020* is a subset of the digital book. This smaller guide highlights content areas that the authors regard as high-yield—that is, content areas that are especially likely to be tested. For example, Chapter 2: Infectious Diseases appears in both the digital book and the print book, while Chapter 19: Special Populations appears in the digital book only.

Within the chapters, the print book focuses on types of information that can be studied on-the-go. For instance, all drug tables appear in the print book, because they are ideal for piecemeal study. Each disease state chapter in the print book presents only the following:

- Disease state
- Guidelines summary
- Summary of treatment recommendations
- Overview of treatment (if applicable)
- Treatment algorithm (if applicable)
- Drug tables

Step 4: Take the First Online Practice Test

You should take Practice Test 1 before the beginning of your study period. Take the exam in a quiet area with a good Internet connection, and dedicate 6 hours to the test. This is the same per-question allotment as on the current 250-question NAPLEX exam. The goal is to simulate exam conditions, so eliminate distractions like your cell phone.

When the test is completed, you will receive immediate feedback on your performance as the software analyzes your strengths and weaknesses in various content areas. Use the results to identify your areas of strength and weakness and tailor an individualized study plan for yourself. For example, if you score below average on questions related to oncology therapeutics, plan to spend additional time studying this subject, whereas if cardiovascular therapeutics was the area in which you scored the highest, you might opt to leave this section for last when studying.

As you review the results of Practice Test 1, pay particular attention to the answer explanations. Studying the answer explanations is often one of the most valuable study methods. Note that explanations provide the reasoning for *not* choosing the incorrect answer choices. Use this information to understand the rationale behind eliminating each distracter.

Step 5: Start Your Content Review

Kaplan recommends that you begin your study in the areas that you have determined are your weakest; in this way, you can spend additional review time on difficult concepts. Each chapter in the digital book gives a suggested study time, prepared by the authors. Adjust these times based on the results of Practice Test 1 and the overall amount of time in your study-time "budget." Be sure to take each end-of-chapter practice quiz to assess how well you have retained the material.

Step 6: Take the Second Online Practice Test

You should take Practice Test 2 once you have completed the majority of your study—a week or two prior to your exam date. It is also a full-length online exam with 250 unique questions. Take Practice Test 2 in a quiet, distraction-free area with a good Internet connection, and dedicate 6 hours to the test.

Best of luck to you on your journey toward a successful career as a pharmacist!

TEST CHANGES OR LATE-BREAKING DEVELOPMENTS

kaptest.com/publishing

The material in this book is up-to-date at the time of publication. However, the NABP® may have instituted changes in the test after this book was published. Be sure to carefully read the materials you receive when you register for the test. If there are any important late-breaking developments—or any changes or corrections to the Kaplan test preparation materials in this book—we will post that information online at kaptest.com/publishing.

Part Two

Review of Therapeutics

Cardiovascular Disorders

1

This chapter covers the following topics:

- **Hypertension**
- **Dyslipidemia**
- **Heart failure**
- **Antiarrhythmic drugs**
- **Antithrombotic drugs**
- **Ischemic heart disease**
- **Acute pharmacologic management of UA/NSTEMI**
- **Acute pharmacologic management of STEMI**
- **Secondary prevention of MI**

HYPERTENSION

Guidelines Summary

- BP treatment thresholds (i.e., when to start antihypertensive medications) (AHA/ACC guidelines)
    - Secondary prevention of cardiovascular disease (CVD): ≥130/80 mmHg
    - Primary prevention of CVD in patients with a 10-year atherosclerotic cardiovascular (ASCVD) risk score ≥10%: ≥130/80 mmHg
    - Primary prevention of CVD in patients with a 10-year ASCVD risk score <10%: ≥140/90 mmHg

Treatment Recommendations (AHA/ACC Guidelines)

BP Category	Treatment Recommendation	Time to Follow-Up
Normal (BP <120/80 mmHg)	Encourage optimal lifestyle habits	1 yr
Elevated (BP 120–129/<80 mmHg)	Nonpharmacological therapy	3–6 mo
Stage 1 HTN (BP 130–139/80–89 mmHg) with clinical ASCVD or 10-yr ASCVD risk score ≥10%	Nonpharmacological therapy + antihypertensive medication	1 mo; if BP goal met, reassess in 3–6 mo; if BP goal not met, optimize adherence and consider therapy intensification and reassess in 1 mo (once goal met can reassess in 3–6 mo)
Stage 1 HTN (BP 130–139/80–89 mmHg) without clinical ASCVD or 10-yr ASCVD risk score <10%	Nonpharmacological therapy	3–6 mo
Stage 2 HTN (BP ≥140/90 mmHg)	Nonpharmacological therapy + antihypertensive medication (2 medications of different classes)	1 mo; if BP goal met, reassess in 3–6 mo; if BP goal not met, optimize adherence and consider therapy intensification and reassess in 1 mo (once goal met, can reassess in 3–6 mo)

- BP goals
  - CVD or 10-year ASCVD risk score ≥10%: <130/80 mmHg (recommended) (AHA/ACC HTN guidelines)
  - Without additional markers of CVD: <130/80 mmHg (reasonable) (AHA/ACC HTN guidelines)
  - Older adults (≥65 years old): SBP <130 mmHg (AHA/ACC Guidelines)
  - Stable ischemic heart disease (SIHD): <130/80 mmHg (AHA/ACC HTN guidelines)
  - HF
    » HFrEF: <130/80 mmHg (AHA/ACC HTN guidelines)
    » HFpEF: SBP <130 mmHg (AHA/ACC HTN guidelines)
    » SBP <130 mmHg (ACC/AHA/Heart Failure Society of America focused update)
  - CKD
    » <130/80 mmHg (AHA/ACC HTN guidelines)
    » Urine albumin excretion <30 mg/day: <140/90 mmHg (KDIGO guidelines)
    » Urine albumin excretion ≥30 mg/day: <130/80 mmHg (KDIGO guidelines)
  - Stroke/TIA: <130/80 mmHg (AHA/ACC HTN guidelines)
  - Diabetes mellitus (DM)
    » <130/80 mmHg (AHA/ACC HTN guidelines)
    » <140/90 mmHg (American Diabetes Association guidelines)

- Lifestyle modifications: Weight loss (goal body mass index [BMI] 18.5–24.9 kg/m^2), diet rich in fruits, vegetables, and low-fat dairy products with ↓ saturated and total fat, ↓ sodium (Na$^+$) intake (<1,500 mg/day), potassium (K+) supplementation (3,500–5,000 mg/day) (unless with CKD), ↑ physical activity (90–150 minutes/week), moderation of alcohol use (≤2 drinks/day [men], ≤1 drink/day [women]), smoking cessation
- Pharmacologic therapy
  - Initial antihypertensive drug selection (AHA/ACC guidelines)
    » First-line agents: Thiazide diuretic, calcium channel blocker (CCB), angiotensin-converting enzyme inhibitor (ACEI), angiotensin II receptor blocker (ARB)
    » Black patients (with or without DM; without HF or CKD): Thiazide diuretic, CCB
  - Presence of other comorbidities may warrant selection of other agents as first-line antihypertensive therapy (based on AHA/ACC guidelines and hypertension guidelines for each of these conditions).
    » HFrEF: Diuretic, ACEI (or ARB), β-blocker (carvedilol, metoprolol succinate, or bisoprolol), aldosterone receptor antagonist (ARA), angiotensin receptor–neprilysin inhibitor
    » HFpEF: Diuretic, ACEI (or ARB), β-blocker
    » SIHD: β-blocker, ACEI (or ARB)
    » CKD (≥Stage 3 or Stage 1 or 2 with albuminuria [≥300 mg/day or ≥300 mg/g albumin-to-creatinine ratio]): ACEI (or ARB)
    » Secondary stroke prevention: Thiazide diuretic, ACEI, ARB
    » DM, no albuminuria: Thiazide diuretic, CCB (dihydropyridine as per American Diabetes Association guidelines), ACEI, ARB
    » DM with albuminuria: ACEI or ARB
  - Three approaches for initiation and titration of antihypertensive therapy:
    » Initiate one antihypertensive drug → Titrate to maximum dose to achieve goal BP → If goal BP not achieved, add second antihypertensive drug → Titrate dose of second drug to maximum → If goal BP still not achieved, add third antihypertensive drug
      – Avoid concomitant use of ACEI, ARB, and/or renin inhibitor
    » Initiate one antihypertensive drug → If goal BP not achieved, add second antihypertensive drug before maximum dose of initial drug achieved → If goal BP not achieved, titrate doses of both drugs up to maximum → If goal BP still not achieved, add third antihypertensive drug
      – Avoid concomitant use of ACEI and ARB

» Initiate two antihypertensive drugs at same time (avoid concomitant use of ACEI and ARB) → If goal BP not achieved, titrate doses of both drugs up to maximum → If goal BP still not achieved, add third antihypertensive drug

– Initiate two antihypertensive agents of different classes in patients with stage 2 HTN and an average BP >20/10 mmHg above their BP goal

Diuretics

Generic • Brand • Dose	Contra-indications	Primary Side Effects	Key Monitoring	Pertinent Drug Interactions	Med Pearl
Thiazide Diuretics – inhibit Na$^+$ reabsorption in the distal convoluted tubule					
Chlorothiazide • Diuril • 500–2,000 mg/day • Chlorthalidone ☆ • Only available generically • 12.5–100 mg/day Hydrochlorothiazide ☆ • Microzide • 12.5–50 mg/day Indapamide • Only available generically • 1.25–5 mg/day Metolazone ☆ • Zaroxolyn • 2.5–5 mg/day	Sulfa allergy	• Hypokalemia • Hypomagnesemia • Hyponatremia • Hypercalcemia • Hyperglycemia • Hyperuricemia • Photosensitivity	• BP • Electrolytes • Blood urea nitrogen (BUN)/serum creatinine (SCr) • Blood glucose • Uric acid	• May ↑ risk of lithium toxicity • May ↓ effect of antidiabetic agents • NSAIDs ↓ antihypertensive effects	• Often used as first-line therapy for HTN • Synergistic effect with other antihypertensives • Not effective (except metolazone) when creatinine clearance (CrCl) <30 mL/min; use loop diuretics • Have ceiling dose (unlike loop diuretics) • Chlorothiazide also available as injection
Loop Diuretics – inhibit Na$^+$ reabsorption in the ascending limb of loop of Henle (should only be used for HTN in patients with renal impairment [maintain efficacy when CrCl <30 mL/min], severe edema, or HF) (see HF section for further details)					
Potassium-Sparing Diuretics – inhibit Na$^+$ reabsorption in the collecting ducts					
Amiloride • Only available generically • 5–10 mg/day Triamterene • Dyrenium • 50–100 mg/day	• Hyperkalemia • CKD	Hyperkalemia	• BP • K$^+$ • BUN/SCr	Use with K$^+$ supplements, ACEIs, ARBs, ARAs, or NSAIDs may ↑ risk of hyperkalemia	• Not used often as monotherapy (weak antihypertensives) • Often used with hydrochlorothiazide to ↓ K$^+$ loss

Combination products:
    Triamterene/hydrochlorothiazide (Dyazide, Maxzide)
    Amiloride/hydrochlorothiazide (only available generically)					

Aldosterone Receptor Antagonists – have similar mechanism of action to K$^+$-sparing diuretics (also block the effects of aldosterone) (not used often for HTN) (see HF section for further details)					
Combination products: Spironolactone/hydrochlorothiazide (Aldactazide)					

β-Blockers

Generic • Brand • Dose	Contraindications	Primary Side Effects	Key Monitoring	Pertinent Drug Interactions	Med Pearl

Mechanism of action – ↓ cardiac output (CO) by negative inotropic (↓ contractility) and negative chronotropic (↓ heart rate [HR]) effects
• Cardioselective – bind more to β$_1$ than β$_2$ receptors (at low doses); less likely to cause bronchoconstriction or vasoconstriction at low doses (safer to use in patients with asthma, chronic obstructive pulmonary disease [COPD], PAD, or DM); cardioselectivity may be lost at higher doses
    – Bisoprolol, atenolol, metoprolol, betaxolol, acebutolol, nebivolol (BAMBAN)
• Intrinsic sympathomimetic activity (ISA) – have partial β-receptor agonist activity
    – Carteolol, acebutolol, pindolol, penbutolol (CAPP)
• Lipophilic vs. hydrophilic – lipophilic (propranolol, metoprolol, carvedilol, labetalol, pindolol, nebivolol) more likely to cause central nervous system (CNS) side effects (e.g., depression, fatigue) than hydrophilic (atenolol)					

Cardioselective					
Acebutolol • Only available generically • 200–1,200 mg/day Atenolol ☆ • Tenormin • 25–100 mg/day Betaxolol • Only available generically • 5–20 mg/day Bisoprolol • Only available generically • 2.5–20 mg/day Metoprolol ☆ • Tartrate: Lopressor (2 × daily), Succinate: Kapspargo Sprinkle, Toprol XL (1 × daily) • 25–400 mg/day Nebivolol ☆ • Bystolic • 5–40 mg/day	• ≥2nd degree heart block (in absence of pacemaker) • HF (except metoprolol succinate or bisoprolol)	• Bradycardia/heart block • HF exacerbation • Bronchospasm • Cold extremities • Fatigue • ↓ exercise tolerance • Depression • Glucose intolerance • Mask hypoglycemia (in patients with DM)	• BP • HR • S/S of HF • Blood glucose (in patients with DM)	Use with other negative chronotropes (e.g., digoxin, verapamil, diltiazem, clonidine, or ivabradine) may ↑ risk of bradycardia	• Abrupt discontinuation may cause angina, MI, or hypertensive emergency; need to taper over 2 wk • Metoprolol tartrate also available as injection • Metoprolol succinate also available as oral capsule sprinkle (Kapspargo)

β-Blockers *(cont'd)*

Generic • Brand • Dose	Contraindications	Primary Side Effects	Key Monitoring	Pertinent Drug Interactions	Med Pearl
Nonselective					
Carvedilol ☆ • Coreg, Coreg CR • Immediate-release (IR): 12.5–50 mg/day (in two divided doses) • Controlled-release (CR): 20–80 mg/day (1 × daily) Labetalol • Trandate • 200–2,400 mg/day Nadolol • Corgard • 20–320 mg/day Pindolol • Only available generically • 5–60 mg/day Propranolol ☆ • Inderal, Inderal LA, InnoPran XL • 80–640 mg/day (IR given 2–3 × daily; extended-release [ER] given 1 × daily) Timolol • Only available generically • 20–60 mg/day	• ≥2nd degree heart block (in absence of pacemaker) • HF (except carvedilol)	Same as with cardioselective β-blockers	Same as with cardioselective β-blockers	Same as with cardioselective β-blockers	• Same as with cardioselective β-blockers • Labetalol and carvedilol also have α_1-blocking properties • Labetalol and propranolol also available as injection

Combination products:

Atenolol/chlorthalidone (Tenoretic)
Bisoprolol/hydrochlorothiazide (Ziac)

Metoprolol tartrate/hydrochlorothiazide (Lopressor HCT)
Metoprolol succinate/hydrochlorothiazide (Dutoprol)

Nadolol/bendroflumethiazide (Corzide)
Nebivolol/valsartan (Byvalson)
Propranolol/hydrochlorothiazide (only available generically)

Angiotensin-Converting Enzyme Inhibitors

Generic • Brand • Dose	Contra-indications	Primary Side Effects	Key Monitoring	Pertinent Drug Interactions	Med Pearl
Mechanism of action – inhibit angiotensin-converting enzyme and prevent the conversion of angiotensin I to angiotensin II → vasodilation, ↓ aldosterone production; also inhibit degradation of bradykinin					
Benazepril☆ • Lotensin • 5–40 mg/day Captopril • Only available generically • 12.5–450 mg/day Enalapril☆ • Epaned, Vasotec • 2.5–40 mg/day Fosinopril☆ • Only available generically • 5–80 mg/day Lisinopril☆ • Prinivil, Qbrelis, Zestril • 2.5–40 mg/day Moexipril • Only available generically • 3.75–30 mg/day Perindopril • Only available generically • 4–16 mg/day Quinapril☆ • Accupril • 10–80 mg/day Ramipril☆ • Altace • 1.25–20 mg/day Trandolapril☆ • Only available generically • 0.5–4 mg/day	• Pregnancy • History of angioedema or renal failure with prior use • Hyperkalemia • Bilateral renal artery stenosis • Concurrent use with aliskiren in DM	• Hyperkalemia • Renal impairment • Cough (dry) • Angioedema	• BP • BUN/SCr • K⁺	• Use with K⁺ supplements, K⁺-sparing diuretics, ARAs, or NSAIDs may ↑ risk of hyperkalemia • Use with ARBs or aliskiren may ↑ risk of hyperkalemia and renal impairment (avoid concurrent use with aliskiren in DM and CrCl <60 mL/min) • May ↑ risk of lithium toxicity • Use with sirolimus, temsirolimus, or everolimus may ↑ risk of angioedema • Use with sacubitril/valsartan may ↑ risk of angioedema; do not use within 36 hr of switching to/from sacubitril/valsartan	• Captopril has shortest duration of action • Enalapril also available as oral solution (Epaned) and injection (enalaprilat) • Lisinopril also available as oral solution (Qbrelis) • If patient has intolerable dry cough, may switch to ARB • Hyperkalemia and renal impairment also likely to occur with ARBs (risk of angioedema cross-sensitivity with ARBs controversial)

Combination products:
 	
   Benazepril/amlodipine (Lotrel)
   Benazepril/hydrochlorothiazide (Lotensin HCT)
   Captopril/hydrochlorothiazide (only available generically)
		Enalapril/hydrochlorothiazide (Vaseretic)
		Fosinopril/hydrochlorothiazide (only available generically)
		Lisinopril/hydrochlorothiazide (Zestoretic)
				Moexipril/hydrochlorothiazide (only available generically)
				Perindopril/amlodipine (Prestalia)
				Quinapril/hydrochlorothiazide (Accuretic)
				Trandolapril/verapamil (Tarka)	

Angiotensin II Receptor Blockers

Generic • Brand • Dose	Contra-indications	Primary Side Effects	Key Monitoring	Pertinent Drug Interactions	Med Pearl
Mechanism of action – inhibit the binding of angiotensin II to the angiotensin type 1 (AT_1) receptor → vasodilation, ↓ aldosterone production; no effect on bradykinin					
Azilsartan • Edarbi • 40–80 mg/day	Same as for ACEIs	• Same as for ACEIs (except no cough) • Sprue-like enteropathy (olmesartan)	Same as for ACEIs	• Use with K+ supplements, K+- sparing diuretics, ARAs, or NSAIDs may ↑ risk of hyperkalemia • Use with ACEIs or aliskiren may ↑ risk of hyperkalemia or renal impairment (avoid concurrent use with aliskiren in DM and CrCl <60 mL/min) • May ↑ risk of lithium toxicity	• Hyperkalemia and renal impairment also likely to occur with ACEIs (risk of angioedema cross-sensitivity with ACEIs is controversial) • Valsartan also available as oral solution (Prexxartan)
Candesartan • Atacand • 4–32 mg/day					
Eprosartan • Only available generically • 400–800 mg/day					
Irbesartan ☆ • Avapro • 75–300 mg/day					
Losartan ☆ • Cozaar • 25–100 mg/day					
Olmesartan ☆ • Benicar • 20–40 mg/day					
Telmisartan ☆ • Micardis • 20–80 mg/day					
Valsartan ☆ • Diovan, Prexxartan • 80–320 mg/day					

Combination products:

Azilsartan/chlorthalidone (Edarbyclor)
Candesartan/hydrochlorothiazide (Atacand HCT)
Irbesartan/hydrochlorothiazide (Avalide)
Losartan/hydrochlorothiazide (Hyzaar)

Olmesartan/amlodipine (Azor)
Olmesartan/amlodipine/hydrochlorothiazide (Tribenzor)
Olmesartan/hydrochlorothiazide (Benicar HCT)
Telmisartan/amlodipine (Twynsta)

Telmisartan/hydrochlorothiazide (Micardis HCT)
Valsartan/amlodipine (Exforge)
Valsartan/hydrochlorothiazide (Diovan HCT)
Valsartan/amlodipine/hydrochlorothiazide (Exforge HCT)

Renin Inhibitor

Generic • Brand • Dose	Contra-indications	Primary Side Effects	Key Monitoring	Pertinent Drug Interactions	Med Pearl
Mechanism of action – inhibits renin and prevents the conversion of angiotensinogen to angiotensin I, which then ↓ production of angiotensin II					
Aliskiren ☆ • Tekturna • 150–300 mg/day	• Pregnancy • History of ACEI- or ARB-induced angioedema • Hyperkalemia • Bilateral renal artery stenosis • Use with ACEIs or ARBs in DM	• Headache • Dizziness • Diarrhea • Hyperkalemia • Renal impairment	• BP • BUN/SCr • K+	• Use with K+ supplements, K+-sparing diuretics, ARAs, or NSAIDs may ↑ risk of hyperkalemia • Use with ACEIs or ARBs may ↑ risk of hyperkalemia or renal impairment (avoid concurrent use in DM and CrCl <60 mL/min) • Itraconazole or cyclosporine may ↑ effects; avoid concurrent use • May ↓ effects of furosemide	• Use with caution in patients with CrCl <30 mL/min • Avoid taking with high-fat meals
Combination products: Aliskiren/hydrochlorothiazide (Tekturna HCT)					

Calcium Channel Blockers

Generic • Brand • Dose	Contra-indications	Primary Side Effects	Key Monitoring	Pertinent Drug Interactions	Med Pearl
Mechanism of action – bind to L-type channels in heart and coronary/peripheral arteries to block inward movement of calcium (Ca^{2+}) $\longrightarrow$ vascular smooth-muscle relaxation (vasodilation); all (except for amlodipine and felodipine) have negative inotropic effects ($\downarrow$ contractility) • Dihydropyridines (DHPs) – more selective to vasculature; more potent vasodilators; have no effect on cardiac conduction • Non-DHPs – cause less peripheral vasodilation than DHPs; have negative chronotropic properties ($\downarrow$ HR)					
DHPs					
Amlodipine ☆ • Norvasc • 2.5–10 mg/day Felodipine ☆ • Only available generically • 2.5–20 mg/day Isradipine • Only available generically • 5–10 mg/day Nicardipine • Cardene • 60–120 mg/day Nifedipine ☆ • Adalat CC, Afeditab CR, Procardia XL • 30–180 mg/day Nisoldipine • Sular • ER: 10–40 mg/day • Geomatrix: 17–34 mg/day	None	• Reflex tachycardia • Headache • Flushing • Peripheral edema • Gingival hyperplasia • HF exacerbation (except amlodipine and felodipine)	• BP • HR • S/S of HF	• Cytochrome P450 (CYP) 3A4 substrates • CYP3A4 inhibitors may ↑ effects • CYP3A4 inducers may ↓ effects	• Sublingual nifedipine should not be used → may ↑ risk of MI, death • Do not use grapefruit juice • Nicardipine also available as injection
Non-DHPs					
Diltiazem ☆ • Cardizem, Cardizem CD, Cardizem LA, Cartia XT, Taztia XT, Tiazac • 120–540 mg/day Verapamil ☆ • Calan, Calan SR, Verelan, Verelan PM • 120–360 mg/day (IR given 2–3 × daily, sustained-release [SR] given 1–2 × daily)	• ≥2nd degree heart block (in absence of pacemaker) • HFrEF	• Bradycardia/heart block • Constipation • Peripheral edema • Gingival hyperplasia • HF exacerbation	Same as for DHPs	• CYP3A4 substrates and inhibitors • CYP3A4 inhibitors may ↑ effects • CYP3A4 inducers may ↓ effects • May ↑ effect/toxicity of CYP3A4 substrates • Use with other negative chronotropes (e.g., digoxin, β-blockers, clonidine, or ivabradine) may ↑ risk of bradycardia • May ↑ risk of digoxin toxicity	• Do not use grapefruit juice • Verapamil and diltiazem also available as injection
Combination products: Amlodipine/celecoxib (Consensi)					

α_1-Receptor Antagonists

Generic • Brand • Dose	Contra-indications	Primary Side Effects	Key Monitoring	Pertinent Drug Interactions	Med Pearl
Mechanism of action – block the α_1 receptor on peripheral blood vessels $\rightarrow$ arterial and venous vasodilation					
Doxazosin☆ • Cardura • 1–16 mg/day Prazosin • Minipress • 1–20 mg/day Terazosin☆ • Only available generically • 1–20 mg/day	Should not be used with phosphodi-esterase (PDE)-5 inhibitors (e.g., avanafil, sildenafil, tadalafil, varde-nafil) $\rightarrow$ ↑ risk of hypotension	• Orthostatic hypotension • Reflex tachycardia • Peripheral edema • Headache • Drowsiness • Priapism	• BP • HR	↑ risk of hypoten-sion with PDE-5 inhibitors (avoid concurrent use)	• Take dose at bedtime to minimize risk of orthostatic hypotension • ALLHAT trial $\rightarrow$ 25% ↑ in cardiovascular events with doxazosin • ↑ risk of intraoperative floppy iris syndrome in patients undergoing cataract surgery • Also used for benign prostatic hyperplasia (BPH) • Cardura XL not indicated for HTN; used for BPH

Central α_2-Receptor Agonists

Generic • Brand • Dose	Contra-indications	Primary Side Effects	Key Monitoring	Pertinent Drug Interactions	Med Pearl
Mechanism of action – stimulate α_2 receptors in brain $\longrightarrow$ ↓ sympathetic outflow (release of norepinephrine) $\rightarrow$ ↓ BP and HR					
Clonidine☆ • Catapres, Catapres-TTS • Oral: 0.2–2.4 mg/day • Transdermal: 0.1–0.3 mg weekly Methyldopa • Only available generically • 250–1,000 mg/day	Methyldopa: Liver disease	• Sedation • Orthostatic hypotension • Depression • Peripheral edema • Dry mouth • Bradycardia • Hepatitis (methyldopa)	• BP • HR • Liver function tests (LFTs) (methyldopa)	Use with other negative chronotropes (e.g., digoxin, verapamil, diltiazem, β-blockers, or ivabradine) may ↑ risk of bradycardia	• Clonidine patch should be applied once weekly • Abrupt discontinuation (especially in presence of β-blockers) may cause angina, MI, or hypertensive emergency; need to taper over 2 wk • When starting clonidine patch, overlap with oral for 2–3 days, then discontinue oral • Should not be used as first-line therapy • Clonidine also available as epidural injection (for pain) • Clonidine also used to treat attention-deficit/hyperactivity disorder • Methyldopa also available as injection • Methyldopa safe to use in pregnant women with HTN

Direct Vasodilators

Generic • Brand • Dose	Contra-indications	Primary Side Effects	Key Monitoring	Pertinent Drug Interactions	Med Pearl
Mechanism of action – ↑ cyclic GMP → arterial vasodilation					
Hydralazine • Only available generically • 25–300 mg/day Minoxidil • Only available generically • 2.5–100 mg/day	• Acute MI • Aortic dissection	• Reflex tachycardia • Orthostatic hypotension • Peripheral edema • Lupus-like syndrome (hydralazine) • Hirsutism (minoxidil)	• BP • HR • S/S of lupus (e.g., stabbing chest pain, joint pain, fever, rash)	None	• Should not be used as first-line therapy • Minoxidil is usually absolutely last-line therapy (because of side effects) • Hydralazine also available as injection • Minoxidil also available as topical solution/foam to stimulate hair growth

DYSLIPIDEMIA

Guidelines Summary

- Achievement of specific LDL-C goals is *no longer* recommended in the most recent dyslipidemia guidelines.
- Four groups most likely to benefit from statin therapy are:
  - Clinical ASCVD (secondary prevention)
  - LDL-C ≥190 mg/dL (primary prevention)
  - Age 40–75 yr with DM **AND** LDL-C 70–189 mg/dL (primary prevention)
  - Age 40–75 yr without clinical ASCVD or DM, and with LDL-C 70–189 mg/dL and 10-yr ASCVD risk ≥7.5%
- Heart-healthy lifestyle habits should be encouraged for all patients.
- Pharmacologic therapy
  - Statin therapy recommendations for four major benefit groups:

Major Benefit Groups	Statin Therapy Recommendations
Clinical ASCVD	• Age ≤75 yr → High-intensity statin therapy • Age >75 yr **OR** if not a candidate for high-intensity statin therapy → Moderate-intensity statin therapy
LDL-C ≥190 mg/dL	High-intensity statin therapy (moderate-intensity if not candidate for high-intensity therapy)
Age 40–75 yr with DM **AND** LDL-C 70–189 mg/dL	• 10-yr ASCVD risk <7.5% → Moderate-intensity statin therapy • 10-yr ASCVD risk ≥7.5% → High-intensity statin therapy
Age 40–75 yr without clinical ASCVD or DM, and with LDL-C 70–189 mg/dL and 10-yr ASCVD risk ≥7.5%	Moderate–high intensity statin therapy

- High-intensity versus moderate-intensity statin therapy
  - » High-intensity: ↓ LDL-C by ≥50%
    - Atorvastatin 40–80 mg daily
    - Rosuvastatin 20–40 mg daily
  - » Moderate-intensity: ↓ LDL-C by 30–<50%
    - Atorvastatin 10–20 mg daily
    - Rosuvastatin 5–10 mg daily
    - Simvastatin 20–40 mg daily
    - Pravastatin 40–80 mg daily
    - Lovastatin 40 mg daily
    - Fluvastatin XL 80 mg daily
    - Fluvastatin 40 mg twice daily
    - Pitavastatin 2–4 mg daily
- Nonstatin therapy can be considered in selected high-risk patients (clinical ASCVD, LDL-C ≥190 mg/dL, or age 40–75 yr with DM and LDL-C 70–189 mg/dL) who are/have:
  - » Less than anticipated response to statin therapy
  - » Unable to tolerate a less than recommended intensity of statin therapy
  - » Completely intolerant to statin therapy

Lipid-Lowering Effects of Various Drug Classes

Drug Class	Effect on LDL-C	Effect on HDL-C	Effect on TGs
Bile acid resins	↓ 15–30%	↑ 3–5%	↑ 1–10%
Niacin	↓ 5–25%	↑ 15–35%	↓ 20–50%
Fibric acid derivatives	↓/↑ 5–20%	↑ 10–20%	↓ 20–50%
Statins	↓ 18–55%	↑ 5–15%	↓ 7–30%
Cholesterol absorption inhibitors	↓ 15–20%	↑ 1%	↓ 8%
PCSK9 inhibitors	↓ 40–75%	↑ 4–9%	↓ 2–16%

Bile Acid Resins

Generic • Brand • Dose	Contra-indications	Primary Side Effects	Key Monitoring	Pertinent Drug Interactions	Med Pearl
Mechanism of action – bind bile acids in intestines, forming insoluble complex that is excreted in feces → ↓ in bile acids causes liver to convert cholesterol into bile acids, which then ↓ cholesterol stores → ↑ demand for cholesterol in liver → upregulation of LDL receptors → ↑ LDL-C clearance from bloodstream					
Cholestyramine • Prevalite • 4–24 g/day Colesevelam ☆ • Welchol • 3.75 g/day Colestipol • Colestid • Granules: 5–30 g/day • Tablets: 2–16 g/day	Complete biliary obstruction	• Constipation • Bloating • Abdominal pain • Nausea/vomiting (N/V) • Flatulence • ↑ TGs	Lipid panel	Bind to and ↓ absorption of many drugs (e.g., warfarin, digoxin, thiazides, levothyroxine, mycophenolate)	• Used to ↓ LDL-C • Can be used in patients with liver disease • Do not use in patients with ↑ TGs • Colesevelam has fewer gastrointestinal (GI) side effects and drug interactions

Niacin

Generic • Brand • Dose	Contra-indications	Primary Side Effects	Key Monitoring	Pertinent Drug Interactions	Med Pearl
Mechanism of action – ↓ production of very low density lipoproteins (VLDL) in liver → ↓ synthesis of LDL-C					
Niacin ☆ • Niaspan; also available as over-the-counter (OTC) product • 500–3,000 mg/day	• Hepatic impairment • Active gout • Active peptic ulcer disease	• Flushing/itching • Nausea • Orthostatic hypotension • ↑ LFTs • Myopathy • Hyperuricemia • Hyperglycemia	• Lipid panel • LFTs • Creatine kinase (CK) (if muscle aches) • Uric acid • Blood glucose (if patient has DM)	None significant	• Used to ↓ LDL-C, ↓ TGs, and ↑ HDL-C • Most effective drug for ↑ HDL-C • Do not ↑ dose by >500 mg in 4 wk period • Avoid use of OTC SR products (↑ risk of hepatotoxicity)

Fibric Acid Derivatives

Generic • Brand • Dose	Contra-indications	Primary Side Effects	Key Monitoring	Pertinent Drug Interactions	Med Pearl
Mechanism of action – ↑ activity of lipoprotein lipase → ↑ catabolism of VLDL → ↓ TGs					
Fenofibrate/ fenofibric acid☆ • Antara, Fenoglide, Fibricor, Lipofen, Tricor, Triglide, Trilipix • 30–200 mg/day (depending on brand) Gemfibrozil☆ • Lopid • 1,200 mg/day	• Hepatic impairment • Severe renal impairment • Gallbladder disease • Concurrent use with statins, repaglinide, dasabuvir, or selexipag (gemfibrozil)	• Nausea/vomiting/ diarrhea (N/V/D) • Abdominal pain • ↑ LFTs • Myopathy • Severe rash • Anaphylaxis/ angioedema	• Lipid panel • LFTs • CK (if muscle aches)	• Gemfibrozil is CYP2C8 inhibitor • Avoid using gemfibrozil with statins (↑ risk of myopathy), repaglinide (↑ risk of hypoglycemia), dasabuvir (↑ risk of QT interval prolongation), and selexipag (↑ levels) • ↑ effects of warfarin and sulfonylureas • ↓ cyclosporine levels	• Used to ↓ TGs and/ or ↑ HDL-C • Fenofibrate preferred with statins • Adjust dose in renal impairment

Omega-3 Fatty Acids (Fish Oil)

Generic • Brand • Dose	Contra-indications	Primary Side Effects	Key Monitoring	Pertinent Drug Interactions	Med Pearl
Mechanism of action – ↓ production of TGs in the liver					
Icosapent ethyl • Vascepa • 4 g/day	Fish allergy	Arthralgia	Lipid panel	May ↑ risk of bleed-ing with antithrom-botic agents	• Used to ↓ TGs • Minimal effect on LDL-C • Take with meals
Omega-3-Acid Ethyl Esters☆ • Lovaza; also available as OTC product • 2–4 g/day	Fish allergy	• Belching ("fishy taste") • Dyspepsia	Lipid panel	May ↑ risk of bleeding with antithrombotic agents	• Used to ↓ TGs • May ↑ LDL-C

HMG-CoA Reductase Inhibitors (Statins)

Generic • Brand • Dose	Contra-indications	Primary Side Effects	Key Monitoring	Pertinent Drug Interactions	Med Pearl
Mechanism of action – inhibit HMG-CoA reductase → prevent the conversion of HMG-CoA to mevalonate (rate-limiting step in cholesterol synthesis)					
Atorvastatin ☆ • Lipitor • 10–80 mg/day Fluvastatin • Lescol XL • 20–80 mg/day Lovastatin ☆ • Altoprev • 20–80 mg/day Pitavastatin • Livalo, Zypitamag • 1–4 mg/day Pravastatin ☆ • Pravachol • 10–80 mg/day Rosuvastatin ☆ • Crestor • 5–40 mg/day Simvastatin ☆ • FloLipid, Zocor • 10–40 mg/day	• Hepatic impairment • Pregnancy • Concomitant use with cyclosporine (pitavastatin and atorvastatin) • Concomitant use with strong CYP3A4 inhibitors (lovastatin) • Concomitant use with strong CYP3A4 inhibitors, cyclosporine, or danazol (simvastatin)	• ↑ LFTs • Myopathy • N/V • Constipation	• Lipid panel • LFTs • CK (if muscle aches)	• Atorvastatin, lovastatin, and simvastatin are CYP3A4 substrates; CYP3A4 inhibitors may ↑ risk of side effects; may ↑ effects of warfarin • Fluvastatin and pitavastatin are CYP2C9 substrates; may ↑ effects of warfarin • Pravastatin not metabolized by CYP enzymes	• Most effective drugs for ↓ LDL-C • Lower maximum dosage of atorvastatin when used with clarithromycin, darunavir/ritonavir, fosamprenavir, fosamprenavir/ritonavir, itraconazole, nelfinavir, or saquinavir/ritonavir • Lower maximum dosage of fluvastatin when used with cyclosporine or fluconazole • Lower maximum dosage of lovastatin when used with amiodarone, dronedarone, verapamil, diltiazem, danazol, or lomitapide • Lower maximum dosage of pitavastatin when used with erythromycin or rifampin • Lower maximum dosage of pravastatin when used with clarithromycin • Lower maximum dosage of rosuvastatin when used with cyclosporine, gemfibrozil, lopinavir/ritonavir, atazanavir/ritonavir, or simeprevir • Lower maximum dosage of simvastatin when used with amiodarone, amlodipine, diltiazem, dronedarone, niacin, ranolazine, verapamil, or lomitapide • Adjust dose of pitavastatin and rosuvastatin in renal impairment • Simvastatin also available as oral suspension (FloLipid)
Combination products:		Atorvastatin/amlodipine (Caduet)		Simvastatin/ezetimibe (Vytorin)	

Cholesterol Absorption Inhibitor

Generic • Brand • Dose	Contra-indications	Primary Side Effects	Key Monitoring	Pertinent Drug Interactions	Med Pearl
Mechanism of action – prevents absorption of cholesterol from small intestine					
Ezetimibe ☆ • Zetia • 10 mg/day	None	• Headache • Diarrhea	Lipid panel	• Cyclosporine and fibrates may ↑ effects • ↑ cyclosporine levels • ↑ effects of warfarin	• Used to ↓ LDL-C • Can add to statin to further ↓ LDL-C or if dose-limiting side effects occur with statin

Microsomal Triglyceride Transfer Protein (MTP) Inhibitor

Generic • Brand • Dose	Contra-indications	Primary Side Effects	Key Monitoring	Pertinent Drug Interactions	Med Pearl
Mechanism of action – inhibits MTP and prevents the assembly of apo-B containing lipoproteins, which results in ↓ LDL-C					
Lomitapide • Juxtapid • 5–60 mg/day	• Pregnancy • Concomitant use with moderate or strong CYP3A4 inhibitors • Hepatic impairment	• ↑ LFTs • N/V/D	• Lipid panel • LFTs (monitor before every dose ↑)	• CYP3A4 substrate • CYP3A4 inhibitors may ↑ risk of side effects • May ↑ effects of warfarin • May ↑ risk of side effects with simvastatin and lovastatin (limit statin dose) • May ↑ effect/toxicity of P-glycoprotein (P-gp) substrates	• Used to ↓ LDL-C in patients with homozygous familial hypercholesterolemia • Has REMS program • Lower maximum dosage when used with weak CYP3A4 inhibitor (alprazolam, amiodarone, amlodipine, atorvastatin, bicalutamide, cilostazol, cimetidine, cyclosporine, fluoxetine, fluvoxamine, isoniazid, lapatinib, nilotinib, oral contraceptives, pazopanib, ranitidine, ranolazine, ticagrelor, or zileuton) • Take ≥2 hr after evening meal with glass of water (food ↑ GI side effects) • Take daily vitamin supplement (containing 400 IU vitamin E and ≥200 mg linoleic acid, 210 mg alpha-linoleic acid, 110 mg eicosapentaenoic acid, and 80 mg docosahexaenoic acid)

PCSK9 Inhibitors

Generic • Brand • Dose	Contra-indications	Primary Side Effects	Key Monitoring	Pertinent Drug Interactions	Med Pearl
Mechanism of action – inhibit binding of proprotein convertase subtilisin kexin type 9 (PCSK9) to LDL receptors on the surface of the hepatocyte, which ↑ number of LDL receptors available to clear circulating LDL and lowers LDL-C					
Alirocumab • Praluent • 75–150 mg subcut q2wk	None	• Hypersensitivity reactions • ↑ LFTs • Diarrhea	Lipid panel	None	Used to ↓ LDL-C (by up to 60%)
Evolocumab • Repatha • 140 mg subcut q2wk or 420 mg subcut monthly	None	Hypersensitivity reactions	Lipid panel	None	• Used to ↓ LDL-C (by up to 60%) • Also indicated to reduce the risk of MI, stroke, and coronary revascularization in patients with CVD • To administer 420-mg dose, give 3 consecutive injections within 30 min

HEART FAILURE

Guidelines Summary

The goals of therapy are to relieve symptoms, improve quality of life, improve survival, reduce hospitalizations, and slow the progression of disease.

- Nonpharmacologic therapy: Regular low-intensity physical activity, ↓ Na⁺ (≤3 g/day), ↓ fluid intake (<2 L/day), weight loss (if obese), alcohol restriction, and smoking cessation
- Pharmacologic therapy
  - Stage A: Modify risk factors and control HTN, DM, CAD, and dyslipidemia; ACEI or ARB in patients with risk factors for vascular disease
  - Stage B: ACEI + β-blocker
  - Stage C: ACEI (or ARB or sacubitril/valsartan) + β-blocker + diuretic
    - » Other drugs to be considered:
      - Sacubitril/valsartan: NYHA class II-III patients who tolerate an ACEI or ARB (to be used in place of ACEI or ARB)
      - ARA: NYHA class II-IV patients who are already receiving ACEI (or ARB) and β-blocker; NYHA class II patients should have history of prior cardiovascular hospitalization or ↑ BNP level to be considered for ARA therapy
      - ARBs: Patients who cannot tolerate an ACEI due to intractable cough or angioedema
      - Digoxin: Patients who remain symptomatic despite optimal therapy with ACEI (or ARB), β-blocker, and diuretic
      - Hydralazine/isosorbide dinitrate (HDZ/ISDN): Patients with intolerance or contraindications (renal insufficiency, hyperkalemia) to ACEI or ARB; African-American patients with NYHA class III or IV symptoms who remain symptomatic despite optimal therapy with ACEI (or ARB) and β-blocker
      - Ivabradine: NYHA class II-III patients with stable HFrEF (LVEF ≤35%) and in sinus rhythm who are receiving a β-blocker at a maximally tolerated dose and having a resting heart rate ≥70 bpm
  - Stage D: Chronic positive inotrope therapy (e.g., dobutamine, milrinone), mechanical circulatory support (e.g., LV assist device), heart transplant, end-of-life care/hospice

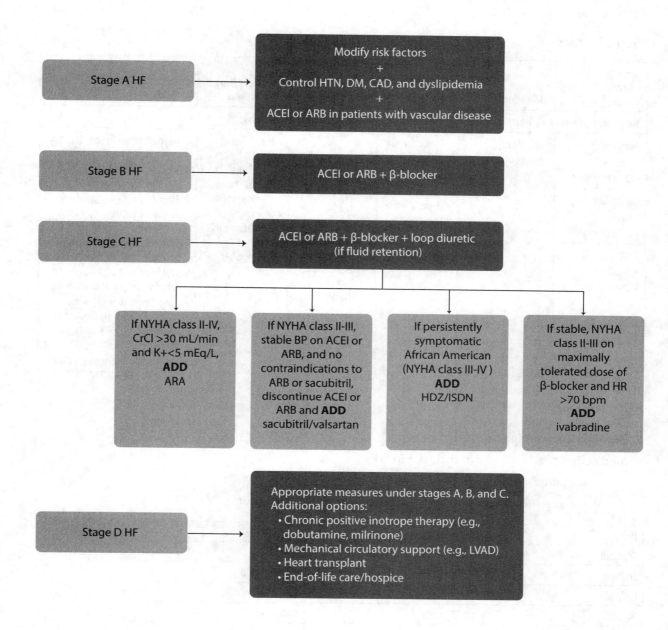

Stage A HF → Modify risk factors
+
Control HTN, DM, CAD, and dyslipidemia
+
ACEI or ARB in patients with vascular disease

Stage B HF → ACEI or ARB + β-blocker

Stage C HF → ACEI or ARB + β-blocker + loop diuretic
(if fluid retention)

If NYHA class II-IV, CrCl >30 mL/min and K+<5 mEq/L, **ADD** ARA

If NYHA class II-III, stable BP on ACEI or ARB, and no contraindications to ARB or sacubitril, discontinue ACEI or ARB and **ADD** sacubitril/valsartan

If persistently symptomatic African American (NYHA class III-IV) **ADD** HDZ/ISDN

If stable, NYHA class II-III on maximally tolerated dose of β-blocker and HR >70 bpm **ADD** ivabradine

Stage D HF → Appropriate measures under stages A, B, and C. Additional options:
• Chronic positive inotrope therapy (e.g., dobutamine, milrinone)
• Mechanical circulatory support (e.g., LVAD)
• Heart transplant
• End-of-life care/hospice

Loop Diuretics

Generic • Brand • Dose	Contra-indications	Primary Side Effects	Key Monitoring	Pertinent Drug Interactions	Med Pearl
Mechanism of action – inhibit Na$^+$ reabsorption in the ascending limb of loop of Henle; ↓ preload					
Bumetanide • Bumex • 0.5–10 mg/day Furosemide ☆ • Lasix • 20–600 mg/day Torsemide • Demadex • 10–200 mg/day	Sulfa allergy	• Hypocalcemia • Hypokalemia • Hypomagne-semia • Hyponatremia • Hyperglycemia • Hyperuricemia • Metabolic alkalosis • Azotemia	• BP • Electrolytes • BUN/SCr • Blood glucose • Uric acid • Jugular venous pressure • Urine output • Weight (↓ by 0.5–1 kg/day initially)	• May ↑ risk of lithium toxicity • May ↑ risk of ototoxicity with aminoglycosides • May ↓ effect of antidiabetic agents • NSAIDs ↓ effects	• ↓ symptoms; effect on mortality unknown • Bumetanide and furosemide also available IV • If initial dose inadequate, double dose, dose 2× daily, add metolazone, or use IV • Similar side effects as thiazides (except loops cause hypocalcemia) • BUN/SCr ratio >20:1 → dehydration (prerenal azotemia) • 1 mg bumetanide = 20 mg torsemide = 40 mg furosemide • Furosemide PO dose = 2× IV dose • Bumetanide PO dose = IV dose

ACE Inhibitors

- See HTN monograph for further details.
- Medication pearls specific to their use in HF
  - ↓ mortality; ↓ preload and afterload
  - Strive to achieve target dose, if possible (titrate dose to symptoms, not BP).

Drug	Initial Dose	Target Dose
Captopril	6.25 mg TID	50 mg TID
Enalapril	2.5 mg BID	10–20 mg BID
Lisinopril	2.5 mg daily	20–40 mg daily
Ramipril	1.25 mg daily	10 mg daily
Trandolapril	1 mg daily	4 mg daily
Fosinopril	5 mg daily	40 mg daily
Quinapril	5 mg BID	20 mg BID
Perindopril	2 mg daily	8–16 mg daily

β-Blockers

Generic • Brand • Dose	Contra-indications	Primary Side Effects	Key Monitoring	Pertinent Drug Interactions	Med Pearl
Mechanism of action – ↓ activation of the sympathetic nervous system; slow and potentially reverse detrimental effects (e.g., ventricular remodeling) of catecholamines					
Bisoprolol • Zebeta • 1.25–10 mg/day • Target dose: 10 mg daily Carvedilol ☆ • Coreg, Coreg CR • IR: 6.25–100 mg/day (in two divided doses) • Target dose: <85 kg = 25 mg BID; >85 kg = 50 mg BID • CR: 10–80 mg/day (1× daily) • Target dose: 80 mg daily Metoprolol succinate ☆ • Kapspargo Sprinkle, Toprol XL • 12.5–200 mg/day • Target dose: 200 mg daily	• Symptomatic bradycardia • ≥2nd-degree heart block (in absence of pacemaker) • SBP <85 mmHg • Severe asthma • Decompensated HF	See HTN section	• BP • HR • S/S of HF • Weight	Carvedilol may ↑ digoxin levels	• ↓ mortality • Metoprolol succinate (not tartrate) approved for HF • Patient should be fairly euvolemic before starting • Strive to achieve target dose, if possible • Dose can be doubled every 2–4 wk to achieve target dose (unless side effects) • Manage worsening HF by ↑ diuretic dose • If hypotension occurs, may ↓ dose of ACEI, ARB, or other vasodilator (more common with carvedilol) • If bradycardia occurs, ↓ dose • Abrupt discontinuation may cause worsening HF

Angiotensin II Receptor Blockers

- See HTN monograph for further details.
- Medication pearls specific to their use in HF
  - Only candesartan, losartan, or valsartan recommended for the management of HF (only candesartan and valsartan approved for HF)
  - Should not be considered equivalent or superior to ACEIs

Drug	Initial Dose	Target Dose
Candesartan	4–8 mg daily	32 mg daily
Losartan	25–50 mg daily	50–150 mg daily
Valsartan	20–40 mg BID	160 mg BID

Sacubitril/Valsartan

Generic • Brand • Dose	Contra-indications	Primary Side Effects	Key Monitoring	Pertinent Drug Interactions	Med Pearl
Mechanism of action – sacubitril: prodrug, inhibits neprilysin (neutral endopeptidase) → ↑ levels of peptides (including natriuretic peptides); valsartan: ARB					
Sacubitril/valsartan • Entresto • Sacubitril 49–97 mg/valsartan 51–103 mg BID • New or previously low-dose user of ACEI/ARB: Start with sacubitril 24 mg/valsartan 26 mg BID • Target dose: sacubitril 97 mg/valsartan 103 mg BID	• Pregnancy • History of angioedema with prior ACEI/ARB use • Concurrent use with ACEI • Concurrent use with aliskiren in DM	• Angioedema • Hypotension • Renal impairment • Hyperkalemia	• BP • BUN/SCr • K^+	• Use with K^+ supplements, K^+-sparing diuretics, ARAs, or NSAIDs may ↑ risk of hyperkalemia • Use with ACEI ↑ risk of angioedema (contraindicated) • Use with aliskiren may ↑ risk of hyperkalemia and renal impairment (avoid concurrent use in DM and CrCl <60 mL/min) • May ↑ risk of lithium toxicity	• ↓ cardiovascular death and hospitalizations • Do not give within 36 hr of switch from/to ACEI • Double dose every 2–4 wk to achieve target dose (unless side effects) • Adjust dose in renal or hepatic impairment

Digoxin

Generic • Brand • Dose	Contra-indications	Primary Side Effects	Key Monitoring	Pertinent Drug Interactions	Med Pearl
Mechanism of action – inhibits Na^+/K^+ ATPase pump → ↑ intracellular Ca^{2+} → ↑ myocardial contractility; also ↓ neurohormonal activation					
Digoxin ☆ • Lanoxin • 0.125–0.25 mg/day (loading doses not necessary in HF)	≥2nd-degree heart block (in absence of pacemaker)	• Bradycardia/heart block • S/S of digoxin toxicity (visual disturbances, N/V, confusion, anorexia, arrhythmias)	• HR • Electrolytes (predisposed to toxicity if hypokalemia, hypomagnesemia, or hypercalcemia) • BUN/SCr • Digoxin concentrations	• P-gp substrate • Amiodarone, dronedarone, quinidine, verapamil, clarithromycin, lapatinib, propafenone, and ritonavir may ↑ levels • Antacids may ↓ levels (separate by 1–2 hours) • Use with other negative chronotropes (e.g., β-blockers, verapamil, diltiazem, clonidine, or ivabradine) may ↑ risk of bradycardia	• Improves symptoms, ↓ hospitalizations; no effect on mortality • Used to ↑ contractility in HFrEF and to ↓ HR in atrial fibrillation (AF) • Abrupt discontinuation may cause worsening HF • ↓ dose by 50% when starting amiodarone or dronedarone • Adjust dose in renal impairment • Target level: 0.5–0.9 ng/mL (↑ mortality if >0.9 ng/mL)

Aldosterone Receptor Antagonists

Generic • Brand • Dose	Contra-indications	Primary Side Effects	Key Monitoring	Pertinent Drug Interactions	Med Pearl
Mechanism of action – inhibit the effects of aldosterone → ↓ remodeling and Na$^+$/water retention • Spironolactone is nonselective ARA (also blocks androgen and progesterone receptors → associated with endocrine side effects) • Eplerenone is selective ARA (not associated with endocrinologic side effects)					
Eplerenone • Inspra • 25–50 mg/day Spironolactone • Aldactone, CaroSpir • 12.5–25 mg/day	• K$^+$ >5 mEq/L • SCr >2.5 mg/dL (men) or >2 mg/dL (women) (or CrCl ≤30 mL/min) • Concomitant ACEI **and** ARB use • Concurrent use of eplerenone with strong CYP3A4 inhibitors (e.g., ritonavir, ketoconazole, itraconazole, nefazodone, clarithromycin, nelfinavir)	• Hyperkalemia • Also for spironolactone: Gynecomastia, breast tenderness, menstrual changes, hirsutism	• BP • K$^+$ • BUN/SCr	• Eplerenone is CYP3A4 substrate • CYP3A4 inhibitors may ↑ effects • Use with ACEIs, ARBs, K$^+$ supplements, or NSAIDs may ↑ risk of hyperkalemia	• ↓ mortality • Should consider discontinuing or ↓ dose of K$^+$ supplements • Spironolactone also available as oral suspension (CaroSpir) • Eplerenone tends to be used in patients who develop endocrine side effects (i.e., gynecomastia) with spironolactone • Lower maximum dosage of eplerenone when used with erythromycin, saquinavir, verapamil, or fluconazole

Hydralazine/Isosorbide Dinitrate

Generic • Brand • Dose	Contra-indications	Primary Side Effects	Key Monitoring	Pertinent Drug Interactions	Med Pearl
Mechanism of action: • Hydralazine – causes arterial vasodilation (↓ afterload) • Isosorbide dinitrate – causes venous vasodilation (↓ preload)					
Hydralazine • Only available generically • 40–300 mg/day	None	• Headache • Dizziness • Reflex tachycardia • Peripheral edema (hydralazine) • Lupus-like syndrome (hydralazine)	• BP • HR	None	• ↓ mortality (when used together) • Combination often used in patients who cannot tolerate ACEIs or ARBs due to renal impairment, hyperkalemia, or angioedema • Do not use hydralazine alone (↑ mortality)
Isosorbide dinitrate ☆ • Isordil • 30–120 mg/day	None				
Combination product: Hydralazine/isosorbide dinitrate (BiDil) – approved for African-American patients with NYHA class III or IV HF due to LV systolic dysfunction (LVEF ≤40%) who are receiving an ACEI (or ARB) and a β-blocker (can also use individual products together if there are financial concerns)					

I$_f$ Channel Inhibitor

Generic • Brand • Dose	Contra-indications	Primary Side Effects	Key Monitoring	Pertinent Drug Interactions	Med Pearl
Mechanism of action – blocks hyperpolarization-activated cyclic nucleotide-gated channel responsible for cardiac pacemaker I$_f$ current in sinoatrial node, resulting in ↓ in HR					
Ivabradine • Corlanor • 2.5–7.5 mg BID	• ADHF • BP <90/50 mmHg • Sick sinus syndrome or 3rd-degree heart block (in absence of pacemaker) • HR <60 bpm (at baseline) • Severe hepatic impairment • Pacemaker dependence • Concurrent use of strong CYP3A4 inhibitors	• Bradycardia • Heart block • AF • Phosphenes	• HR • Electrocardio-gram (ECG)	• CYP3A4 substrate • CYP3A4 inhibitors may ↑ effects • CYP3A4 inducers may ↓ effects (avoid use) • Use with other negative chronotropes (e.g., β-blockers, verapamil, diltiazem, digoxin, or clonidine) may ↑ risk of bradycardia	• ↓ hospitalizations; no effect on mortality • Titrate dose by 2.5 mg BID to achieve target resting HR of 50–60 bpm

Intravenous Drugs for Treatment of ADHF

Drug	Mechanism of Action	Primary Side Effects	Med Pearl
Vasodilators			
Nitroglycerin (NTG)	• Venous vasodilation → ↓ preload • Can cause arterial vasodilation at higher doses	• Hypotension • Tachycardia • Headache • Tolerance	• Especially useful in patients with myocardial ischemia • Tolerance can develop (overcome by ↑ infusion rate)
Nitroprusside	Arterial and venous vasodilation → ↓ preload and afterload	• Hypotension • N/V • Cyanide/thiocyanate toxicity (risk ↑ if infusion >24 hours)	Avoid in patients with renal impairment

Intravenous Drugs for Treatment of ADHF *(cont'd)*

Drug	Mechanism of Action	Primary Side Effects	Med Pearl
Positive Inotropes			
Dopamine	• 0.5–3 mcg/kg/min → Stimulates dopamine receptors → ↑ urine output • 3–10 mcg/kg/min → Stimulates β_1 receptors → ↑ CO, ↑ HR • >10 mcg/kg/min → Stimulates α_1 receptors → ↑ BP	• Arrhythmias • Tachycardia • Myocardial ischemia • N/V	Avoid in patients with myocardial ischemia
Dobutamine	β_1 and β_2 receptor agonist and weak α_1 receptor agonist → ↑ CO and vasodilation	• Arrhythmias • Tachycardia • Myocardial ischemia • Hypokalemia • Tremor	• Avoid in patients with myocardial ischemia • Should not be used in patients receiving chronic β-blocker therapy • Tolerance can develop
Milrinone	PDE III inhibitor → ↑ CO and vasodilation	• Hypotension • Arrhythmias	• Can be used in patients receiving chronic β-blocker therapy, or in those not responding to or tolerating dobutamine • Tolerance does not develop • Use lower initial dose in patients with renal impairment

ANTIARRHYTHMIC DRUGS

Class IA

Generic • Brand • Dose	Contra-indications	Primary Side Effects	Key Monitoring	Pertinent Drug Interactions	Med Pearl
Mechanism of action – Na^+ channel blockers; slow conduction velocity, prolong refractoriness, ↓ automaticity					
Disopyramide • Norpace, Norpace CR • 400–1,600 mg/day	• HF • ≥2nd-degree heart block (in absence of pacemaker) • Long QT syndrome	• Dry mouth • Urinary retention • Blurred vision • Constipation • HF exacerbation • Hypotension • Torsade de pointes (TdP)	• ECG (QTc interval, QRS duration) • BP • S/S of HF • Electrolytes • Disopyramide concentrations	• CYP3A4 substrate • CYP3A4 inhibitors and anticholinergics may ↑ risk of side effects • CYP3A4 inducers may ↓ effects • ↑ risk of TdP with other drugs that prolong QT interval	• Used for atrial and ventricular arrhythmias • Therapeutic range: 2–5 mcg/mL • Adjust dose in renal impairment

Class IA   *(cont'd)*

Generic • Brand • Dose	Contra-indications	Primary Side Effects	Key Monitoring	Pertinent Drug Interactions	Med Pearl

Procainamide
• Only available generically
• IV:
  • *Loading dose:* 15–17 mg/kg over 25–60 min
  • *Maintenance dose:* 1–4 mg/min continuous infusion
	• ≥2nd-degree heart block (in absence of pacemaker)
	• Long QT syndrome
		• Lupus-like syndrome
		• TdP
		• Hypotension
		• Agranulocytosis
			• ECG (QTc interval, QRS duration)
			• BP
			• S/S of lupus (e.g., stabbing chest pain, joint pain, rash)
			• Procainamide/N-acetylprocainamide (NAPA) concentrations
			• Complete blood count (CBC) with differential
			• Electrolytes
				↑ risk of TdP with other drugs that prolong QT interval	• Used for atrial and ventricular arrhythmias
					• Therapeutic range: 4–10 mcg/mL (procainamide); 15–25 mcg/mL (NAPA); 10–30 mcg/mL (total)
					• Use with caution, if at all, in renal impairment

Quinidine • Only available generically • Sulfate: 800–2,400 mg/day • Gluconate: 648–2,916 mg/day	• ≥2nd-degree heart block (in absence of pacemaker) • Long QT syndrome • Concurrent use of ritonavir	• Diarrhea • Stomach cramps • TdP • Hypotension • Cinchonism (tinnitus, blurred vision, headache) • Thrombocytopenia	• ECG (QTc interval, QRS duration) • BP • Quinidine-concentrations • CBC with differential • LFTs • Electrolytes	• CYP3A4 substrate and CYP2D6 inhibitor • CYP3A4 inhibitors may ↑ risk of side effects • CYP3A4 inducers may ↓ effects • May ↑ toxicity of CYP2D6 substrates • ↑ risk of digoxin toxicity • ↑ risk of TdP with other drugs that prolong QT interval	• Used for atrial and ventricular arrhythmias • Therapeutic range: 2–5 mcg/mL • Administer with food to minimize GI effects

■ Avoid all Class IA antiarrhythmics in patients with structural heart disease (i.e., HF, CAD, left ventricular hypertrophy, valvular disease).

Class IB

Generic • Brand • Dose	Contra- indications	Primary Side Effects	Key Monitoring	Pertinent Drug Interactions	Med Pearl
Mechanism of action – Na$^+$ channel blockers; little effect on conduction velocity, shorten refractoriness, ↓ automaticity					

Lidocaine
• Xylocaine
• IV:
  • *Loading dose:* 1–1.5 mg/kg, up to 3 mg/kg (total)
  • *Maintenance dose:* 1–4 mg/min
	≥2nd-degree heart block (in absence of pacemaker)	CNS toxicity (dizziness, blurred vision, slurred speech, confusion, paresthesias, seizures)	• ECG (QRS duration)
			• BP
			• Neurologic exam
			• Lidocaine concentrations (if duration of therapy >24 hours)
				Amiodarone may ↑ risk of toxicity	• Used only for ventricular arrhythmias
					• Therapeutic range: 1.5–5 mcg/mL
					• Use lower infusion rate in elderly, HF or hepatic impairment

Mexiletine • Only available generically • 600–1,200 mg/day	Same as for lidocaine	• CNS toxicity (same as lidocaine) • N/V	• ECG (QRS duration) • BP • LFTs • Neurologic exam	• CYP1A2 and CYP2D6 substrate • ↑ risk of theophylline toxicity • CYP1A2 and CYP2D6 inhibitors may ↑ risk of toxicity	• Used only for ventricular arrhythmias • Take with food to minimize GI effects • ↓ dose in HF or hepatic impairment

- Class IB antiarrhythmics do not cause TdP.

Class IC

Generic • Brand • Dose	Contra-indications	Primary Side Effects	Key Monitoring	Pertinent Drug Interactions	Med Pearl
Mechanism of action — Na$^+$ channel blockers (most potent); markedly slow conduction velocity, no effect on refractoriness, ↓ automaticity; propafenone also has nonselective β-blocking properties					
Flecainide • Only available generically • *Loading dose (for AF conversion):* 200–300 mg × 1 dose • *Maintenance dose:* 100–400 mg/day	• ≥2nd-degree heart block (in absence of pacemaker) • History of MI • HF	• Dizziness • Tremor • HF exacerbation • Ventricular tachycardia (VT)	• ECG (QRS duration) • Echocardiogram (at baseline to evaluate LV function) • Electrolytes	↑ risk of digoxin toxicity	• Used for atrial and ventricular arrhythmias • Adjust dose in renal impairment

Propafenone
• Rythmol, Rythmol SR
• IR:
  • *Loading dose (for AF conversion):* 450–600 mg × 1
  • *Maintenance dose:* 450–900 mg/day (in 3 divided doses)
• SR:
  • *Maintenance dose:* 450–950 mg/day (in 2 divided doses)
	• ≥2nd-degree heart block (in absence of pacemaker)
	• Bradycardia
	• Bronchospastic disorders
	• HF
	• History of MI
		• Bradycardia/heart block
		• HF exacerbation
		• Bronchospasm
		• Taste disturbances
		• VT
			• ECG (QRS duration, PR interval)
			• BP
			• HR
			• Echocardiogram (at baseline to evaluate LV function)
			• Electrolytes
				• ↑ risk of digoxin toxicity
				• ↑ effects of warfarin
				• Use with other negative chronotropes (e.g., β-blockers, digoxin, verapamil, diltiazem, clonidine, or ivabradine) may ↑ risk of bradycardia
					• Used for atrial and ventricular arrhythmias

- Avoid Class IC antiarrhythmics in patients with structural heart disease.
- Class IC antiarrhythmics do not cause TdP.

Class II

(See medication chart in HTN section for discussion on β-blockers.)

Class III

Generic • Brand • Dose	Contra-indications	Primary Side Effects	Key Monitoring	Pertinent Drug Interactions	Med Pearl
Mechanism of action – K⁺ channel blockers; no effect on conduction velocity or automaticity; amiodarone and dronedarone also have Na⁺-channel blocking, β-blocking, and CCB properties; sotalol also has nonselective β-blocking properties					

Amiodarone☆
• Nexterone, Pacerone
• Loading dose (IV):
  • *Stable VT:* 150 mg over 10 min
  • *Pulseless VT/ventricular fibrillation:* 300 mg IV push
  • *AF:* 5 mg/kg over 30–60 min
• Loading dose (PO):
  • *Ventricular arrhythmias:* 1,200–1,600 mg/day (in 2–3 divided doses)
  • *Atrial arrhythmias:* 800–1,200 mg/day (in 2–3 divided doses) until 10 g total
• Maintenance dose:
  • IV: 1 mg/min × 6 hr, then 0.5 mg/min
  • PO: 100–400 mg/day
	≥2nd-degree heart block (in absence of pacemaker)	IV:
		• Hypotension
		• Bradycardia/heart block
		• Phlebitis
		PO:
		• Hypo-/hyperthyroidism
		• Pulmonary fibrosis
		• Bradycardia/heart block
		• Corneal microdeposits
		• Optic neuritis
		• N/V
		• ↑ LFTs
		• Ataxia
		• Paresthesias
		• Photosensitivity
		• Blue-gray skin discoloration
			• ECG (QTc interval, QRS duration, PR interval)
			• BP
			• HR
			• Chest x-ray (baseline; then every 12 months)
			• Pulmonary function tests (baseline; then if symptoms develop)
			• High-resolution chest CT scan (if symptoms develop)
			• Thyroid function tests (TFTs) (baseline; then every 6 months)
			• LFTs (baseline; then every 6 months)
			• Ophthalmologic exam (baseline if visual impairment present; then if symptoms develop)
				• CYP2C8 and CYP3A4 substrate
				• CYP1A2, CYP2C9, CYP2D6, and CYP3A4 inhibitor
				• CYP3A4 inhibitors may ↑ risk of side effects
				• CYP3A4 inducers may ↓ effects
				• ↑ risk of digoxin toxicity (↓ digoxin dose by 50%)
				• ↑ effects of warfarin (↓ warfarin dose by 30%)
				• Use with other negative chronotropes (e.g., β-blockers, digoxin, verapamil, diltiazem, clonidine, or ivabradine) or sofosbuvir-containing regimens may ↑ risk of bradycardia
				• May ↑ cyclosporine or phenytoin levels
				• May ↑ risk of side effects of simvastatin and lovastatin
					• Used for atrial and ventricular arrhythmias
					• Safe to use in HF
					• Half-life = 40–60 days
					• If pulmonary fibrosis or blurred vision occur, discontinue therapy
					• If TFTs abnormal, treat thyroid disorder
					• If ↑ LFTs occur, ↓ amiodarone dose or discontinue therapy if LFTs >2x upper limit of normal
					• Take with food to minimize GI effects
					• Advise patients to wear sunscreen

Class III (cont'd)

Generic • Brand • Dose	Contra-indications	Primary Side Effects	Key Monitoring	Pertinent Drug Interactions	Med Pearl
Dronedarone • Multaq • 400 mg BID with meals	• Permanent AF • NYHA class IV HF or NYHA class II–III HF with recent decompensation requiring hospitalization or referral to specialized HF clinic • ≥2nd-degree heart block (in absence of pacemaker) • Bradycardia • Concurrent use of strong CYP3A4 inhibitors or strong CYP3A4 inducers • Concurrent use of other drugs that prolong QT interval • QTc interval ≥500 msec • PR interval >280 msec • Severe hepatic impairment • Liver or lung toxicity related to previous amiodarone use • Pregnancy	• N/V/D • ↑ SCr/acute renal failure • Bradycardia • ↑ LFTs • New-onset or worsening HF	• ECG (QTc interval, PR interval) • HR • BUN/SCr • S/S of HF • LFTs	• CYP3A4 substrate • CYP2D6 and CYP3A4 inhibitor • May ↑ toxicity of CYP2D6 and CYP3A4 substrates • CYP3A4 inhibitors may ↑ risk of side effects • CYP3A4 inducers may ↓ effects • ↑ risk of digoxin toxicity (↓ digoxin dose by 50% or consider discontinuing) • Use with other negative chronotropes (e.g., β-blockers, digoxin, verapamil, diltiazem, clonidine, or ivabradine) may ↑ risk of bradycardia • ↑ effects of dabigatran (↓ dose of dabigatran to 75 mg BID if CrCl 30–50 mL/min) • May ↑ risk of side effects of simvastatin and lovastatin	• Used only for atrial arrhythmias • Structurally related to amiodarone (does not have iodine component); less likely to cause thyroid toxicity; also has shorter half-life
Dofetilide • Tikosyn • 500 mcg BID	• CrCl <20 mL/min • QTc interval >440 msec • Hypokalemia/hypomagnesemia • Concurrent use of verapamil, ketoconazole, cimetidine, trimethoprim, prochlorperazine, hydrochlorothiazide, dolutegravir, megestrol, or other drugs that prolong QT interval	TdP	• ECG (QTc interval) • SCr • Electrolytes	↑ risk of TdP with other drugs that prolong QT interval	• Used only for atrial arrhythmias • Adjust dose based on renal function and QT interval • Must be initiated in hospital • Safe to use in HF

Class III *(cont'd)*

Generic • Brand • Dose	Contra-indications	Primary Side Effects	Key Monitoring	Pertinent Drug Interactions	Med Pearl
Ibutilide • Corvert • IV: 1 mg over 10 min; repeat × 1, if needed	• QTc interval >440 msec • Hypokalemia/hypomagnesemia • Concurrent use of other drugs that prolong QT interval	TdP	• ECG (QTc interval) • Electrolytes	↑ risk of TdP with other drugs that prolong QT interval	Used only for atrial arrhythmias
Sotalol • Betapace, Betapace AF, Sorine, Sotylize • PO: 160–640 mg/day (in 2 divided doses)	• ≥2nd-degree heart block (in absence of pacemaker) • Concurrent use of other drugs that prolong QT interval • CrCl <40 mL/min (for AF) • Long QT syndrome • HF	• TdP • Bradycardia/heart block • Bronchospasm • HF exacerbation	• ECG (QTc interval, PR interval) • HR • SCr • Electrolytes	• ↑ risk of TdP with other drugs that prolong QT interval • Use with other negative chronotropes (e.g., β-blockers, digoxin, verapamil, diltiazem, clonidine, or ivabradine) may ↑ risk of bradycardia	• Used for atrial and ventricular arrhythmias • Adjust dosing interval in renal impairment • Also available as oral solution and injection

Class IV Antiarrhythmics

(See medication chart in HTN section for discussion on non-DHP CCBs.)

ANTITHROMBOTIC DRUGS

Vitamin K Antagonist

Generic • Brand • Dose	Contra-indications	Primary Side Effects	Key Monitoring	Pertinent Drug Interactions	Med Pearl
Mechanism of action – interferes with synthesis of vitamin-K-dependent clotting factors of the liver (II, VII, IX, and X) as well as protein C and S					
Warfarin • Coumadin, Jantoven • Usual initial dose: 5–10 mg daily (2.5–10 mg daily in older adults)	• Pregnancy • Recent surgery	• Bleeding • Skin necrosis (especially in patients with protein C deficiency) • Purple toe syndrome	• Prothrombin time (PT)/international normalized ratio (INR) • Hemoglobin (Hgb)/hematocrit (Hct) • Bleeding	• CYP2C9 and CYP3A4 substrate • CYP2C9 and CYP3A4 inhibitors may ↑ effects and risk of bleeding • CYP3A4 inducers may ↓ effects and ↑ risk of clotting	• Vitamin K is antidote (PO preferred) • Full effect of a particular dose not seen for 3–4 days

Direct Thrombin Inhibitor (Oral)

Generic • Brand • Dose	Contra-indications	Primary Side Effects	Key Monitoring	Pertinent Drug Interactions	Med Pearl
Mechanism of action – direct thrombin inhibitor					
Dabigatran • Pradaxa • AF: • CrCl >30 mL/min: 150 mg BID • CrCl 15–30 mL/min: 75 mg BID • CrCl <15 mL/min: Not recommended • Treatment of deep venous thrombosis (DVT)/ pulmonary embolism (PE): • CrCl >30 mL/min: 150 mg BID (after 5–10 days of parenteral anticoagulation) • CrCl ≤30 mL/min: No dosing recommendations • Prevention of recurrent DVT/PE: • CrCl >30 mL/min: 150 mg BID • CrCl ≤30 mL/min: No dosing recommendations • Prevention of DVT/PE after hip replacement surgery: • CrCl >30 mL/min: 110 mg 1–4 hr after surgery, then 220 mg daily × 28–35 days • CrCl ≤30 mL/min: No dosing recommendations	• Active bleeding • Mechanical prosthetic heart valve	• Bleeding • Dyspepsia	• Hgb/Hct • Bleeding	• P-gp substrate • P-gp inhibitors may ↑ effects and risk of bleeding • Rifampin ↓ effects and ↑ risk of clotting (avoid concurrent use) AF: • ↓ dabigatran dose to 75 mg BID when used with dronedarone or ketoconazole if CrCl 30–50 mL/min (avoid concurrent use with P-gp inhibitors if CrCl <30 mL/min) DVT/PE treatment/prevention (including after hip replacement surgery): • Avoid concurrent use with P-gp inhibitors if CrCl <50 mL/min	• When converting from warfarin, discontinue warfarin and start dabigatran when INR <2 • When converting to warfarin, adjust starting time of warfarin based on CrCl • When converting from parenteral anticoagulant, start dabigatran 0–2 hr before time of next dose of or at time of discontinuation of parenteral anticoagulant • When converting to parenteral anticoagulant, wait 12–24 hr (based on CrCl) after last dose of dabigatran before starting therapy with parenteral anticoagulant • Antidote = idarucizumab (Praxbind); 2.5 g IV; repeat dose in 15 min

Factor Xa Inhibitors (Oral)

Generic • Brand • Dose	Contra-indications	Primary Side Effects	Key Monitoring	Pertinent Drug Interactions	Med Pearl
Mechanism of action – factor Xa inhibitor					

Apixaban
• Eliquis
• AF:
  • 5 mg BID
  • If patient has ≥2 of the following (age ≥80 yr, weight ≤60 kg, SCr ≥1.5 mg/dL): 2.5 mg BID
• Postoperative DVT/PE prophylaxis:
  • 2.5 mg BID (× 35 days for hip replacement; × 12 days for knee replacement)
• Treatment of DVT/PE:
  • 10 mg BID × 7 days, then 5 mg BID
• Prevention of recurrent DVT/PE in patients at continued risk for recurrent DVT/PE after completion of initial therapy lasting ≥6 mo:
  • 10 mg daily with or without food
	Active bleeding	Bleeding	• Hgb/Hct
			• Bleeding
				• CYP3A4 and P-gp substrate
				• CYP3A4 and P-gp inhibitors may ↑ effects and risk of bleeding (if receiving 5 mg BID or 10 mg BID dose, ↓ apixaban dose by 50% when used with strong dual inhibitors of CYP3A4 and P-gp; if receiving 2.5 mg BID dose, avoid concurrent use with strong dual inhibitors of CYP3A4 and P-gp)
				• CYP3A4 and P-gp inducers ↓ effects and ↑ risk of clotting (avoid concurrent use)
					• When converting from warfarin, discontinue warfarin and start apixaban when INR <2
					• When converting to warfarin, discontinue apixaban and start parenteral anticoagulant and warfarin at the time the next dose of apixaban would have been taken; discontinue parenteral anticoagulant when desired INR achieved
					• When converting from parenteral anticoagulant, discontinue parenteral anticoagulant and start apixaban at the usual time of the next dose of parenteral anticoagulant
					• When converting to parenteral anticoagulant, discontinue apixaban and initiate parenteral anticoagulant at time the next dose of apixaban would have been taken
					• Antidote = Coagulation factor Xa (inactivated) (Andexxa); dose is dependent on apixaban dose and time since last dose of apixaban

Factor Xa Inhibitors (Oral) *(cont'd)*

Generic • Brand • Dose	Contra-indications	Primary Side Effects	Key Monitoring	Pertinent Drug Interactions	Med Pearl
Betrixaban • Bevyxxa • DVT/PE prophylaxis in at-risk hospital-ized patients: • CrCl ≥30 mL/min: 160 mg × 1, then 80 mg daily with food (treatment duration = 35–42 days) • CrCl 15–29 mL/min: 80 mg × 1, then 40 mg daily with food (treat-ment duration = 35–42 days)	Active bleeding	Bleeding	• Hgb/Hct • Bleeding	• P-gp substrate • P-gp inhibitors may ↑ effects and risk of bleeding (↓ betrixaban dose to 80 mg × 1, then 40 mg daily when used with P-gp inhibitors)	No antidote currently available

Factor Xa Inhibitors (Oral) *(cont'd)*

Generic • Brand • Dose	Contra-indications	Primary Side Effects	Key Monitoring	Pertinent Drug Interactions	Med Pearl

Edoxaban
• Savaysa
• AF:
  • CrCl >95 mL/min: Avoid use
  • CrCl 51–95 mL/min: 60 mg daily
  • CrCl 15–50 mL/min: 30 mg daily
• Treatment of DVT/PE:
  • CrCl ≥51 mL/min: 60 mg daily (after 5–10 days of parenteral anticoagulation)
  • CrCl 15–50 mL/min or weight ≤60 kg: 30 mg daily (after 5–10 days of parenteral anticoagulation)
	Active bleeding	Bleeding	• Hgb/Hct
			• Bleeding
				• P-gp substrate
				• P-gp inhibitors may ↑ effects and risk of bleeding
				• Rifampin may ↓ effects and ↑ risk of clotting (avoid concurrent use)
				Treatment of DVT/PE:
				• ↓ edoxaban dose to 30 mg daily when used with verapamil, quinidine, azithromycin, clarithromycin, erythromycin, itraconazole, or ketoconazole
					• When converting from warfarin, discontinue warfarin and start edoxaban when INR ≤2.5
					• When converting to warfarin, ↓ dose of edoxaban (60 mg to 30 mg daily; 30 mg to 15 mg daily) and begin warfarin concurrently; discontinue edoxaban when desired INR achieved; may also discontinue edoxaban and start parenteral anticoagulant and warfarin at the time the next dose of edoxaban would have been taken; discontinue parenteral anticoagulant when desired INR achieved
					• When converting from low molecular weight heparin (LMWH), start edoxaban at the time of the next dose of LMWH (and discontinue LMWH); for unfractionated heparin (UFH), discontinue infusion and start edoxaban 4 hr later
					• When converting to parenteral anticoagulant, discontinue edoxaban and initiate parenteral anticoagulant at time the next dose of edoxaban would have been taken
					• No antidote currently available

Factor Xa Inhibitors (Oral)   *(cont'd)*

Generic • Brand • Dose	Contra-indications	Primary Side Effects	Key Monitoring	Pertinent Drug Interactions	Med Pearl
Rivaroxaban • Xarelto • AF: • CrCl >50 mL/min: 20 mg daily with evening meal • CrCl 15–50 mL/min: 15 mg daily with evening meal • Postoperative DVT/PE prophylaxis: • 10 mg daily (× 35 days for hip replacement; × 12 days for knee replacement) • Treatment of DVT/PE: • 15 mg BID with food × 21 days, then 20 mg daily with food • Prevention of recurrent DVT/PE in patients at continued risk for recurrent DVT/PE after completion of initial therapy lasting ≥6 mo: • 10 mg daily with or without food	Active bleeding	Bleeding	• Hgb/Hct • Bleeding	• CYP3A4 and P-gp substrate • CYP3A4 and P-gp inhibitors may ↑ effects and risk of bleeding (avoid concurrent use with combined P-gp and strong CYP3A4 inhibitors) • CYP3A4 and P-gp inducers ↓ effects and ↑ risk of clotting (avoid concurrent use with combined P-gp and strong CYP3A4 inducers)	• When converting from warfarin, discontinue warfarin and start rivaroxaban when INR <3 • When converting to warfarin, discontinue rivaroxaban and start parenteral anticoagulant and warfarin at the time the next dose of rivaroxaban would have been taken; discontinue parenteral anticoagulant when desired INR achieved • When converting from parenteral anticoagulant, start rivaroxaban 0–2 hr before time of next dose of parenteral anticoagulant (and discontinue parenteral anticoagulant); for UFH, discontinue infusion and start rivaroxaban • When converting to parenteral anticoagulant, discontinue rivaroxaban and initiate parenteral anticoagulant at time the next dose of rivaroxaban would have been taken • Antidote = Coagulation factor Xa (inactivated) (Andexxa); dose is dependent on rivaroxaban dose and time since last dose of rivaroxaban

ISCHEMIC HEART DISEASE

Findings	UA	NSTEMI	STEMI
Cardiac enzymes (troponin, CK-MB)	Negative	Positive	Positive
ECG changes	ST-segment depression, T-wave inversion, or no ECG changes (any changes are usually transient)	ST-segment depression, T-wave inversion, or no ECG changes	ST-segment elevation

ACUTE PHARMACOLOGIC MANAGEMENT OF UA/NSTEMI

Anti-Ischemic and Analgesic Therapy

Morphine

- May be reasonable for patients who continue to have chest discomfort despite maximally tolerated anti-ischemic medications
- Dose: 1–5 mg IV every 5–30 minutes as needed for pain

NTG

- Can be given to patients with ongoing chest discomfort (0.4 mg sublingually every 5 min × 3 doses); following these doses, give IV NTG within the initial 48 hours if patients continue to have ischemia, or if they present with HF or are hypertensive
- Dose: 5–10 mcg/min continuous infusion; can be titrated up to 100 mcg/min for relief of symptoms
- Adverse effects: Reflex tachycardia, hypotension, headache

β-Blockers

- Oral β-blockers: Given within the first 24 hours to patients who **do not** have signs/symptoms of HF, risk factors for developing cardiogenic shock (age >70 years, SBP <120 mmHg, HR >110 bpm, or prolonged duration since presenting with UA/NSTEMI), PR interval >0.24 sec, ≥2nd-degree heart block, or severe reactive airway disease
- IV β-blockers no longer recommended

CCBs

- A non-DHP CCB (verapamil or diltiazem) can be used alternatively if the patient has a contraindication to β-blocker therapy and does not have evidence of LV dysfunction.
- A long-acting non-DHP CCB can be used in patients who have recurrent ischemia despite being on a β-blocker and nitrate therapy.

ACEIs

- Should be given to all patients with LVEF ≤40% and in those with HTN, DM, or stable CKD, provided they have no contraindications
- May be reasonable in all other patients with cardiac or other vascular disease
- An ARB can be used alternatively in patients who cannot tolerate ACEIs.

Antiplatelet Therapy

Aspirin

- All patients should receive 162–325 mg (non–enteric-coated) at the onset of chest pain (should be chewed and swallowed).
- Patients should continue to receive 81–325 mg daily indefinitely (regardless of whether the patient undergoes PCI).

Clopidogrel (Plavix)

- Prodrug; must be converted via CYP2C19 to active drug
- The following loading and maintenance doses should be given (**with** aspirin):
  - Early invasive strategy (PCI ± stent)
    - » Loading dose = 600 mg × 1
    - » Maintenance dose = 75 mg daily
    - » Continue for ≥12 months
  - Ischemia-guided strategy
    - » Loading dose = 300 mg × 1
    - » Maintenance dose = 75 mg daily
    - » Continue for up to 12 months
- Can also be used as an alternative to aspirin in patients who are allergic or have a major GI intolerance to aspirin
- Drug interactions
  - Avoid concurrent use of omeprazole or esomeprazole (use pantoprazole if PPI needed).
  - Opioids may ↓ levels (use IV antiplatelet during ACS if opioid needed).
- Discontinue ≥5 days before CABG.

Prasugrel (Effient)

- Prodrug
- Alternative to clopidogrel in patients with ACS managed with early invasive strategy
- Initiate only in patients with known coronary artery anatomy (after angiography, but before PCI).

- Achieves faster inhibition of platelet aggregation than clopidogrel
- Administered as a loading dose of 60 mg prior to PCI, followed by maintenance dose of 10 mg daily ($\downarrow$ dose to 5 mg daily in patients <60 kg)
- Not recommended for patients ≥75 years unless they have DM or history of MI ($\uparrow$ risk of bleeding), in patients with prior history of stroke or TIA, or in patients requiring triple antithrombotic therapy
- Drug interactions: Opioids may $\downarrow$ levels (use IV antiplatelet during ACS if opioid needed).
- Continue for ≥12 months.
- Discontinue ≥7 days before CABG.

Ticagrelor (Brilinta)

- NOT a thienopyridine
  - Reversibly binds to the P2Y12 receptor
  - Does not require conversion to an active metabolite (NOT a prodrug)
- Alternative to clopidogrel in patients with ACS managed with early invasive or ischemia-guided strategy
- Contraindicated in severe hepatic impairment
- Drug interactions
  - CYP3A4 substrate; CYP3A4 and P-gp inhibitor
  - Avoid concurrent use with strong CYP3A4 inhibitors or inducers.
  - Avoid simvastatin or lovastatin doses >40 mg/day.
  - May $\uparrow$ digoxin levels
  - Opioids may $\downarrow$ levels (use IV antiplatelet during ACS if opioid needed).
- Administered as a loading dose of 180 mg prior to PCI, followed by maintenance dose of 90 mg BID (dose of aspirin during maintenance therapy should not exceed 100 mg/day); if continued >12 months, $\downarrow$ dose to 60 mg BID
- Continue for ≥12 months (early invasive strategy) or up to 12 months (ischemia-guided strategy).
- Discontinue ≥5 days before CABG.

Glycoprotein IIb/IIIa Receptor Blockers (GPBs)

- PCI planned: Clopidogrel (or ticagrelor) and/or GPB (eptifibatide or tirofiban) can be initiated prior to angiography. Do not need GPB if bivalirudin + 300 mg loading dose of clopidogrel (given ≥6 hours before angiography) are used.
- Conservative strategy: Adding eptifibatide or tirofiban to clopidogrel or ticagrelor can be considered (especially if patient has recurrent ischemia and requires angiography).

Anticoagulant Therapy

- Early invasive strategy: UFH, enoxaparin, fondaparinux, or bivalirudin should be added to antiplatelet therapy.
- Ischemia-guided strategy: UFH, enoxaparin, or fondaparinux should be added to antiplatelet therapy.

ACUTE PHARMACOLOGIC MANAGEMENT OF STEMI

Anti-Ischemic and Analgesic Therapy

Morphine, NTG, β-Blockers, ACEIs

- Same recommendations as for UA/NSTEMI

Antiplatelet Therapy

Aspirin

- Same recommendations as for UA/NSTEMI

Clopidogrel

- The following loading and maintenance doses should be given:
  - Patients undergoing primary PCI
    - » Loading dose = 600 mg × 1
    - » Maintenance dose = 75 mg daily
  - Patients receiving fibrinolytic therapy and patients who do not receive reperfusion therapy
    - » Loading dose = 300 mg × 1 (no loading dose in patients age ≥75 years)
    - » Maintenance dose = 75 mg daily
- Can also be used as an alternative to aspirin in patients who are allergic or have a major GI intolerance to aspirin
- Clopidogrel should be continued (**with** aspirin) for the following durations of time:
  - Bare metal stent (BMS) or drug-eluting stent (DES): 12 months
  - No stent: At least 14 days (can be considered for up to 1 year)
- Discontinue ≥ 5 days before CABG.

Prasugrel

- Same recommendations as for UA/NSTEMI

Ticagrelor

- Same recommendations as for UA/NSTEMI

GPBs

- Can be used if patient undergoing primary PCI

Fibrinolytic Therapy

- Should be used in patients presenting to a hospital without the capability to perform PCI or cannot perform PCI within 120 minutes of first medical contact ("door-to-balloon" time)
- Should be initiated within 30 minutes of presenting to the hospital ("door-to-needle" time)

Anticoagulant Therapy

- Fibrinolytic administered: UFH, enoxaparin, or fondaparinux can be used; should be continued for up to 8 days; UFH should only be used if the treatment duration is <48 hours because of risk for heparin-induced thrombocytopenia (HIT) with prolonged therapy.
- Primary PCI: UFH or bivalirudin can be used.

SECONDARY PREVENTION OF MI

- **Aspirin:** See recommendation above regarding dosing and duration of therapy.
- **Clopidogrel, prasugrel, or ticagrelor:** See recommendations in respective NSTEMI and STEMI sections regarding dosing and duration of therapy.
- **β-blockers:** Continue indefinitely.
- **ACEIs:** Should be given and continued indefinitely in all patients; ARB can be used in patients intolerant of ACEIs.
- **ARAs:** Should be given to patients with LVEF ≤40% receiving optimal ACEI and β-blocker therapy who have DM or HF.
- **Statins:** Should be given and continued indefinitely in all patients.

Glycoprotein IIb/IIIa Receptor Blockers

Generic • Brand • Dose	Contra-indications	Primary Side Effects	Key Monitoring	Pertinent Drug Interactions	Med Pearl
Mechanism of action — block the glycoprotein IIb/IIIa receptor on platelets to prevent the binding of fibrinogen → Inhibit platelet aggregation					
Abciximab • ReoPro • *Loading dose:* 0.25 mg/kg IV bolus • *Maintenance dose:* 0.125 mcg/kg/min (max of 10 mcg/min); continue for 12 hr after PCI Eptifibatide • Integrilin • *Loading dose:* 180 mcg/kg (max of 22.6 mg) IV bolus × 2 (given 10 min apart) • *Maintenance dose:* 2 mcg/kg/min (max of 15 mg/hr); continue for 18–24 hr after PCI Tirofiban • Aggrastat • NSTEMI: 　• *Loading dose:* 25 mcg/kg IV over ≤5 min 　• *Maintenance dose:* 0.15 mcg/kg/min; continue for up to 18 hr after PCI • STEMI (with PCI): 　• *Loading dose:* 25 mcg/kg IV bolus 　• *Maintenance dose:* 0.15 mcg/kg/min; continue for 18–24 hr after PCI	• Active bleeding • Prior stroke within past 30 days or any hemorrhagic stroke • History of intracranial neoplasms or aneurysm • Thrombocytopenia • BP >180/110 mmHg • Dialysis-dependent (for eptifibatide)	• Bleeding • Thrombocytopenia	• CBC • PT/activated partial thromboplastin time (aPTT) • Activated clotting time (ACT) (with PCI) • S/S bleeding • SCr (baseline)	Anticoagulants and other antiplatelets may ↑ risk of bleeding	Adjust dose of maintenance infusion of tirofiban and eptifibatide in renal impairment

Anticoagulants

Generic • Brand • Dose	Contra-indications	Primary Side Effects	Key Monitoring	Pertinent Drug Interactions	Med Pearl
Mechanism of action: • UFH: Potentiates the action of antithrombin III, which inactivates the clotting factors, IIa (thrombin), IXa, Xa, XIa, and XIIa, and ultimately prevents the conversion of fibrinogen to fibrin • Enoxaparin: LMWH; similar mechanism as UFH, but primarily inhibits factor Xa • Fondaparinux: Selective inhibitor of factor Xa • Bivalirudin: Direct thrombin inhibitor					
UFH • Only available generically • *Loading dose:* 60 units/kg IV bolus (max = 4,000 units) • *Maintenance dose:* 12 units/kg/hr (max = 1,000 units/hr)	• Active bleeding • History of HIT (within the past 100 days or in the presence of circulating antibodies for enoxaparin) • Recent stroke	• Bleeding • Thrombocytopenia (UFH and LMWH)	• PT/aPTT (only for UFH) • CBC • Anti-Xa levels (for enoxaparin) (consider in obese or renal impairment) • S/S bleeding	Antiplatelets and other anticoagulants may ↑ risk of bleeding	• If platelets <100,000 or ↓ by >50% from baseline, test for HIT; discontinue UFH and start direct thrombin inhibitor (e.g., argatroban, bivalirudin) • Protamine can be used to reverse effects
Enoxaparin • Lovenox • *Loading dose:* 30 mg IV × 1 (for STEMI only) • *Maintenance dose:* 1 mg/kg subcut every 12 hr					• ↓ enoxaparin dose to 1 mg/kg every 24 hr if CrCl <30 mL/min • Protamine only partially reverses effects
Fondaparinux • Arixtra • 2.5 mg subcut daily	• Active bleeding • CrCl <30 mL/min				For STEMI, can give initial dose IV
Bivalirudin • Angiomax • *Loading dose:* 0.75 mg/kg IV bolus • *Maintenance dose:* 1.75 mg/kg/hr	Active bleeding		• PT/aPTT • ACT		Can also be used during PCI in patients with HIT

Fibrinolytic Agents

Generic • Brand • Dose	Contra-indications	Primary Side Effects	Key Monitoring	Pertinent Drug Interactions	Med Pearl
Mechanism of action – activate and convert plasminogen into plasmin, which then degrades fibrin (lyses the clot) to form fibrin degradation products					
Alteplase • Activase • 15 mg IV bolus, then 0.75 mg/kg (max = 50 mg) over 30 min, then 0.5 mg/kg (max = 35 mg) over 60 min	• Active bleeding • Any history of intracranial hemorrhage • Known intracranial neoplasm or arteriovenous malformation • Suspected aortic dissection • Significant closed head or facial trauma within 3 months	Bleeding	• CBC • ECG (for signs of reperfusion) • S/S bleeding	Antiplatelets and other anticoagulants may ↑ risk of bleeding	Alteplase also approved for treatment of acute ischemic stroke and pulmonary embolism
Reteplase (rPA) • Retavase • 10 units IV × 2 doses (separated by 30 min)					
Tenecteplase (TNK) • TNKase • All doses given as IV bolus: • <60 kg: 30 mg • 60–69.9 kg: 35 mg • 70–79.9 kg: 40 mg • 80–89.9 kg: 45 mg • ≥90 kg: 50 mg					

Infectious Diseases

2

This chapter reviews various antibiotic agents, including antibacterial, antifungal, and antiviral agents. A brief overview of the recommended pharmacologic treatments of the following infections is also provided:

- **Urinary tract infections**
- **Pneumonia**
- **Meningitis**
- **Infective endocarditis**
- **Infectious diarrhea**
- **Otitis media**
- **Sexually transmitted diseases**
- **Skin and soft tissue infections**
- **Invasive fungal infections**
- **Human immunodeficiency virus**
- **Tuberculosis**

PRINCIPLES OF ANTIBIOTIC THERAPY

Factors to Consider When Selecting Antibiotic Therapy

- Identity/susceptibility of bacteria
  - Important to know which bacteria may be causing the infection
    - » Can begin empiric antibiotic therapy without knowing the actual identity (or sensitivities) of the organism; select antibiotic(s) (usually broad-spectrum) based on the organism(s) *most* likely to cause a particular infection.
    - » Once organism (and sensitivities) identified, adjust/narrow antibiotic therapy, as needed, to cover this organism.

- Site of infection
  - Especially important for meningitis, urinary tract infections (UTIs), prostatitis, and osteomyelitis
    - » Only certain antibiotics can penetrate into these areas to target the infection; these drugs may need to be used at higher doses, especially for meningitis, prostatitis, and osteomyelitis.
- Patient allergies
- Concomitant medications
  - May need to be concerned with potential drug interactions when selecting an antibiotic
- Hepatic and renal function
  - May need to adjust antibiotic dosages if hepatic or renal dysfunction present
- Past medical history
  - Certain antibiotics may need to be avoided in particular disease states (e.g., seizure disorders).
- Patient age
  - Some antibiotics are contraindicated in pediatric patients.
- Pregnancy/breastfeeding
  - Some antibiotics are contraindicated in these patients.

URINARY TRACT INFECTIONS

Guidelines Summary

Acute Uncomplicated Cystitis

First-line therapy	Nitrofurantoin 100 mg PO BID × 5 days
Second-line therapy	Trimethoprim/sulfamethoxazole (TMP/SMX) 160/800 mg (double-strength [DS]) PO BID × 3 days
Third-line therapy	Fosfomycin 3 g PO × 1 dose

- *Alternative agents*
  - Fluoroquinolone (FQ) × 3 days
    - » Only use when other agents cannot be used.
  - β-lactams (i.e., amoxicillin-clavulanate, cefdinir, cefaclor, cefpodoxime) × 3–7 days
    - » Avoid unless other agents are not appropriate.

Acute Pyelonephritis (Outpatient Therapy)

- First-line therapy
  - Ciprofloxacin 500 mg PO BID × 7 days
  - Cipro XR 1 g PO daily × 7 days
  - Levofloxacin 750 mg PO daily × 5 days
  - May be combined with either of the following:
    - Ceftriaxone 1 g IV × 1 day **OR**
    - Gentamicin 5–7 mg/kg IV × 1 day
- Second-line therapy: TMP/SMX DS PO BID × 14 days
  - May be combined with either of the following:
    - Ceftriaxone 1 g IV × 1 day **OR**
    - Gentamicin 5–7 mg/kg IV × 1 day
- Third-line therapy: Oral β-lactam (i.e., amoxicillin-clavulanate) × 10–14 days AND one-time dose of ceftriaxone 1 g IV or gentamicin 5–7 mg/kg IV

Acute Pyelonephritis (Inpatient Therapy)

- IV FQ
- Aminoglycoside +/– IV ampicillin
- IV extended-spectrum cephalosporin or penicillin +/– aminoglycoside
- IV carbapenem (e.g., imipenem/cilastatin)

Complicated UTIs

- Duration of therapy: 10–14 days

PNEUMONIA

Guidelines Summary

Diagnosis	Treatment	Duration
Community-acquired (ambulatory)	*Previously healthy and no antibiotic therapy in past 3 months:* Macrolide (clarithromycin or azithromycin) **OR** Doxycycline	≥5 days
	With comorbidities (see table notes)[1] that place patient at risk for drug-resistant Streptococcus pneumoniae or antibiotic use in past 3 months: FQ (moxifloxacin, gemifloxacin, or levofloxacin) **OR** Macrolide (or doxycycline) *plus* one of the following: • High-dose amoxicillin • Amoxicillin/clavulanate • Cephalosporin (ceftriaxone, cefuroxime, or cefpodoxime)	
Community-acquired (hospitalized)	*Not in Intensive Care Unit (ICU):* FQ (moxifloxacin, gemifloxacin, or levofloxacin) **OR** Macrolide (or doxycycline) *plus* one of the following: • Ampicillin • Ceftriaxone • Cefotaxime	
	In ICU: FQ (moxifloxacin, gemifloxacin, or levofloxacin) *plus* one of the following: • Ampicillin/sulbactam • Ceftriaxone • Cefotaxime **OR** Azithromycin *plus* one of the following: • Ampicillin/sulbactam • Ceftriaxone • Cefotaxime	

Guidelines Summary *(cont'd)*

Diagnosis	Treatment	Duration
Hospital-acquired	*Not at high risk for mortality (see below)[2]* **AND** *no factors increasing likelihood of methicillin-resistant S. aureus (MRSA) (see below)[3] (select one of the following drugs):* • Piperacillin/tazobactam • Cefepime • Levofloxacin • Imipenem/cilastatin or meropenem	7 days
	Not at high risk for mortality (see below)[2] but **WITH** *factors increasing the likelihood of MRSA (see below)[3]:* Vancomycin **OR** Linezolid **PLUS** one of the following: • Piperacillin/tazobactam • Ceftazidime • Cefepime • Levofloxacin or ciprofloxacin • Imipenem/cilastatin or meropenem • Aztreonam	
	High risk for mortality (see below)[2] or receipt of IV antibiotics in the past 90 days: Vancomycin **OR** Linezolid **PLUS** 2 of the following (avoid 2 β-lactams): • Piperacillin/tazobactam • Ceftazidime • Cefepime • Levofloxacin or ciprofloxacin • Imipenem/cilastatin or meropenem • Aztreonam • Amikacin, or gentamicin, or tobramycin	

[1] *Comorbidities: Chronic obstructive pulmonary disease (COPD), diabetes, chronic renal failure, chronic liver failure, heart failure (HF), cancer, asplenia, immunosuppressed*

[2] *Risk factors for mortality: Need for ventilatory support due to pneumonia and septic shock*

[3] *Risk factors for MRSA infection: Prior IV antibiotic use in past 90 days, hospitalization in a unit where >20% of S. aureus isolates are methicillin-resistant or the prevalence of MRSA is unknown*

MENINGITIS

Guidelines Summary

Empiric Treatment

Age Group	Treatment
<1 mo	Ampicillin + aminoglycoside **OR** Ampicillin + cefotaxime
1–23 mo	Third-generation cephalosporin (cefotaxime or ceftriaxone) + vancomycin
2–50 yr	Third-generation cephalosporin (cefotaxime or ceftriaxone) + vancomycin
>50 yr	Third-generation cephalosporin (cefotaxime or ceftriaxone) + vancomycin + ampicillin

- Dexamethasone may be considered as adjunctive therapy for the following:
  - Infants and children: *H. influenzae* meningitis
  - Adults: *Streptococcus pneumoniae* meningitis

INFECTIVE ENDOCARDITIS

Guidelines Summary, Empiric Treatment

Viridans Group Streptococci and *Streptococcus bovis* Highly Susceptible to Penicillin (MIC ≤0.12 mcg/mL): Native Valve IE

Treatment Regimen	Duration	Clinical Pearls
Penicillin G 12–18 million units/day IV in 4–6 divided doses **OR** Ceftriaxone 2 g IV/IM q24h	4 wk 4 wk	If patient has NO β-lactam allergy
Penicillin G 12–18 million units/day IV in 6 divided doses **OR** ceftriaxone 2 g IV/IM q24h **PLUS** Gentamicin 3 mg/kg IV q24h or 1 mg/kg IV q8h	2 wk 2 wk	Should not be used if patients have: • Cardiac or extracardiac abscess • Creatinine clearance <20 mL/min For gentamicin q8h dosing: • Target peak concentration = 3–4 mcg/mL • Target trough concentration <1 mcg/mL
Vancomycin 15 mg/kg IV q12h	4 wk	• For patients with β-lactam allergy • Target trough concentration = 10–15 mcg/mL

Viridans Group Streptococci and *Streptococcus bovis* Relatively Resistant to Penicillin (MIC >0.12 and <0.5 mcg/mL): Native Valve IE

Treatment Regimen	Duration	Clinical Pearls
Penicillin G 24 million units/day IV in 4–6 divided doses **PLUS** Gentamicin 3 mg/kg IV q24h or 1 mg/kg IV q8h	4 wk 2 wk	If organism susceptible to ceftriaxone, may use ceftriaxone monotherapy For gentamicin q8h dosing: • Target peak concentration = 3–4 mcg/mL • Target trough concentration <1 mcg/mL
Vancomycin 15 mg/kg IV q12h	4 wk	• For patients with β-lactam allergy • Target trough concentration = 10–15 mcg/mL

Viridans Group Streptococci and *Streptococcus bovis* Resistant to Penicillin (MIC ≥0.5 mcg/mL): Native Valve IE

- Treat as enterococcal IE

Viridans Group Streptococci and *Streptococcus bovis* Susceptible to Penicillin (MIC ≤0.12 mcg/mL): Prosthetic Valve IE

Treatment Regimen	Duration	Clinical Pearls
Penicillin G 24 million units/day IV in 4–6 divided doses **OR** ceftriaxone 2 g IV/IM q24h **WITH OR WITHOUT** Gentamicin 3 mg/kg IV q24h or 1 mg/kg IV q8h	6 wk 2 wk	Do NOT give gentamicin if patient's CrCl <30 mL/min For gentamicin q8h dosing: • Target peak concentration = 3–4 mcg/mL • Target trough concentration <1 mcg/mL
Vancomycin 15 mg/kg IV q12h	6 wk	• For patients with β-lactam allergy • Target trough concentration = 10–15 mcg/mL

Viridans Group Streptococci and *Streptococcus bovis* Relatively or Fully Resistant to Penicillin (MIC >0.12 mcg/mL): Prosthetic Valve IE

Treatment Regimen	Duration	Clinical Pearls
Penicillin G 24 million units/day IV in 4–6 divided doses **OR** ceftriaxone 2 g IV/IM q24h **PLUS** Gentamicin 3 mg/kg IV q24h or 1 mg/kg IV q8h	6 wk 6 wk	For gentamicin q8h dosing: • Target peak concentration = 3–4 mcg/mL • Target trough concentration <1 mcg/mL
Vancomycin 15 mg/kg IV q12h	6 wk	• For patients with β-lactam allergy • Target trough concentration = 10–15 mcg/mL

Staphylococci: Native Valve IE

Treatment Regimen	Duration	Clinical Pearls
Oxacillin-Susceptible Strains		
Nafcillin or oxacillin 12 g/day IV in 4–6 divided doses	6 wk (complicated, right-sided IE and uncomplicated, left-sided IE); ≥6 wk (complicated, left-sided IE); 2 wk (uncomplicated, right-sided IE)	
Cefazolin 2 g IV q8h	6 wk	For patients with non-anaphylactoid-type β-lactam allergy
Vancomycin 15 mg/kg IV q12h	6 wk	• For patients with anaphylactoid-type β-lactam allergy • Target trough concentration = 10–20 mcg/mL
Oxacillin-Resistant Strains		
Vancomycin 15 mg/kg IV q12h	6 wk	Target trough concentration = 10–20 mcg/mL
Daptomycin ≥8 mg/kg/dose	6 wk	

Staphylococci: Prosthetic Valve IE

Treatment Regimen	Duration	Clinical Pearls
Oxacillin-Susceptible Strains		
Nafcillin or oxacillin 2 g IV q4h **PLUS**	≥6 wk	Cefazolin may be substituted for nafcillin/oxacillin in patients with non-anaphylactoid-type β-lactam allergy
Rifampin 300 mg IV/PO q8h **PLUS**	≥6 wk	Vancomycin may be substituted for nafcillin/oxacillin in patients with anaphylactoid-type β-lactam allergy
Gentamicin 3 mg/kg/day IV in 2–3 divided doses	2 wk	For gentamicin: • Target peak concentration = 3–4 mcg/mL • Target trough concentration <1 mcg/mL
Oxacillin-Resistant Strains		
Vancomycin 15 mg/kg IV q12h **PLUS**	≥6 wk	Target vancomycin trough concentration = 10–20 mcg/mL For gentamicin:
Rifampin 300 mg IV/PO q8h **PLUS**	≥6 wk	• Target peak concentration = 3–4 mcg/mL
Gentamicin 3 mg/kg/day IV in 2–3 divided doses	2 wk	• Target trough concentration <1 mcg/mL

Enterococcus Species Susceptible to Penicillin and Gentamicin in Patients Who Can Tolerate β-Lactam Therapy: Native or Prosthetic Valve IE

Treatment Regimen	Duration	Clinical Pearls
Ampicillin 2 g IV q4h **OR** penicillin G 18–30 million units IV in 6 divided doses **PLUS**	4–6 wk	Recommended for patients with CrCl >50 mL/min 4 wk of therapy recommended for patients with native valve IE with symptoms <3 mo
Gentamicin 3 mg/kg/day IV in 2–3 divided doses	4–6 wk	6 wk of therapy recommended for patients with native valve IE with symptoms >3 mo **OR** prosthetic valve IE For gentamicin: • Target peak concentration = 3–4 mcg/mL • Target trough concentration <1 mcg/mL
Ampicillin 2 g IV q4h **PLUS**	6 wk	Recommended for patients with CrCl <50 mL/min
Ceftriaxone 2 g IV q12h	6 wk	

Enterococcus Species Susceptible to Vancomycin and Gentamicin and Resistant to Penicillin in Patients Who Cannot Tolerate β-Lactam Therapy: Native or Prosthetic Valve IE

Treatment Regimen	Duration	Clinical Pearls
Vancomycin 15 mg/kg IV q12h **PLUS** Gentamicin 1 mg/kg IV q8h	6 wk 6 wk	Target vancomycin trough concentration = 10–20 mcg/mL For gentamicin: • Target peak concentration = 3–4 mcg/mL • Target trough concentration <1 mcg/mL

Enterococcus Species Resistant to Penicillin, Aminoglycosides, and Vancomycin: Native or Prosthetic Valve IE

Treatment Regimen	Duration
Linezolid 600 mg IV/PO q12h **OR** Daptomycin 10–12 mg/kg per dose	>6 wk >6 wk

INFECTIOUS DIARRHEA

Guidelines Summary

Organism	First-Line Treatment
Shigella	Azithromycin or ciprofloxacin or ceftriaxone
Salmonella (non-typhoidal)	Usually not indicated if uncomplicated (if treatment needed, use ceftriaxone or ciprofloxacin or TMP/SMX or amoxicillin)
Campylobacter	Azithromycin
Yersinia	TMP/SMX
E.coli, enterohemorrhagic (STEC)	Avoid antimotility drugs and antibiotics
C. difficile	• Discontinue antibiotics and avoid antimotility agents • Initial episode (nonsevere) (WBC ≤15,000 cells/mm^3 and SCr <1.5 mg/dL): Vancomycin 125 mg PO 4 times daily × 10 days **OR** fidaxomicin 200 mg PO BID × 10 days (metronidazole should be considered only if vancomycin and fidaxomicin unavailable) • Initial episode (severe) (WBC >15,000 cells/mm^3 or SCr >1.5 mg/dL): Vancomycin 125 mg PO 4 times daily × 10 days **OR** fidaxomicin 200 mg PO BID × 10 days • First recurrence: Vancomycin 125 mg PO 4 times daily × 10 days (if metronidazole was used for initial episode) **OR** prolonged vancomycin taper (if standard regimen used for initial episode) **OR** fidaxomicin 200 mg PO BID (if vancomycin was used for initial episode) • Bezlotoxumab (Zinplava), a monoclonal antibody that binds *C. difficile* toxin B, can be used in patients who are receiving antibacterial therapy for *C. difficile* infection and are at risk for recurrence of disease (age ≥65 years, history of *C. difficile* infection in previous 6 mo, immunocompromised, severe *C. difficile* infection, or *C. difficile* ribotype 027)
Giardia	Tinidazole or nitazoxanide
Cryptosporidium	Nitazoxanide
Isospora	TMP/SMX
Cyclospora	TMP/SMX

OTITIS MEDIA

Guidelines Summary

Initial Management of Uncomplicated AOM

Age	Otorrhea with AOM	Unilateral or Bilateral AOM with Severe Symptoms	Bilateral AOM without Otorrhea	Unilateral AOM without Otorrhea
• 6 months–2 years	• Antibiotic therapy	• Antibiotic therapy	• Antibiotic therapy	• Antibiotic therapy **OR** additional observation
• ≥2 years	• Antibiotic therapy	• Antibiotic therapy	• Antibiotic therapy **OR** additional observation	• Antibiotic therapy **OR** additional observation

Recommended Antibiotic Therapy for Management of Uncomplicated AOM

	First-Line Therapy	Alternative Therapy
Initial Immediate or Delayed Treatment	Amoxicillin (high-dose) 80–90 mg/kg/day PO in 2 divided doses **OR** *If history of amoxicillin use in past 90 days, concurrent purulent conjunctivitis, or history of recurrent AOM unresponsive to amoxicillin:* Amoxicillin-clavulanate (high-dose) 90 mg/kg/day of amoxicillin + 6.4 mg/kg/day of clavulanate PO in 2 divided doses	*If penicillin allergy:* Cefdinir **OR** Cefuroxime **OR** Cefpodoxime **OR** Ceftriaxone × 1 or 3 days
Treatment after 48–72 Hours of Failure of Initial Antibiotic Treatment	Amoxicillin-clavulanate (high-dose) 90 mg/kg/day of amoxicillin + 6.4 mg/kg/day of clavulanate PO in 2 divided doses **OR** Ceftriaxone 50 mg IM or IV for 3 days	Clindamycin

Duration of Therapy

Age/Characteristic of Symptoms	Duration
<2 yr or severe symptoms	10 days
2–5 yr with mild–moderate symptoms	7 days
≥6 yr with mild–moderate symptoms	5–7 days

SEXUALLY TRANSMITTED DISEASES

Guidelines Summary

Disease	Treatment
Chlamydia	Azithromycin 1 g PO × 1 dose **OR** Doxycycline 100 mg PO q12h × 7 days
Gonorrhea	Ceftriaxone 250 mg IM × 1 dose **PLUS** Azithromycin 1 g PO × 1 dose
Syphilis	*Primary, secondary, or early latent syphilis (<1 yr in duration):* • Benzathine penicillin G 2.4 million units IM × 1 dose *Late latent syphilis (>1 yr in duration), latent syphilis of unknown duration, or tertiary syphilis (not neurosyphilis):* • Benzathine penicillin G 2.4 million units IM once weekly × 3 weeks *Neurosyphilis:* • Aqueous penicillin G 3–4 million units IV q4h or as continuous infusion × 10–14 days

SKIN AND SOFT TISSUE INFECTIONS

Guidelines Summary

Infection	Empiric Treatment
Purulent SSTIs	
Mild	Incision and drainage; no antibiotics
Moderate (with systemic signs of infection*)	Incision and drainage **PLUS** antibiotics: TMP/SMX **OR** Doxycycline
Severe (failed incision and drainage plus PO antibiotics **OR** have systemic signs of infection,* **OR** are immunocompromised)	Incision and drainage **PLUS** antibiotics: Vancomycin **OR** Daptomycin **OR** Dalbavancin **OR** Linezolid **OR** Oritavancin **OR** Telavancin **OR** Tedizolid **OR** Ceftaroline
Nonpurulent SSTIs	
Mild	Penicillin VK **OR** Cephalosporin (PO) **OR** Dicloxacillin **OR** Clindamycin (PO)

Guidelines Summary   *(cont'd)*

Infection	Empiric Treatment
Moderate (with systemic signs of infection*)	Penicillin (IV) **OR** Ceftriaxone **OR** Cefazolin **OR** Clindamycin (IV)
Severe (failed PO antibiotics **OR** signs of systemic infection,* **OR** immunocompromised **OR** signs of deeper infection [e.g., bullae, skin sloughing, hypotension, evidence of organ dysfunction])	Emergent surgical inspection/debridement **PLUS** antibiotics: Vancomycin **AND** Piperacillin/tazobactam

* Signs of systemic infection: Temperature >38°C, heart rate >90 beats/minute, respiratory rate >24 breaths/minute, WBCs >12,000 cells/μL or <400 cells/μL

INVASIVE FUNGAL INFECTIONS

Drugs of Choice for Selected Invasive Fungal Infections

Organism	Disease	First-Line Therapy	Duration
Candida albicans, C. glabrata, C. krusei, C. tropicalis	Candidemia	*Nonneutropenic:* Echinocandin **OR** Fluconazole (if not critically ill) *Neutropenic:* Echinocandin **OR** Lipid amphotericin B **OR** Fluconazole (if not critically ill and no prior azole exposure) If *C. krusei:* Echinocandin, lipid amphotericin B, or voriconazole	14 days after first negative blood culture
	Urinary candidiasis	*Asymptomatic:* Eliminate predisposing factor (i.e., remove urinary catheter) Treat only if high-risk for dissemination: • Neutropenic: Treat as for candidemia (see above) • Undergoing urologic manipulation: Fluconazole (PO) **OR** amphotericin B *Symptomatic:* Fluconazole-susceptible organism: Fluconazole (PO) • Fluconazole-resistant *C. glabrata:* Amphotericin B **OR** flucytosine • *C. krusei:* Amphotericin B	*Asymptomatic:* Treatment for urologic manipulation: Several days before and after procedure *Symptomatic:* • Fluconazole-susceptible organisms: 14 days • Fluconazole-resistant *C. glabrata:* 7–10 days • *C. krusei:* 1–7 days

Drugs of Choice for Selected Invasive Fungal Infections *(cont'd)*

Organism	Disease	First-Line Therapy	Duration
Blastomyces dermatitidis	Pulmonary blastomycosis	*Mild to moderate:* Itraconazole *Moderately severe to severe:* Amphotericin B × 1–2 wk, then itraconazole × 6–12 mo	6–12 mo
	Disseminated blastomycosis	*Mild to moderate:* Itraconazole *Moderately severe to severe:* Amphotericin B × 1–2 wk, then itraconazole × 12 mo	*Mild to moderate:* 6–12 mo *Moderately severe to severe* 12 mo
	Immunosuppressed	Amphotericin B × 1–2 wk, then itraconazole × 12 mo	12 mo
Aspergillus fumigatus, A. flavus, A. niger	Pulmonary aspergillosis	Voriconazole	6–12 wk
Coccidioides immitis	Pulmonary coccidioidomycosis	High-dose fluconazole	3–6 mo
	Disseminated (nonmeningeal) coccidioidomycosis	Fluconazole or itraconazole	≥6–12 mo
	Disseminated (meningeal) coccidioidomycosis	Fluconazole	Lifelong
Histoplasma capsulatum	Pulmonary histoplasmosis	*Mild to moderate:* Symptoms <4 wk: No treatment Symptoms >4 wk: Itraconazole *Moderately severe to severe:* Amphotericin B × 1–2 wk, then itraconazole × total of 12 wk	*Mild to moderate:* 6–12 wk *Moderately severe to severe:* 12 wk
Cryptococcus neoformans	Cryptococcal meningoencephalitis (in HIV-infected patients)	*Induction:* Amphotericin B + flucytosine *Consolidation:* Fluconazole	*Induction:* ≥2 wk *Consolidation:* ≥8 wk

Antibacterial Agents

Penicillins (β-Lactams)

Generic • Brand • Dose/Dosage Forms	Spectrum of Activity	Contraindications	Primary Side Effects	Pertinent Drug Interactions	Med Pearl
Mechanism of action – inhibit bacterial cell wall synthesis; bactericidal					
Natural Penicillins					
Penicillin G • Only available generically • 2–4 million units IV q4–6h • Injection Penicillin G benzathine • Bicillin LA • 1.2–2.4 million units IM at specified intervals • Injection Penicillin G procaine • Only available generically • 1.2–4.8 million units IM/day at specified intervals • Injection Penicillin VK☆ • Only available generically • 250–500 mg PO q6h • Solution, tabs	• *Strep. viridans* • *Strep. pyogenes* • *Strep. pneumoniae* (↑ resistance) • Mouth anaerobes	Allergy to penicillins, cephalosporins, or carbapenems	• Hypersensitivity reaction (rash, hives, dyspnea, throat swelling) • Nausea/vomiting/diarrhea (N/V/D) • Interstitial nephritis • Hemolytic anemia (with prolonged administration) • Stevens-Johnson syndrome, toxic epidermal necrolysis	• Probenecid may ↑ effects (may be used for this purpose) • May ↓ effects of oral contraceptives	• Adjust dose in renal impairment • Penicillin G benzathine or procaine used for syphilis; benzathine also used for Strep throat • Take penicillin VK 1 hr before or 2 hr after meals
Penicillinase-Resistant Penicillins					
Dicloxacillin • Only available generically • 125–500 mg PO q6h • Caps Nafcillin • Only available generically • 500 mg–2 g IV q4–6h • Injection Oxacillin • Bactocill • 250 mg–2 g IV q4–6h • Injection	• *Staph aureus* (methicillin-sensitive, MSSA) • *Streptococcus*	Same as natural penicillins	Same as natural penicillins	Same as natural penicillins	• No need to adjust dose in renal impairment (cleared by biliary excretion) • Take dicloxacillin 1 hr before or 2 hr after meals • Patients on nafcillin (IV) or oxacillin (IV) can be switched to dicloxacillin (PO)

Penicillins (β-Lactams) *(cont'd)*

Generic • Brand • Dose/Dosage Forms	Spectrum of Activity	Contraindications	Primary Side Effects	Pertinent Drug Interactions	Med Pearl
Aminopenicillins					
Amoxicillin ☆ • Moxatag • Immediate-release (IR): 250–500 mg PO q8h or 500–875 mg PO q12h. Extended release (ER): 775 mg PO daily • Caps, chewable tabs, suspension, tabs (ER and IR)	• *Strep pneumoniae* • *H. influenzae* • *E. coli* • *Proteus mirabilis* • *Salmonella* • *Shigella*	Same as natural penicillins	Same as natural penicillins	Same as natural penicillins	• Amoxicillin can be used in 3-drug regimen for *H. pylori* • Adjust dose in renal impairment • Take ampicillin 1 hr before or 2 hr after meals
Ampicillin • Only available generically • 250–500 mg PO q6h • 250 mg–2 g IV q4–6h • Caps, injection, suspension					
Aminopenicillins + β-Lactamase Inhibitors					
Amoxicillin-clavulanate ☆ • Augmentin • IR: 250–500 mg PO q8h or 500–875 mg PO q12h • ER: 2,000 mg PO q12h • Chewable tabs, suspension, tabs (ER and IR)	• β-lactamase producing *Staph. aureus* (MSSA), *H. influenzae*, *M. catarrhalis*, *E. coli*, and *K. pneumoniae* • Anaerobes	Same as natural penicillins	Same as natural penicillins	Same as natural penicillins	• Adjust dose in renal impairment • Patients on ampicillin sulbactam (IV) can be switched to amoxicillin-clavulanate (PO) • Good anaerobic coverage
Ampicillin-sulbactam • Unasyn • 1.5–3 g IV q6h • Injection					
Antipseudomonal Penicillin + β-Lactamase Inhibitor					
Piperacillin-tazobactam • Zosyn • 3.375 IV q6h or 4.5 g IV q6–8h • Injection	• Same as amoxicillin-clavulanate and ampicillin-sulbactam • *Pseudomonas aeruginosa*	Same as natural penicillins	Same as natural penicillins	• Same as natural penicillins • ↑ risk of nephrotoxicity when used with vancomycin	• Adjust dose in renal impairment • Primarily used for *Pseudomonas* infections • Good anaerobic coverage • Contains Na+ (use with caution in volume-overloaded patients)

Cephalosporins (β-Lactams)

Generic • Brand • Dose/Dosage Forms	Spectrum of Activity	Contraindications	Primary Side Effects	Pertinent Drug Interactions	Med Pearl
Mechanism of action – inhibit bacterial cell wall synthesis; bactericidal • As drugs move from 1st through 4th generation, ↑ activity against Gram (−) organisms and ↓ activity against Gram (+) organisms					
First-Generation					
Cefadroxil • Only available generically • 500 mg–1 g PO q12h • Caps, suspension, tabs Cefazolin • Ancef • 250 mg–1 g IV q8h • Injection Cephalexin ☆ • Keflex • 250–500 mg PO q6h • Caps, suspension, tabs	• *Staph. aureus* (MSSA) • *Staph. epidermidis* • *Strep. pyogenes* • *Strep. pneumoniae* • *E. coli* • *P. mirabilis* • *K. pneumoniae*	Allergy to penicillins, cephalosporins, or carbapenems (up to 10% risk of cross-sensitivity)	Same as natural penicillins	Same as natural penicillins	• Adjust dose in renal impairment • Patients on cefazolin (IV) can be switched to cephalexin (PO) • Cefazolin often used for surgical prophylaxis
Second-Generation					
Cefaclor • Only available generically • 250–500 mg PO q8h • Caps, ER tabs, suspension Cefotetan • Cefotan • 1–2 g IV q12h • Injection Cefoxitin • Mefoxin • 1–2 g IV q6–8h • Injection Cefprozil • Only available generically • 250–500 mg q12–24h • Suspension, tabs Cefuroxime • Ceftin, Zinacef • 250–500 mg PO q12h • 500 mg–1.5 g IV q8h • Injection, suspension, tabs	• Gram (+) activity similar to 1st-generation agents • Same Gram (−) activity as 1st-generation agents, but with added activity against *Acinetobacter, Citrobacter, Enterobacter, Neisseria, Serratia,* and *H. influenzae* • Anaerobes (cefotetan and cefoxitin only)	Same as 1st-generation agents	• Same as natural penicillins • Bleeding/bruising (with cefotetan and cefoxitin)	• Same as natural penicillins • Disulfiram-like reaction may occur if alcohol is used during treatment with cefotetan • Cefotetan and cefoxitin may ↑ risk of bleeding with warfarin	• Adjust dose in renal impairment • Take cefaclor ER tabs and cefuroxime suspension with food to ↑ absorption

Cephalosporins (β-Lactams) *(cont'd)*

Generic • Brand • Dose/Dosage Forms	Spectrum of Activity	Contraindications	Primary Side Effects	Pertinent Drug Interactions	Med Pearl
Third-Generation					
Cefdinir☆ • Only available generically • 300 mg PO q12h or 600 mg PO daily • Caps, suspension	• Limited Gram (+) activity • More extensive Gram (−) activity vs. 2nd-generation agents • *Pseudomonas aeruginosa* (ceftazidime and ceftazidime-avibactam only)	• Same as 1st-generation agents • Ceftriaxone should be avoided in neonates (↑ risk of hyperbilirubinemia, kernicterus)	Same as natural penicillins	• Same as natural penicillins • Antacids and iron may ↓ absorption of cefdinir • Antacids and H₂ antagonists may ↓ absorption of cefpodoxime • Ceftriaxone may cause precipitation if given with Ca²⁺-containing solutions	• Adjust dose for all, except cefoperazone and ceftriaxone, in renal impairment • Take cefpodoxime tabs with food to ↑ absorption • Ceftriaxone often used for meningitis and sexually transmitted diseases (STDs) • Ceftazidime-avibactam indicated for complicated intra-abdominal infections (with metronidazole), complicated UTIs, and hospital-acquired/ventilator-associated bacterial pneumonia • Avibactam is β-lactamase inhibitor • ↓ efficacy of ceftazidime-avibactam in patients with CrCl 30–50 mL/min
Cefixime • Suprax • 400 mg PO daily • Caps, chewable tabs, suspension, tabs					
Cefotaxime • Only available generically • 1–2 g IV q8h • Injection					
Cefpodoxime • Only available generically • 100–400 mg PO q12h • Suspension, tabs					
Ceftazidime • Fortaz, Tazicef • 1–2 g IV q8–12h • Injection					
Ceftazidime-avibactam • Avycaz • 2.5 g IV q8h • Injection					
Ceftriaxone • Only available generically • 1–2 g IV daily • Injection					

Cephalosporins (β-Lactams) *(cont'd)*

Generic • Brand • Dose/Dosage Forms	Spectrum of Activity	Contraindications	Primary Side Effects	Pertinent Drug Interactions	Med Pearl
Fourth-Generation					
Cefepime • Maxipime • 1–2 g IV q8–12h • Injection	• Gram (+) activity better than 3rd-generation agents • More extensive Gram (−) activity vs. 3rd-generation agents • *Pseudomonas aeruginosa*	Same as 1st-generation agents	Same as natural penicillins	Same as natural penicillins	Adjust dose in renal impairment
Fifth-Generation					
Ceftaroline • Teflaro • 600 mg IV q12h • Injection	• *Staph. aureus* (MSSA and MRSA [for skin infections only]) • *Strep. pyogenes* • *Strep. pneumoniae* • *Klebsiella* • *E. coli* • *H. influenzae*	Same as 1st-generation agents	Same as natural penicillins	Same as natural penicillins	• Indicated for SSTIs and community-acquired pneumonia • Adjust dose in renal impairment
Ceftolozane-tazobactam • Zerbaxa • 1.5 g IV q8h • Injection	• Gram (+) and Gram (−) organisms, including drug-resistant organisms • *Pseudomonas aeruginosa* • Some activity against anaerobes (*Bacteroides fragilis*) • No activity against *Staph. aureus*				• Indicated for complicated intra-abdominal infections (with metronidazole) and complicated UTIs • Tazobactam is β-lactamase inhibitor • Adjust dose in renal impairment • ↓ efficacy in patients with CrCl 30–50 mL/min

Carbapenems (β-Lactams)

Generic • Brand • Dose/Dosage Forms	Spectrum of Activity	Contraindications	Primary Side Effects	Pertinent Drug Interactions	Med Pearl
Mechanism of action – inhibit bacterial cell wall synthesis; bactericidal					
Ertapenem • Invanz • 1 g IV daily • Injection	• Broad-spectrum (active against Gram [+], Gram [−], and anaerobic organisms) • All, except ertapenem, are active against *Pseudomonas aeruginosa*	Allergy to penicillins, cephalosporins, or carbapenems	• Same as natural penicillins • Seizures (esp. in patients with renal impairment or history of seizure disorder)	• Same as natural penicillins • May ↓ valproic acid levels	• Adjust dose in renal impairment • Risk of seizures is highest with imipenem/cilastatin
Imipenem-cilastatin • Primaxin • 250 mg–1 g IV q6–12h • Injection					
Meropenem • Merrem • 500 mg–1 g IV q8h • Injection					
Meropenem/vaborbactam • Vabomere • 4 g IV q8h • Injection	Gram (−) organisms, including *Pseudomonas aeruginosa*				• Indicated for complicated UTIs • Vaborbactam is β-lactamase inhibitor • Adjust dose in renal impairment

Monobactam (β-Lactam)

Generic • Brand • Dose/Dosage Forms	Spectrum of Activity	Contraindications	Primary Side Effects	Pertinent Drug Interactions	Med Pearl
Mechanism of action – inhibits bacterial cell wall synthesis; bactericidal					
Aztreonam • Azactam, Cayston • IV: 500 mg–2 g IV q6–12h • Nebs: 75 mg via nebulization 3× daily (at least 4 hr apart) × 28 days • Injection, nebulizer solution	Only effective against Gram (−) organisms, including *Pseudomonas aeruginosa*	None	Same as natural penicillins	None	• Can be used in patients allergic to penicillins, cephalosporins, or carbapenems • Adjust dose for IV in renal impairment • Cayston used for patients with cystic fibrosis (*Pseudomonas*); do not repeat for 28 days after completion

Aminoglycosides

Generic • Brand • Dose/Dosage Forms	Spectrum of Activity	Contraindications	Primary Side Effects	Pertinent Drug Interactions	Med Pearl
Mechanism of action – inhibit bacterial protein synthesis by binding to the 30S subunit of the bacterial ribosome; bactericidal					
Amikacin • Only available generically • 15 mg/kg IV q24h or 5–7.5 mg/kg IV q8h • Injection Gentamicin • Gentak • 5–7 mg/kg IV q24h or 1–2.5 mg/kg IV q8–12h • Injection, ophthalmic ointment/solution, topical cream/ointment Neomycin • Only available generically • 500 mg–2 g PO q6–8h • Tabs Plazomicin • Zemdri • 15 mg/kg IV q24h • Injection Streptomycin • Only available generically • 15 mg/kg/day IM • Injection Tobramycin • Bethkis, Kitabis Pak, TOBI, Tobrex • 5–7 mg/kg IV q24h or 1–2.5 mg/kg IV q8–12h • Caps for inhalation, injection, nebulizer solution, ophthalmic ointment/solution	• Primarily used for Gram (−) organisms (*E. coli, Klebsiella, P. mirabilis, Enterobacter, Acinetobacter, Serratia*) • Amikacin, gentamicin, and tobramycin active against *Pseudomonas aeruginosa* • Amikacin, gentamicin, and tobramycin provide synergistic activity against *Staph., Strep.,* or *Enterococcus* when used with penicillins or vancomycin • Streptomycin and amikacin active against *Mycobacteria* • Neomycin used as prep for bowel surgery or for hepatic encephalopathy	None	• Nephrotoxicity • Ototoxicity (both related to dose and duration of therapy; may be reversible) • Bronchospasm (inhalation only)	• May ↑ effects of neuromuscular blocking agents • ↑ risk of nephrotoxicity when used with amphotericin B, loop diuretics, tacrolimus, cyclosporine, or cisplatin	• Bactericidal effect is concentration-dependent • Adjust dose of amikacin, gentamicin, plazomicin, and tobramycin in renal impairment • Target serum concentrations (for traditional dosing): *Amikacin:* Peak = Life-threatening infections: 25–40 mcg/mL; serious infections: 20–25 mcg/mL, UTIs: 15–20 mcg/mL; Trough <8 mcg/mL (The American Thoracic Society [ATS] recommends trough levels of <4–5 mcg/mL for patients with hospital-acquired pneumonia) *Tobramycin and gentamicin:* Peak = 4–10 mcg/mL, depending on the infection; Trough = 0.5–2 mcg/mL for serious infections; <1 mcg/mL for hospital-acquired pneumonia • Target serum concentrations (for extended-interval dosing) (peaks not routinely monitored): *Amikacin:* Trough <8 mcg/mL (The ATS recommends trough levels of <4–5 mcg/mL for patients with hospital-acquired pneumonia) *Tobramycin and gentamicin:* Trough = 0.5–2 mcg/mL for serious infections, <1 mcg/mL for hospital-acquired pneumonia *Plazomicin:* Trough <3 mcg/mL • Bethkis, Kitabis Pak, and TOBI used for patients with cystic fibrosis (*Pseudomonas*) Plazomicin indicated for complicated UTIs

Macrolides

Generic • Brand • Dose/Dosage Forms	Spectrum of Activity	Contraindications	Primary Side Effects	Pertinent Drug Interactions	Med Pearl
Mechanism of action – inhibit bacterial protein synthesis by binding to the 50S subunit of the bacterial ribosome; bacteriostatic					
Macrolides					
Azithromycin☆ • AzaSite, Zithromax • 250–500 mg PO/IV q24h • Injection, ophthalmic solution, suspension, tabs Clarithromycin☆ • Biaxin • IR: 250–500 mg PO q12h • ER: 1,000 mg PO q24h • Suspension, tabs (IR and ER) Erythromycin • E.E.S., Erygel, EryPed, Ery-Tab, Erythrocin • 250–500 mg PO q6h • 500 mg–1 g IV q6h • Caps, injection, ophthalmic ointment, suspension, tabs, topical gel/ointment/solution Fidaxomicin • Dificid • 200 mg PO q12h • Tabs	• Gram (+) organisms (esp. *Streptococcus*); azithromycin and clarithromycin have better activity against *Streptococcus* than erythromycin • Gram (−) organisms • Atypical organisms (e.g., *Chlamydia pneumoniae*, *Legionella*, *Mycoplasma pneumoniae*) • Azithromycin and clarithromycin active against *Mycobacteria* • Fidaxomicin active against *Clostridium difficile*	• QT interval prolongation or concurrent use with other drugs that prolong QT interval (azithromycin, clarithromycin, and erythromycin) • Concurrent use with lovastatin or simvastatin (erythromycin)	• Prolonged QT interval (azithromycin, clarithromycin, and erythromycin) • N/V/D • Phlebitis (erythromycin IV) • Stevens-Johnson syndrome, toxic epidermal necrolysis	• Clarithromycin and erythromycin are major substrates and inhibitors of CYP3A4 (azithromycin less affected by CYP interactions) • CYP3A4 inhibitors may ↑ risk of side effects of clarithromycin and erythromycin • CYP3A4 inducers may ↓ effects of clarithromycin and erythromycin • Clarithromycin and erythromycin may ↑ effect/toxicity of CYP3A4 substrates • ↑ risk of torsade de pointes (TdP) with other drugs that prolong QT interval (azithromycin, clarithromycin, and erythromycin) • Azithromycin, clarithromycin, and erythromycin may ↑ risk of bleeding with warfarin • Azithromycin, clarithromycin, and erythromycin may ↑ risk of digoxin toxicity	• 400 mg erythromycin ethylsuccinate (EES) = 250 mg erythromycin base or stearate • Azithromycin, clarithromycin, and erythromycin are good alternatives for patients allergic to penicillin • Take with food to ↓ gastrointestinal (GI) effects • Clarithromycin can be used in 3-drug regimen for *H. pylori* • Erythromycin can be used for diabetic gastroparesis and acne • Take ER clarithromycin tabs with food to ↑ absorption • Azithromycin or erythromycin preferred in pregnancy • Use clarithromycin with caution in patients with coronary artery disease (↑ mortality) • Fidaxomicin used to treat *Clostridium difficile*

Tetracyclines

Generic • Brand • Dose/Dosage Forms	Spectrum of Activity	Contraindications	Primary Side Effects	Pertinent Drug Interactions	Med Pearl
Mechanism of action – inhibit bacterial protein synthesis by binding to the 30S subunit of the bacterial ribosome; bacteriostatic					
Demeclocycline • Only available generically • 150 mg PO q6h or 300 mg PO q12h • Tabs Doxycycline ☆ • Acticlate, Doryx, Monodox, Oracea, Vibramycin • 100 mg IV/PO q12h • Caps, delayed-release caps/tabs, injection, suspension, syrup, tabs Minocycline ☆ • Minocin, Minolira, Solodyn • 100 mg PO q12h • Caps, injection, tabs (IR and ER) Tetracycline • Only available generically • 250–500 mg PO q6–12h • Caps	• Gram (+) organisms • Gram (−) organisms • Atypical organisms	Children ≤8 yr and pregnant/breast-feeding women (may cause permanent teeth discoloration and impaired teeth/bone growth)	• N/V/D • Photosensitivity • Phlebitis (IV) • Vertigo (minocycline) • Intracranial hypertension (pseudotumor cerebri) • Stevens-Johnson syndrome, toxic epidermal necrolysis	• Absorption ↓ with antacids, dairy products, and products containing iron, magnesium, aluminum, calcium, or zinc (separate by 2 hr) • Tetracycline is a CYP3A4 substrate • CYP3A4 inhibitors may ↑ risk of side effects of tetracycline • CYP3A4 inducers may ↓ effects • May ↑ risk of bleeding with warfarin • May ↓ effects of oral contraceptives • Use with isotretinoin may ↑ risk of intracranial hypertension	• Good alternative for patients allergic to penicillin • Demeclocycline also used to treat syndrome of inappropriate antidiuretic hormone secretion (SIADH) • Tetracycline can be used in 4-drug regimen for *H. pylori* • All except demeclocycline can be used for acne • Doxycycline is drug of choice for Lyme disease • Take demeclocycline and tetracycline 1 hr before or 2 hr after meals • Do not use after expiration date (can cause Fanconi syndrome) • Adjust dose for all, except doxycycline, in renal impairment

Glycylcyclines

Generic • Brand • Dose/Dosage Forms	Spectrum of Activity	Contraindications	Primary Side Effects	Pertinent Drug Interactions	Med Pearl
Mechanism of action – inhibits bacterial protein synthesis by binding to the 30S subunit of the bacterial ribosome (mechanism similar to tetracyclines); bacteriostatic					
Tigecycline • Tygacil • 100 mg IV × 1, then 50 mg IV q12h • Injection	• Gram (+) organisms (MSSA, MRSA, vancomycin-sensitive *Enterococcus faecalis*) • Gram (−) organisms (*E. coli, Enterobacter, H. influenzae, Klebsiella, Legionella*)	Children ≤8 yr and pregnant/breast-feeding women (may cause permanent teeth discoloration and impaired teeth/bone growth)	• N/V/D • Infusion site reaction • Photosensitivity • Hepatotoxicity • Pancreatitis	May ↑ risk of bleeding with warfarin	• Indicated for complicated SSTIs, complicated intra-abdominal infections, and community-acquired pneumonia • Structurally similar to tetracyclines

Oxazolidinones

Generic • Brand • Dose/Dosage Forms	Spectrum of Activity	Contraindications	Primary Side Effects	Pertinent Drug Interactions	Med Pearl
Mechanism of action – inhibit bacterial protein synthesis by binding to the 50S subunit of the bacterial ribosome; bacteriostatic					
Linezolid ☆ • Zyvox • 400–600 mg IV/PO q12h • Injection, suspension, tabs	Gram (+) organisms (vancomycin-resistant *Enterococcus faecium* [VRE], MRSA, resistant *Strep. pneumoniae*)	• Concurrent or recent (within 2 wk) use of MAO inhibitors (MAOI) • Patients with uncontrolled hypertension, pheochromocytoma, thyrotoxicosis, and/or taking sympathomimetic agents (e.g., pseudoephedrine), vasopressor agents (e.g., epinephrine), or dopaminergic agents (e.g., dopamine) • Concurrent use of selective serotonin reuptake inhibitors, tricyclic antidepressants, 5-HT$_1$ receptor agonists (triptans), meperidine, or buspirone	• N/V/D • Headache • Myelosuppression (more common if therapy >2 wk) • Peripheral/optic neuropathy (more common if therapy >4 wk) • Seizures	• Avoid taking with foods or beverages with high tyramine content (may ↑ risk of hypertensive crises) • Use with serotonergic agents may ↑ risk of serotonin syndrome; avoid concurrent use • Use with adrenergic agents (e.g., dopamine, epinephrine) may ↑ risk of hypertensive crises • Use with tramadol may ↑ risk of seizures • Use with insulin or oral hypoglycemic agents may ↑ risk of hypoglycemia	• Indicated for nosocomial/community-acquired pneumonia, SSTIs, and VRE • Weak MAOI • Monitor complete blood count (CBC) weekly if therapy >2 wk
Tedizolid • Sivextro • 200 mg IV/PO q24h × 6 days • Injection, tabs	Gram (+) organisms (MSSA, MRSA, *Enterococcus faecalis, Streptococcus*)	None	• N/V/D • Headache • Dizziness	None	• Indicated for SSTIs • Weak MAOI

Streptogramin

Generic • Brand • Dose/Dosage Forms	Spectrum of Activity	Contraindications	Primary Side Effects	Pertinent Drug Interactions	Med Pearl
Mechanism of action – inhibits bacterial protein synthesis by binding to the 50S subunit of the bacterial ribosome; bactericidal					
Quinupristin-dalfopristin • Synercid • 7.5 mg/kg IV q8–12h • Injection	Gram (+) organisms (MSSA and *Strep. pyogenes*)	None	• N/V/D • Infusion site reactions (pain, phlebitis) • Muscle/joint pain • ↑ bilirubin	• CYP3A4 inhibitor • May ↑ effect/toxicity of CYP3A4 substrates	• Indicated for complicated SSTIs • Flush line with D5W before and after infusion • If infusion reaction occurs, can ↑ volume of diluent or administer via central line

Fluoroquinolones

Generic • Brand • Dose/Dosage Forms	Spectrum of Activity	Contraindications	Primary Side Effects	Pertinent Drug Interactions	Med Pearl
Mechanism of action – inhibit bacterial DNA topoisomerase and gyrase → inhibit bacterial DNA replication; bactericidal					
Besifloxacin • Besivance • 1 drop TID • Ophthalmic solution Ciprofloxacin ☆ • Cetraxal, Ciloxan, Cipro, Cipro XR, Otiprio • IR: 250–750 mg PO q12h • ER: 500 mg–1 g PO q24h • IV: 200–400 mg IV q8–12h • Injection, ophthalmic ointment/solution, suspension, otic solution/suspension, tabs (ER and IR) Delafloxacin • Baxdela • 300 mg IV q12h • 450 mg PO q12h • Injection, tabs Gatifloxacin • Zymaxid • 1 drop q2h while awake on day 1, then 1 drop 2–4 times/day while awake • Ophthalmic solution Gemifloxacin • Factive • 320 mg PO q24h • Tabs Levofloxacin ☆ • Levaquin • 250–750 mg IV/PO q24h • Injection, ophthalmic solution, solution, tabs Moxifloxacin ☆ • Avelox, Moxeza, Vigamox • 400 mg IV/PO q24h • Injection, ophthalmic solution, tabs Ofloxacin • Ocuflox • 200–400 mg PO q12h • Ophthalmic solution, otic solution, tabs	• Gram (+) organisms (levofloxacin, gemifloxacin, and moxifloxacin have greatest activity against *Streptococcus*; delafloxacin active against MRSA) • Gram (−) organisms • Ciprofloxacin, delafloxacin, and levofloxacin active against *Pseudomonas aeruginosa* • Atypical organisms (except delafloxacin)	• Children <18 yr and pregnant/breastfeeding women (may cause impaired bone growth) • Concurrent use with other drugs that prolong QT interval • Myasthenia gravis	• N/D • Photosensitivity • Tendinitis/tendon rupture • Hyper-/hypoglycemia • Peripheral neuropathy • Seizures • Prolonged QT interval	• Absorption ↓ with antacids, dairy products, and products containing iron, magnesium, aluminum, calcium, or zinc (separate by 2 hr) • Use with corticosteroids may ↑ risk of tendon rupture • Use with nonsteroidal anti-inflammatory drugs (NSAIDs) may ↑ risk of seizures • Ciprofloxacin and ofloxacin are strong CYP1A2 inhibitors • Ciprofloxacin and ofloxacin may ↑ effects of CYP1A2 substrates • Ciprofloxacin may ↓ phenytoin levels • May ↑ risk of bleeding with warfarin • Use with antidiabetic agents may ↑ risk of hypoglycemia • ↑ risk of TdP with other drugs that prolong QT interval	• Should only be used when patients have no other alternative treatment options for chronic bronchitis, uncomplicated UTI, and acute sinusitis • Ciprofloxacin ER and IR tabs are not interchangeable • Adjust dose for all, except moxifloxacin, in renal impairment (for delafloxacin, only IV needs dose adjustment) • Take levofloxacin oral solution 1 hr before or 2 hr after meals • Patients with diabetes should monitor their blood glucose more frequently • Ciprofloxacin, levofloxacin, and moxifloxacin can be used to treat plague (*Yersinia pestis*) • Ophthalmic preparations used to treat bacterial conjunctivitis

Sulfonamide

Generic • Brand • Dose/Dosage Forms	Spectrum of Activity	Contraindications	Primary Side Effects	Pertinent Drug Interactions	Med Pearl
Mechanism of action – inhibits incorporation of para-aminobenzoic acid (PABA) into DNA → inhibits folic acid production and bacterial growth; bacteriostatic					
Trimethoprim/sulfa-methoxazole ☆ • Bactrim, Septra, Sulfatrim • 1 double-strength tab PO q12h • 10–20 mg/kg/day of TMP IV in divided doses • Injection, suspension, tabs	• Gram (+) organisms (including MSSA, MRSA) • Gram (−) organisms • 1st-line drug to treat/prevent *Pneumocystis jiroveci* pneumonia (PJP)	• Sulfa allergy • Porphyria • Megaloblastic anemia • Infants and pregnant/breast-feeding women (↑ risk of kernicterus) • Glucose-6-phosphate dehydrogenase (G6PD) deficiency	• N/V/D • Rash • Stevens-Johnson syndrome • Photosensitivity • Folate deficiency • Hypoglycemia (in patients with diabetes)	• May ↑ effects/toxicity of methotrexate • May ↑ risk of bleeding with warfarin • Use with antidiabetic agents may ↑ risk of hypoglycemia	• Instruct patients to take with a full glass of water (to prevent crystalluria) • Adjust dose in renal impairment

Cyclic Lipopeptide

Generic • Brand • Dose/Dosage Forms	Spectrum of Activity	Contraindications	Primary Side Effects	Pertinent Drug Interactions	Med Pearl
Mechanism of action – binds to bacterial cell membranes and causes rapid depolarization → inhibits protein, DNA, and RNA synthesis; bactericidal					
Daptomycin • Cubicin • 4–6 mg/kg IV q24h • Injection	Gram (+) organisms (MSSA, MRSA, vancomycin-sensitive *Enterococcus faecalis*)	Children <1 yr (↑ risk of muscular, neuromuscular, and/or central nervous system [CNS] toxicity)	• N/D • Infusion site reactions • Myopathy/rhabdomyolysis • Peripheral neuropathy • Eosinophilic pneumonia	Use with statins may ↑ risk of myopathy; consider discontinuing statin therapy throughout treatment	• Monitor creatine kinase levels weekly • Adjust dose in renal impairment • Indicated for complicated SSTIs and *Staph. aureus* bloodstream infections

Glycopeptides

Generic • Brand • Dose/Dosage Forms	Spectrum of Activity	Contraindications	Primary Side Effects	Pertinent Drug Interactions	Med Pearl
Mechanism of action – inhibit bacterial cell wall synthesis; bactericidal					
Dalbavancin • Dalvance • 1,000 mg IV × 1, then 500 mg IV 1 wk later **OR** 1,500 mg IV × 1 • Injection	Gram (+) organisms (MSSA, MRSA, *Streptococcus*, vancomycin-sensitive *Enterococcus faecalis*)	None	• Hypersensitivity reactions • Headache • N/D • Red-man syndrome (flushing, hypotension, erythema, pruritus)	None	• Indicated for SSTIs • Adjust dose in renal impairment • If red-man syndrome occurs, ↓ infusion rate
Oritavancin • Orbactiv • 1,200 mg IV × 1 • Injection	Gram (+) organisms (MSSA, MRSA, *Streptococcus*, vancomycin-sensitive *Enterococcus faecalis*)	Use of IV unfractionated heparin × 5 days after administration	• Hypersensitivity reactions • Headache • N/V/D • Red-man syndrome	May ↑ risk of bleeding with warfarin	• Indicated for SSTIs • If red-man syndrome occurs, ↓ infusion rate • May falsely ↑ prothrombin time (PT), international normalized ratio (INR), activated partial thromboplastin time (aPTT), and activated clotting time (ACT) (PT/INR effects can last up to 12 hr after discontinuation; aPTT effects can last up to 5 days after discontinuation; ACT effects can last up to 24 hr after discontinuation)

Glycopeptides *(cont'd)*

Generic • Brand • Dose/Dosage Forms	Spectrum of Activity	Contraindications	Primary Side Effects	Pertinent Drug Interactions	Med Pearl
Telavancin • Vibativ • 10 mg/kg IV q24h • Injection	Gram (+) organisms (MSSA, MRSA, *Streptococcus*, vancomycin-sensitive *Enterococcus faecalis*)	• Pregnancy • Concurrent use of IV unfractionated heparin	• Hypersensitivity reactions • Insomnia • Headache • Nephrotoxicity • Red-man syndrome • Metallic taste • N/V/D • QT interval prolongation	• ↑ risk of nephrotoxicity when used with amphotericin B, loop diuretics, tacrolimus, cyclosporine, or cisplatin • ↑ risk of TdP with other drugs that prolong QT interval	• Indicated for complicated SSTIs and hospital-acquired and ventilator-associated pneumonia • ↑ risk of mortality in hospital-acquired and ventilator-associated pneumonia in patients with CrCl ≤50 mL/min • Adjust dose in renal impairment • Monitor renal function • If red-man syndrome occurs, ↓ infusion rate • May falsely ↑ PT, INR, aPTT, and ACT (can last up to 18 hr after discontinuation) • Has REMS program
Vancomycin • Firvanq, Vancocin • 125–250 mg PO q6h • 500 mg–1 g IV q12h • Caps, injection, solution	• Gram (+) organisms (MSSA, MRSA) • *Clostridium difficile*	None	• Red-man syndrome • Nephrotoxicity • Ototoxicity	↑ risk of nephrotoxicity when used with amphotericin B, loop diuretics, tacrolimus, cyclosporine, piperacillin/tazobactam, or cisplatin	• Bactericidal effect is time-dependent • Adjust dose in renal impairment • Often used in patients with penicillin allergy • Use PO (NOT IV) to treat *Clostridium difficile* (PO not effective for any other type of infection) • If red-man syndrome occurs, ↓ infusion rate • Target serum concentrations (peaks not routinely monitored); trough ≥10 mcg/mL (15–20 mcg/mL for complicated infections)

Miscellaneous Antibacterial Agents

Generic • Brand • Dose/Dosage Forms	Spectrum of Activity	Contraindications	Primary Side Effects	Pertinent Drug Interactions	Med Pearl
Mechanism of action – inhibits bacterial protein synthesis by binding to the 50S subunit of the bacterial ribosome; bacteriostatic					
Chloramphenicol • Only available generically • 12.5–25 mg/kg IV q6h • Injection	• Gram (+) organisms (VRE) • Gram (−) organisms	Neonates ($\uparrow$ risk of gray-baby syndrome)	• N/V/D • Myelosuppression (anemia, leukopenia, thrombocytopenia, aplastic anemia) • Gray-baby syndrome (vomiting, lethargy, respiratory depression, death) • Optic neuritis	• Phenobarbital and rifampin may $\downarrow$ effects • May $\uparrow$ effects of warfarin and phenytoin	• Only used for life-threatening infections • Monitor CBC frequently • Target serum concentrations: Peak = 15–25 mcg/mL; Trough = 5–10 mcg/mL
Mechanism of action – inhibits bacterial protein synthesis by binding to the 50S subunit of the bacterial ribosome; bacteriostatic					
Clindamycin☆ • Cleocin, Clindagel, Clindesse, Evoclin • 150–450 mg PO q6h • 300–900 mg IV q8h • Caps, injection, solution, topical foam/gel/lotion/pledgets/solution, vaginal cream/suppository	• Gram (+) organisms • Anaerobes	History of pseudomembranous colitis or ulcerative colitis	• N/V/D • Pseudomembranous colitis (*Clostridium difficile*) (highest incidence) Metallic taste	• CYP3A4 substrate • CYP3A4 inhibitors may $\uparrow$ risk of side effects • CYP3A4 inducers may $\downarrow$ effects	• Also used for acne (topical) • Patients using intravaginally should avoid intercourse ($\downarrow$ efficacy of condoms and diaphragms)
Mechanism of action – interferes with bacterial DNA synthesis; bactericidal					
Metronidazole☆ • Flagyl, Metro, Metrocream, Metrogel, Metrolotion, Noritate, Nuvessa, Vandazole • 250–500 mg PO q8–12h • 500 mg IV q8–12h • Caps, injection, tabs, topical cream/gel/lotion, vaginal gel	• Anaerobes • *Clostridium difficile*	Pregnancy (1st trimester)	• N/D • Confusion • Dizziness • Peripheral neuropathy • Metallic taste	• Disulfiram-like reaction may occur if alcohol is used during treatment • May $\uparrow$ effects of warfarin and lithium • Phenobarbital and phenytoin may $\downarrow$ effects • Cimetidine may $\uparrow$ effects	• Can be used in 4-drug regimen for *H. pylori* • Drug of choice for *Clostridium difficile* • Take ER tabs 1 hr before or 2 hr after meals
Secnidazole • Solosec • 2 g PO × 1 • Oral granules	Anaerobes	None	• Vulvovaginal candidiasis • Headache • N/D	None	To be sprinkled on top of applesauce, yogurt, or pudding

Antifungal Agents

Azole Antifungals

Generic • Brand • Dose/Dosage Forms	Spectrum of Activity	Contraindications	Primary Side Effects	Pertinent Drug Interactions	Med Pearl
Mechanism of action – inhibit synthesis of ergosterol (essential component of fungal cell membrane) • Imidazoles: butoconazole, clotrimazole, econazole, efinaconazole, ketoconazole, luliconazole, miconazole, oxiconazole, sulconazole, tioconazole • Triazoles: fluconazole, itraconazole, isavuconazonium, terconazole, posaconazole, voriconazole					
Fluconazole ☆ • Diflucan • 100–800 mg IV/PO q24h • Injection, suspension, tabs	• *Candida* spp. • *Coccidioides* spp. • *Histoplasma* spp. • *Cryptococcus* spp.	None	• Headache • N/V/D • Abdominal pain • Rash • ↑ liver function tests (LFTs) • Prolonged QT interval	• CYP2C9, CYP2C19, and CYP3A4 inhibitor • May ↑ effect/toxicity of CYP2C9, CYP2C19, and CYP3A4 substrates • Rifampin may ↓ effects • ↑ risk of TdP with other drugs that prolong QT interval	• Adjust dose in renal impairment • Conversion from IV to PO is 1:1 • Monitor LFTs
Isavuconazonium • Cresemba • 372 mg IV/PO q8h × 6 doses (48 hr), then 372 mg IV/PO q24h • Caps, injection	• *Aspergillus* spp. • *Mucormycetes* spp.	• Concurrent use of strong CYP3A4 inhibitors or inducers • Familial short QT syndrome	• ↑ LFTs • Infusion reactions • Rash • N/V/D • Headache • Shortened QT interval	• CYP3A4 substrate and inhibitor • CYP3A4 inhibitors may ↑ risk of side effects • CYP3A4 inducers may ↓ effects • May ↑ effect/toxicity of CYP3A4 substrates • ↑ risk of digoxin toxicity	Monitor LFTs
Itraconazole • Onmel, Sporanox • 100–400 mg/day PO • Caps, solution, tabs	• *Candida* spp. • *Coccidioides* spp. • *Histoplasma* spp. • *Cryptococcus* spp. • *Aspergillus* spp.	• Concurrent use of avanafil, disopyramide, dofetilide, dronedarone, eplerenone, ergot alkaloids, felodipine, irinotecan, isavuconazonium, ivabradine, lomitapide, lovastatin, lurasidone, methadone, midazolam, naloxegol, nisoldipine, pimozide, ranolazine, quinidine, simvastatin, ticagrelor, or triazolam • Concurrent use of colchicine, fesoterodine, or solifenacin in renal or hepatic impairment • HF	• Nausea • Abdominal pain • Rash • ↑ LFTs • Prolonged QT interval	• CYP3A4 substrate and inhibitor • CYP3A4 inhibitors may ↑ risk of side effects • CYP3A4 inducers may ↓ effects • May ↑ effect/toxicity of CYP3A4 substrates • ↑ risk of digoxin toxicity • Absorption ↓ with antacids, H$_2$ antagonists, and proton pump inhibitors (PPIs) (acidic environment required for absorption) (separate by 2 hr) • ↑ risk of TdP with other drugs that prolong QT interval	• Caps and solution cannot be used interchangeably (bioavailability of solution > caps) • Potent negative inotrope • Monitor LFTs

Azole Antifungals *(cont'd)*

Generic • Brand • Dose/Dosage Forms	Spectrum of Activity	Contraindications	Primary Side Effects	Pertinent Drug Interactions	Med Pearl
Ketoconazole☆ • Extina, Nizoral, Xolegel • 200–400 mg PO q24h • Rx: Tabs, topical cream/foam/gel/shampoo • OTC: Shampoo	• *Candida* spp. • *Coccidioides* spp. • *Histoplasma* spp. • *Cryptococcus* spp.	• Concurrent use of ergot alkaloids • Hepatic impairment	• N/V • Gynecomastia • Sexual dysfunction • ↑ LFTs • Prolonged QT interval	Same as itraconazole	• May ↓ testosterone levels • Monitor LFTs
Posaconazole • Noxafil • 300 mg IV/PO (tabs) q12h × 1 day, then 300 mg IV/PO (tabs) q24h • 200 mg PO TID (suspension) (for prophylaxis); 100 mg PO BID × 1 day, then 100 mg PO q24h × 13 days (suspension) (for treatment) • Injection, suspension, tabs	• *Candida* spp. • *Aspergillus* spp.	Concurrent use of ergot alkaloids, quinidine, pimozide, sirolimus, atorvastatin, lovastatin, or simvastatin	• Headache • N/V • Rash • ↑ LFTs • Prolonged QT interval	• CYP3A4 inhibitor • May ↑ effect/toxicity of CYP3A4 substrates • Absorption of suspension ↓ with cimetidine and esomeprazole (avoid concurrent use) • Metoclopramide may ↓ effects of suspension • Efavirenz, fosamprenavir, rifabutin, and phenytoin may ↓ effects • ↑ risk of TdP with other drugs that prolong QT interval	• Tabs and suspension cannot be used interchangeably • Take tabs with food to ↑ absorption • Suspension must be taken with full meal (or liquid nutritional supplement or acidic carbonated beverage) to ↑ absorption • IV and tabs ONLY used for prophylaxis of invasive *Aspergillus* or *Candida* infections • Use PO when CrCl <50 mL/min (diluent in IV can accumulate) • Monitor LFTs
Voriconazole • Vfend • 6 mg/kg IV q12h × 24 hr, then 3–4 mg/kg IV q12h or 100–300 mg PO q12h • Injection, suspension, tabs	• *Candida* spp. • *Aspergillus* spp.	Concurrent use of pimozide, quinidine, long-acting barbiturates, carbamazepine, ergot alkaloids, rifampin, rifabutin, ritonavir (≥ 800 mg/day), efavirenz (≥ 800 mg/day), St. John's wort, or sirolimus	• Visual disturbances (transient) (blurred vision, photophobia, altered perception of color) • Rash • Photosensitivity • ↑ LFTs • Hallucinations • N/V • Prolonged QT interval	• CYP2C9 and CYP2C19 substrate • CYP2C9, CYP2C19, and CYP3A4 inhibitor • May ↑ effect/toxicity of CYP2C9, CYP2C19, and CYP3A4 substrates • CYP2C9 and CYP2C19 inhibitors may ↑ risks of side effects • CYP2C9 and CYP2C19 inducers may ↓ effects • May ↑ efavirenz levels • Efavirenz may ↓ effects • ↑ risk of TdP with other drugs that prolong QT interval	• ↓ dose of cyclosporine by 50% • When using with efavirenz, ↑ voriconazole dose and ↓ efavirenz dose • ↑ dose of voriconazole when using with phenytoin • Use PO when CrCl <50 mL/min (diluent in IV can accumulate) • Take PO 1 hour before or after meals • Monitor LFTs and vision

Echinocandins

Generic • Brand • Dose/Dosage Forms	Spectrum of Activity	Contraindications	Primary Side Effects	Pertinent Drug Interactions	Med Pearl
Mechanism of action – inhibit synthesis of 1,3-β-d-glucan (essential component of fungal cell wall)					
Anidulafungin • Eraxis • 100–200 mg IV on day 1, then 50–100 mg IV q24h • Injection	• *Candida* spp. • *Aspergillus* spp. (caspofungin only)	None	• N/V • Headache • Hypokalemia • Rash • Fever • ↑ LFTs • Phlebitis • Stevens-Johnson syndrome, toxic epidermal necrolysis (caspofungin)	None	Monitor LFTs
Caspofungin • Cancidas • 70 mg IV on day 1, then 50 mg IV q24h • Injection				• Rifampin, carbamazepine, dexamethasone, efavirenz, nevirapine, and phenytoin may ↓ effects • May ↓ tacrolimus levels • Cyclosporine may ↑ risk of side effects	• ↑ dose of caspofungin to 70 mg/day when used with rifampin, carbamazepine, dexamethasone, efavirenz, nevirapine, or phenytoin • Adjust dose in moderate hepatic impairment • Monitor LFTs
Micafungin • Mycamine • 50–150 mg IV q24h • Injection				None	Monitor LFTs

Amphotericin B

Generic • Brand • Dose/Dosage Forms	Spectrum of Activity	Contraindications	Primary Side Effects	Pertinent Drug Interactions	Med Pearl
Mechanism of action – bind to ergosterol in cell membrane → produce a channel in cell membrane (↑ permeability) → allow K$^+$ and Mg^{2+} to leak out of cell ("leaky membrane") → cell death					
Amphotericin B desoxycholate • Only available generically • Test dose of 1 mg IV should be given over 20–30 min (monitor patient for 2–4 hr before starting infusion) • 0.5–1.5 mg/kg/day IV • Injection Amphotericin B lipid complex (ABLC) • Abelcet • 5 mg/kg IV q24h • Injection Liposomal amphotericin B (L-AmB) • AmBisome • 3–6 mg/kg IV q24h • Injection	• *Candida* spp. • *Coccidioides* spp. • *Blastomyces* spp. • *Histoplasma* spp. • *Cryptococcus* spp. • *Aspergillus* spp.	None	• Nephrotoxicity (less common with lipid-based formulations) • Infusion reactions (fever, chills, hypotension, nausea, tachypnea) • Phlebitis • Electrolyte disturbances (i.e., hypokalemia, hypomagnesemia)	↑ risk of nephrotoxicity when used with aminoglycosides, loop diuretics, tacrolimus, cyclosporine, or cisplatin	• May premedicate with acetaminophen, NSAIDs, diphenhydramine, and/or corticosteroid to prevent infusion reactions (give 30–60 min before infusion); meperidine may be used for rigors • Infusion reactions less common with lipid-based formulations (amphotericin B deoxycholate > ABLC > L-Amb) • Infusion reactions ↓ after first few doses • Sodium loading (500 mL of 0.9% NaCl IV before and after infusion) may ↓ risk of nephrotoxicity with amphotericin B desoxycholate • Monitor blood urea nitrogen (BUN)/serum creatinine (SCr), potassium, and magnesium

Other Antifungals

Generic • Brand • Dose/Dosage Forms	Spectrum of Activity	Contraindications	Primary Side Effects	Pertinent Drug Interactions	Med Pearl
Mechanism of action – similar to amphotericin B					
Nystatin ☆ • Nystop • Suspension: 400,000–600,000 units 4 times/day • Topical: Apply 2–3 times daily • Suspension, tabs, topical cream/ointment/powder	*Candida* spp.	None	• N/V/D • Abdominal pain	None	Suspension should be swished and swallowed
Mechanism of action – inhibits squalene epoxidase → inhibits synthesis of ergosterol					
Terbinafine ☆ • Lamisil • PO: 250 mg q24h • Topical: Apply 1–2 times daily • Rx: Granules, tabs, topical solution • OTC: Topical cream/gel/solution	*Trichophyton* spp.	• Hepatic impairment • CrCl <50 mL/min	• Headache • N/V/D • ↑ LFTs	• CYP2D6 inhibitor • May ↑ effect/toxicity of CYP2D6 substrates • May ↓ cyclosporine levels	• Oral used for onychomycosis or tinea capitis (scalp ringworm); topical used for tinea pedis (athlete's foot), tinea corporis (ringworm), or tinea cruris (jock itch) • Give for 6 wk for fingernail infection; 12 wk for toenail infection • Monitor LFTs
Mechanism of action – inhibits fungal protein synthesis					
Tavaborole • Kerydin • Apply once daily × 48 wk • Topical solution	*Trichophyton* spp.	None	Application reactions	None	Indicated for onychomycosis

Other Antifungals *(cont'd)*

Generic • Brand • Dose/Dosage Forms	Spectrum of Activity	Contraindications	Primary Side Effects	Pertinent Drug Interactions	Med Pearl
Mechanism of action – enters fungal cell wall → converted into 5-fluorouracil, which interferes with fungal RNA and protein synthesis					
Flucytosine • Ancobon • 25–37.5 mg/kg PO q6h (administered with amphotericin B) • Caps	• *Candida* spp. • *Cryptococcus* spp.	None	• Confusion • Hallucinations • Ataxia • Headache • N/V/D • ↑ LFTs • Renal impairment • Bone marrow depression	None	• Should not be used as monotherapy • Adjust dose in renal impairment • Monitor LFTs, BUN/SCr, and CBC • Flucytosine concentrations: Peak: 50–100 mcg/mL; Trough: 25–50 mcg/mL
Mechanism of action – inhibits fungal cell mitosis					
Griseofulvin • Gris-PEG • Microsize: 500–1,000 mg/day PO • Ultramicrosize: 375 mg/day PO • Microsize: Suspension, tabs • Ultramicrosize: Tabs	*Trichophyton* spp.	• Hepatic impairment • Porphyria	• Rash/hives • N/V/D • Headache • Confusion • Photosensitivity	• Barbiturates may ↓ effects • May ↓ effects of cyclosporine and warfarin • Disulfiram-like reaction may occur if alcohol is used during treatment	• Monitor LFTs • Administer with high-fat meal to ↑ absorption

Antiviral Agents

Drugs for Treatment of Herpes Simplex Virus and Varicella-Zoster Virus

Generic • Brand • Dose/Dosage Forms	Spectrum of Activity	Contraindications	Primary Side Effects	Pertinent Drug Interactions	Med Pearl
Mechanism of action – inhibit viral DNA polymerase → inhibit replication of viral DNA					
Acyclovir☆ • Sitavig, Zovirax • *Genital herpes (initial episode):* 200 mg PO 5 times/day × 7–10 days **OR** 5 mg/kg IV q8h × 5–7 days • *Herpes labialis (cold sores):* 400 mg PO 5 times/day × 5 days • *Varicella (chickenpox):* 800 mg PO q6h × 5 days **OR** 10 mg/kg IV q8h × 7 days • *Herpes zoster (shingles):* 800 mg PO 5 times/day × 7–10 days **OR** 10 mg/kg IV q8h × 7 days • Buccal tabs, caps, injection, suspension, tabs, topical cream/ointment	• Herpes simplex virus (HSV)-1 (herpes labialis) and HSV-2 (genital herpes) • Varicella zoster virus (causes chickenpox and shingles)	None	• N/V/D • Headache • Phlebitis (IV acyclovir) • Renal impairment (IV acyclovir) • Seizures (esp. in patients with renal impairment)	None	• Adjust dose for all, except penciclovir, in renal impairment • To avoid renal damage with IV acyclovir (can crystallize), infuse slowly and keep patient hydrated • Sitavig is a buccal tab for treatment of recurrent cold sores
Famciclovir☆ (prodrug of penciclovir) • Only available generically • *Genital herpes (initial episode):* 250 mg PO q8h × 7–10 days • *Cold sores:* 1,500 mg PO × 1 • *Herpes zoster:* 500 mg PO q8h × 7 days • Tabs					
Penciclovir • Denavir • *Cold sores:* Apply q2h while awake × 4 days • Topical cream					
Valacyclovir☆ (prodrug of acyclovir) • Valtrex • *Genital herpes (initial episode):* 1 g PO q12h × 10 days • *Genital herpes (recurrence):* 500 mg PO q12h × 3 days • *Cold sores:* 2 g PO q12h × 1 day • *Herpes zoster:* 1 g PO q8h × 7 days • Tabs					

Drugs for Treatment of Cytomegalovirus

Generic • Brand • Dose/Dosage Forms	Spectrum of Activity	Contraindications	Primary Side Effects	Pertinent Drug Interactions	Med Pearl
Mechanism of action – inhibit replication of viral DNA					
Cidofovir • Only available generically • 5 mg/kg IV once weekly × 2 wk, then q2 wk • Injection	• Cytomegalovirus • HSV (foscarnet) • Acute herpetic keratitis (ophthalmic gangiclovir)	• SCr >1.5 mg/dL, CrCl ≤55 mL/min, or proteinuria • Use of other nephrotoxic drugs within 7 days	• Nephrotoxicity • Neutropenia • Metabolic acidosis • ↓ intraocular pressure • Uveitis/iritis	Use of antiretroviral drugs may ↑ risk of side effects	• Monitor BUN/SCr • To minimize renal damage, administer 1 L of 0.9% NaCl before and after each infusion; also give 2 g of probenecid 3 hr before each infusion and then 1 g at 2 hr and 8 hr after each infusion • If SCr ↑ by 0.3–0.4 mg/dL above baseline, ↓ dose to 3 mg/kg; if SCr ↑ by ≥0.5 mg/dL, discontinue • Advise patients to use effective contraception
Foscarnet • Foscavir • 60 mg/kg IV q8h **OR** 90 mg/kg IV q12h × 14–21 days, then 90–120 mg/kg IV q24h • Injection		None	• Nephrotoxicity • N/V • Anemia • Electrolyte disturbances • Genital sores • Seizures	• ↑ risk of nephrotoxicity when used with amphotericin B, aminoglycosides, loop diuretics, tacrolimus, cyclosporine, or cisplatin • Zidovudine may ↑ risk of anemia	• Adjust dose in renal impairment • Monitor BUN/SCr • To minimize renal damage, administer 1 L of 0.9% NaCl IV with each infusion • Rapid infusion associated with seizures and arrhythmias
Ganciclovir • Cytovene, Zirgan • IV: 5 mg/kg q12h × 14 –21 days, then either 5 mg/kg/day 7 times/wk or 6 mg/kg/day 5 times/wk • Ophth: 1 drop 5 times/day until ulcer heals, then 1 drop 3 times/day × 7 days • Injection, ophthalmic gel		• Neutropenia • Thrombocytopenia • Anemia	• Myelosuppression • Fever • Rash • Phlebitis (IV ganciclovir) • ↑ LFTs • Nephrotoxicity • Seizures • N/V/D	• ↑ risk of myelosuppression when used with other immunosuppressive drugs • ↑ risk of nephrotoxicity when used with amphotericin B, aminoglycosides, loop diuretics, tacrolimus, cyclosporine, or cisplatin • May ↑ effects/ toxicity of zidovudine	• Adjust dose in renal impairment • Advise patients to use effective contraception during treatment and for at least 90 days after treatment • Take valganciclovir with food
Valganciclovir (prodrug of ganciclovir) • Valcyte • 900 mg PO q12h × 21 days, then 900 mg PO q24h • Solution, tabs					

Drugs for Treatment of Influenza

Generic • Brand • Dose/Dosage Forms	Spectrum of Activity	Contraindications	Primary Side Effects	Pertinent Drug Interactions	Med Pearl
Mechanism of action – inhibit the enzyme (neuraminidase) responsible for releasing the newly formed mature virus from the host cell					
Oseltamivir • Tamiflu • *Prophylaxis:* 75 mg PO q24h × ≥10 days (6 wk for community outbreak) • *Treatment:* 75 mg PO q12h × 5 days • Caps, suspension	• Influenza A and B • H1N1 influenza	None	• N/V/D • Headache • Rash • Neuropsychiatric events (e.g., confusion, delirium, hallucinations, self-injury)	None	• For prophylaxis, initiate therapy within 2 days of contact with infected person • For treatment, initiate therapy within 2 days of onset of symptoms • Adjust dose in renal impairment • ↓ flu severity and duration by ~ 1 day • Can be used in children ≥1 yr (prophylaxis) or ≥2 wk (treatment)
Peramivir • Rapivab • *Treatment:* 600 mg IV × 1 • Injection			• Rash • Neuropsychiatric events (e.g., confusion, delirium, hallucinations, self-injury)		• Initiate therapy within 2 days of onset of symptoms • Can be used in children ≥2 yr • Adjust dose in renal impairment
Zanamivir • Relenza • *Prophylaxis:* 2 inhalations q24h × 10 days (28 days for community outbreak) • *Treatment:* 2 inhalations q12h × 5 days • Powder for oral inhalation		Asthma/COPD	• Bronchospasm • Cough • Headache • N/D • Rash • Neuropsychiatric events (e.g., confusion, delirium, hallucinations, self-injury)		• For prophylaxis, initiate therapy within 1.5 days (5 days in community setting) of contact with infected person • For treatment, initiate therapy within 2 days of onset of symptoms • ↓ flu severity and duration by ~ 1 day • Can be used in children ≥5 yr (prophylaxis) or ≥7 yr (treatment)

HUMAN IMMUNODEFICIENCY VIRUS

Guidelines Summary

For the NAPLEX, make learning the names of the medications and their respective classes a priority.

- Memorize the non-nucleoside reverse transcriptase inhibitors (NNRTIs)
  - Efavirenz, nevirapine, etravirine, rilpivirine
- All protease inhibitors (PIs) end in "-navir."
  - Examples: Darunavir, atazanavir, ritonavir
- There are only three integrase inhibitors: Dolutegravir, raltegravir, elvitegravir.
- There is only one fusion inhibitor: Enfuvirtide.
- There is only one CCR5 inhibitor: Maraviroc.
- The remaining agents are nucleoside reverse transcriptase inhibitors (NRTIs)
  - Tenofovir, emtricitabine, abacavir, lamivudine, zidovudine, didanosine, stavudine

For the exam, know that antiretroviral therapy is now recommended for ALL HIV-infected patients (regardless of CD4 count). There is increased urgency to initiate anti-retroviral therapy in the following patient populations:

- AIDS-defining condition (including HIV-associated dementia and AIDS-associated malignancies)
- Acute opportunistic infection
- CD4 count <200 cells/mm^3
- HIV-associated nephropathy
- Hepatitis B or hepatitis C coinfection
- Pregnancy
- Acute HIV infection

For the exam, know the signature side effects for the major drug classes (NNRTIs, NRTIs, and PIs) and know the five antiviral regimens that are recommended for starting therapy for most treatment-naïve patients:

- Dolutegravir + abacavir + lamivudine (only for patients who are HLA-B*5701 negative)
- Dolutegravir + tenofovir (disoproxil fumarate or alafenamide) + emtricitabine
- Elvitegravir + cobicistat + tenofovir (disoproxil fumarate or alafenamide) + emtricitabine
- Raltegravir + tenofovir (disoproxil fumarate or alafenamide) + emtricitabine
- Bictegravir + tenofovir (alafenamide) + emtricitabine

A summary of acceptable initial combination regimens for antiretroviral naïve patients follows:

- Integrase inhibitor-based regimen: Integrase inhibitor + 2 NRTIs (recommended for most patients with HIV)
- PI-based regimen: PI (boosted with ritonavir or cobicistat) + 2 NRTIs
- NNRTI-based regimen: NNRTI + 2 NRTIs

Drugs of Choice

Prophylaxis of First-Episode Opportunistic Infections in Patients with HIV

Opportunistic Infection	Indication	First-Line Therapy
PJP	CD4 count <200 cells/mm^3 **OR** CD4% <14% of total lymphocyte count **OR** CD4 count >200 but <250 cells/mm^3, if antiretroviral therapy cannot be initiated, and if CD4 cell count monitoring (e.g., every 3 months) is not possible	TMP/SMX 1 DS tablet PO daily **OR** TMP/SMX 80/400 mg (single-strength [SS]) PO daily
Toxoplasma gondii encephalitis	Toxoplasma IgG (+) with CD4 count <100 cells/mm^3	TMP/SMX 1 DS tablet PO daily
Mycobacterium avium complex (MAC) disease	CD4 count <50 cells/mm^3	Azithromycin 1,200 mg PO 1 × weekly **OR** Clarithromycin 500 mg PO BID **OR** Azithromycin 600 mg PO 2 × weekly

Treatment and Secondary Prophylaxis of AIDS-Associated Opportunistic Infections

Opportunistic Infection	First-Line Therapy/Duration
PJP	*Treatment:* TMP/SMX (IV/PO) ± corticosteroids* × 21 days *Secondary Prophylaxis:* TMP/SMX 1 DS tablet PO daily **OR** TMP/SMX 1 SS tablet PO daily Indication for discontinuing secondary prophylaxis: If CD4 count ↑ from <200 cells/mm^3 to >200 cells/mm^3 for >3 mo due to antiretroviral therapy
Toxoplasma gondii encephalitis	*Initial Treatment:* • Pyrimethamine (PO) + sulfadiazine (PO) + leucovorin† (PO) × ≥6 wk *Chronic Maintenance Therapy:* Pyrimethamine + sulfadiazine + leucovorin† Indication for discontinuing chronic maintenance therapy: Successfully completed initial treatment **AND** no signs/symptoms of *Toxoplasma* encephalitis **AND** CD4 count >200 cells/mm^3 for >6 mo in response to antiretroviral therapy
MAC disease	*Treatment:* Clarithromycin (or azithromycin) (PO) + ethambutol (PO) × ≥12 mo *Secondary Prophylaxis:* Clarithromycin (or azithromycin) + ethambutol Indication for discontinuing secondary prophylaxis: Successfully completed ≥12 months of treatment **AND** no signs/symptoms of MAC disease **AND** CD4 count >100 cells/mm^3 for >6 mo in response to antiretroviral therapy

Treatment and Secondary Prophylaxis of AIDS-Associated Opportunistic Infections (cont'd)

Opportunistic Infection	First-Line Therapy/Duration
Mucocutaneous candidiasis	*Treatment:* Oropharyngeal: Fluconazole (PO) × 7–14 days Esophageal: Fluconazole (IV/PO) **OR** itraconazole (PO) × 14–21 days *Secondary Prophylaxis:* Usually not recommended unless patients have frequent or severe recurrences
Cryptococcal meningitis	*Initial Treatment:* Induction: Liposomal amphotericin B (IV) + flucytosine (PO) × ≥2 wk **OR** amphotericin B desoxycholate (IV) + flucytosine (PO) (if low risk of renal impairment) × ≥2 wk Consolidation: Fluconazole (IV/PO) × ≥8 wk *Maintenance Therapy:* Fluconazole (PO) Indication for discontinuing maintenance therapy: Successfully completed initial (induction, consolidation) therapy and ≥1 year on maintenance therapy **AND** no signs/symptoms from cryptococcal infection **AND** CD4 count ≥100 cells/mm^3 for ≥3 mo and suppressed HIV RNA in response to effective antiretroviral therapy
Cytomegalovirus retinitis	*Treatment:* Ganciclovir (or foscarnet) (via intravitreal injection) × 1–4 doses over 7–10 days + valganciclovir (PO) × 14–21 days *Chronic Maintenance Therapy:* Valganciclovir (PO) Indication for discontinuing chronic maintenance therapy: Chronic maintenance therapy for ≥3–6 mo **AND** lesions are inactive **AND** CD4 count >100 cells/mm^3 for 3–6 mo in response to antiretroviral therapy

* Indications for adjunctive corticosteroid therapy for PJP include PaO$_2$ <70 mmHg (room air) **OR** alveolar-arterial O$_2$ gradient >35 mmHg.

† Leucovorin reduces the risk of bone marrow suppression associated with pyrimethamine.

Non-Nucleoside Reverse Transcriptase Inhibitors (NNRTIs)

Generic • Brand • Dose/Dosage Forms	Contraindications	Primary Side Effects	Key Monitoring	Pertinent Drug Interactions	Med Pearl
Mechanism of action – bind to an allosteric site on reverse transcriptase that results in a conformational change to the enzyme's active site					
Efavirenz • Sustiva • 600 mg PO QHS • Caps, tabs	Concurrent use of elbasvir/grazoprevir	• Rash • ↑ LFTs • Hyperlipidemia • Drowsiness • Dizziness • Insomnia • Abnormal vivid dreaming • Agitation • Depression • Suicidal thoughts • Hallucinations • Fat redistribution • QT interval prolongation	LFTs	• CYP2B6 and CYP3A4 substrate • CYP2C9 and CYP2C19 inhibitor • CYP2B6 and CYP3A4 inducer • ↑ risk of TDP with other drugs that prolong QT interval	• Can cause a false positive cannabinoid or benzodiazepine screening test • Take on an empty stomach
Etravirine • Intelence • 200 mg PO BID • Tabs	None	• Rash • Nausea • Hypersensitivity reaction • ↑ LFTs • Fat redistribution		• CYP3A4, CYP2C9, and CYP2C19 substrate • CYP2C9 and CYP2C19 inhibitor • CYP3A4 inducer	• May disperse tabs in water • Take with food
Nevirapine • Viramune, Viramune XR • IR: 200 mg PO daily × 2 wk, then 200 mg PO BID • ER: 200 mg PO daily (of IR) × 2 wk, then 400 mg PO daily (of ER) • Suspension, tabs (IR and ER)	Moderate or severe hepatic impairment	• Rash • ↑ LFTs • Fat redistribution		CYP2B6 and CYP3A4 substrate and inducer	• Risk of hepatotoxicity in men and women with CD4 count >400 and >250 cells/mm^3, respectively • Hepatotoxicity often associated with a rash • 2-wk lead-in period with IR helps to ↓ rash
Rilpivirine • Edurant • 25 mg PO daily • Tabs	Concurrent use with carbamazepine, oxcarbazepine, phenobarbital, phenytoin, rifampin, rifapentine, PPIs, dexamethasone, and St. John's wort	• Rash • ↑ LFTs • Depression • Insomnia • Headache • Fat redistribution		• CYP3A4 substrate • Does not inhibit or induce CYP450 enzymes • H$_2$-antagonists, PPIs, and antacids may ↓ absorption (avoid concomitant use of PPIs; may use H$_2$-antagonists or antacids [need to space administration])	• Requires ≥500-calorie meal • ↑ virologic failure with high baseline HIV RNA (>100,000 copies/mL)

Nucleoside Reverse Transcriptase Inhibitors (NRTIs)

Generic • Brand • Dose/Dosage Forms	Contraindications	Primary Side Effects	Key Monitoring	Pertinent Drug Interactions	Med Pearl
Mechanism of action – triphosphate moiety competes with natural substrates for incorporation into proviral DNA that is developed by reverse transcriptase					
Abacavir • Ziagen • 300 mg PO BID or 600 mg PO daily • Solution, tabs	• Discontinue drug promptly and do not rechallenge in patients with hypersensitivity • HLA-B*5701 positive • Moderate or severe hepatic impairment	• Hypersensitivity reaction • Lactic acidosis • Hepatomegaly with steatosis	Hypersensitivity symptoms (fever, rash, N/V/D, abdominal pain, malaise, fatigue, dyspnea, cough)	None	Perform HLA-B*5701 test prior to initiating therapy: only use if negative
Didanosine • Videx, Videx EC • ER: ≥60 kg: 400 mg PO daily (250 mg PO daily when used with tenofovir disoproxil fumarate); 25 to <60 kg: 250 mg PO daily (200 mg PO daily when used with tenofovir disoproxil fumarate) • Solution: ≥60 kg: 200 mg PO BID (250 mg PO daily when used with tenofovir disoproxil fumarate); <60 kg: 125 mg PO BID (200 mg PO daily when used with tenofovir disoproxil fumarate) • ER caps, solution	Concurrent use with allopurinol, ribavirin, or stavudine	• Peripheral neuropathy • Pancreatitis • Lactic acidosis • Hepatomegaly with steatosis • Hepatotoxicity • Lipoatrophy • N/V/D • Optic neuritis	LFTs	• Tenofovir ↑ levels (↓ didanosine dose) • Ganciclovir ↑ levels • Methadone ↓ levels (use ER didanosine) • ↓ FQ, ketoconazole, and itraconazole levels (space administration)	• Do not crush or open ER caps • Reconstitute powder for oral solution with water or antacid • Adjust dose in renal impairment • Take on an empty stomach (0.5 hr before or 2 hr after meal)
Emtricitabine • Emtriva • Caps: 200 mg PO daily • Solution: 240 mg PO daily • Caps, solution	None	• N/V/D • Hyperpigmentation of palms/soles • Lactic acidosis • Hepatomegaly with steatosis	None	None	Adjust dose in renal impairment

Nucleoside Reverse Transcriptase Inhibitors (NRTIs) *(cont'd)*

Generic • Brand • Dose/Dosage Forms	Contraindications	Primary Side Effects	Key Monitoring	Pertinent Drug Interactions	Med Pearl
Lamivudine • Epivir • 150 mg PO BID or 300 mg PO daily • Solution, tabs	None	• N/V/D • Pancreatitis • Lactic acidosis • Hepatomegaly with steatosis	Monitor viral load more frequently with oral solution	None	• Also active against hepatitis B (Epivir HBV) • Adjust dose in renal impairment
Stavudine • Zerit • ≥60 kg: 40 mg PO BID • <60 kg: 30 mg PO BID • Caps, solution	Concurrent use of didanosine	• Peripheral neuropathy • Pancreatitis • Lactic acidosis • Hepatomegaly with steatosis • Hepatotoxicity • Lipoatrophy • Hyperlipidemia	LFTs	Additive risk of pancreatitis with concurrent didanosine	Adjust dose in renal impairment
Tenofovir disoproxil fumarate • Viread • 300 mg PO daily • Powder, tabs Tenofovir alafenamide • Vemlidy • 25 mg PO daily (Vemlidy only indicated for hepatitis B; only available in combination products for HIV) • Tabs	CrCl <30 mL/min (alafenamide)	• Renal impairment (> with disoproxil fumarate) • Fanconi syndrome • ↓ bone mineral density (> with disoproxil fumarate) • Lactic acidosis • Hepatomegaly with steatosis • Headache • N/V/D	• SCr • Urine glucose/urine protein • Bone mineral density	• ↓ atazanavir levels • ↑ didanosine levels (↓ didanosine dose) • Lopinavir/ritonavir, atazanavir/ritonavir, darunavir/ritonavir, acyclovir, valacyclovir, ganciclovir, valganciclovir, aminoglycosides, and NSAIDs ↑ levels	• Also active against hepatitis B • Oral powder can be used if patient unable to swallow tabs • Oral powder should be mixed in soft food (NOT liquids) • Adjust dose of disoproxil fumarate in renal impairment • Alafenamide associated with ↓ risk of renal impairment and reduced bone density
Zidovudine • Retrovir • 300 mg PO BID • 1 mg/kg IV q4h until PO can be taken • Caps, injection, solution, tabs	Concurrent ribavirin due to additive toxicity	• Anemia • Neutropenia • Headache • N/V • Myopathy • Lactic acidosis • Hepatomegaly with steatosis • Lipoatrophy • Hyperlipidemia • Nail pigmentation	CBC with differential	None	• Can be used to prevent maternal-fetal HIV transmission • Adjust dose in renal impairment

Protease Inhibitors (PIs)

Generic • Brand • Dose/Dosage Forms	Contraindications	Primary Side Effects	Key Monitoring	Pertinent Drug Interactions	Med Pearl
Mechanism of action – inhibit HIV protease enzyme from processing the gag-pol polyprotein precursor, thereby preventing development and maturation of new HIV particles					
Atazanavir • Reyataz • Therapy naïve: 300 mg PO daily (400 mg PO daily when used with efavirenz) + ritonavir 100 mg PO daily (or cobicistat 150 mg PO daily) **OR** 400 mg PO daily (if unable to tolerate ritonavir) • Therapy experienced: 300 mg PO daily + ritonavir 100 mg PO daily (or cobicistat 150 mg PO daily) • Caps, powder	Concurrent use with alfuzosin, elbasvir/grazoprevir, glecaprevir/pibrentasvir, rifampin, irinotecan, triazolam, ergot derivatives, St. John's wort, lovastatin, simvastatin, pimozide, lurasidone, sildenafil (for pulmonary hypertension), indinavir, and nevirapine	• Indirect hyper-bilirubinemia • PR interval prolongation • Hyperlipidemia • Hepatotoxicity • N/V • Hyperglycemia • Fat redistribu-tion • Cholelithiasis • Nephrolithiasis • Renal impair-ment • Rash	• LFTs • SCr • Urinalysis • Bilirubin • Lipids • Blood glucose • Electro-cardio-gram (ECG)	• CYP3A4 inhibitor and substrate • H_2-antagonists, PPIs, and antacids may ↓ absorption (follow guide-lines for using in combination)	• Oral powder used in children ≥3 mo and 10 to <25 kg • Oral powder can be used in adults if patient unable to swallow tabs • Take with food • Adjust dose in hepatic impairment
Darunavir • Prezista • Therapy naïve or therapy experienced (with no darunavir mutations): 800 mg PO daily + ritonavir 100 mg PO daily (or cobici-stat 150 mg PO daily) • Therapy experienced (with ≥1 darunavir resistance associated substitution): 600 mg PO BID + ritonavir 100 mg PO BID • Suspension, tabs	Concurrent use with alfuzosin, dronedarone, colchicine, ranolazine, rifampin, triazolam, ergot derivatives, St. John's wort, lovastatin, simvastatin, pimozide, lurasidone, and sildenafil (for pulmonary hypertension)	• Hyperlipidemia • Rash • Hepatotoxicity • N/V/D • Headache • Hyperglycemia • Fat redistribu-tion	• LFTs • Lipids • Blood glucose	• CYP3A4 inhibitor and substrate • CYP2C9 inducer	• Perform genotypic and/or phenotypic testing prior to initi-ating therapy • Use with caution in patients with sulfa allergy • Take with food
Fosamprenavir • Lexiva • Therapy naïve: 1,400 mg PO BID **OR** 1,400 mg PO daily + ritonavir 100–200 mg PO daily **OR** 700 mg PO BID + ritonavir 100 mg PO BID • Therapy experienced: 700 mg PO BID + ritonavir 100 mg PO BID • Suspension, tabs	Concurrent use with alfuzosin, flecainide, propafenone, rifampin, triazolam, ergot derivatives, St. John's wort, lovastatin, simvastatin, pimozide, lurasidone, and sildenafil (for pulmonary hypertension)	• Hyperlipidemia • Rash • Headache • Hepatotoxicity • N/V/D • Hyperglycemia • Fat redistribu-tion • Nephrolithiasis	• LFTs • Lipids • Blood glucose	• CYP3A4 inhibitor and substrate • H_2-antagonists ↓ levels	• Use with caution in patients with sulfa allergy • Adjust dose in hepatic impairment • Adults should take suspension without food; children should take suspension with food • Take tabs with meals if taking with ritonavir

Protease Inhibitors (PIs) *(cont'd)*

Generic • Brand • Dose/Dosage Forms	Contraindications	Primary Side Effects	Key Monitoring	Pertinent Drug Interactions	Med Pearl
Indinavir • Crixivan • 800 mg PO q8h **OR** 800 mg PO BID + ritonavir 100–200 mg PO BID • Caps	Concurrent use with alfuzosin, amiodarone, triazolam, alprazolam, ergot derivatives, lovastatin, simvastatin, pimozide, lurasidone, and sildenafil (for pulmonary hypertension)	• Hyperlipidemia • Hepatotoxicity • N/V/D • Nephrolithiasis • Indirect hyper-bilirubinemia • Hyperglycemia • Fat redistribution	• LFTs • Lipids • Bilirubin • Blood glucose	CYP3A4 inhibitor and substrate	• Patients are advised to drink six 8 oz glasses of water per day • Adjust dose in hepatic impairment • If taking *without* ritonavir, take with water 1 hr before or 2 hr after meals
Lopinavir/ritonavir • Kaletra • Lopinavir 400 mg/ ritonavir 100 mg PO BID **OR** lopinavir 800 mg/ ritonavir 200 mg PO daily • BID regimen must be used if patient has ≥3 lopinavir resistance associated substitutions • Solution, tabs	Concurrent use with alfuzosin, dronedarone, elbasvir/grazoprevir, colchicine, rifampin, triazolam, ergot derivatives, elbasvir/ grazoprevir, St. John's wort, lovastatin, simvastatin, ranolazine, pimozide, lurasidone, and sildenafil (for pulmonary hypertension)	• Hyperlipidemia • Pancreatitis • Hepatotoxicity • N/V/D • Hyperglycemia • Fat redistribu-tion • PR interval prolongation • QT interval prolongation	• LFTs • Lipids • Blood glucose • ECG	CYP3A4 substrate and inhibitor	• Recommended PI for pregnant women (BID dosing only) • Oral solution contains alcohol and propylene glycol • Take oral solution with food
Nelfinavir • Viracept • 1,250 mg PO BID **OR** 750 mg PO TID • Tabs	Concurrent use with alfuzosin, amiodarone, quinidine, rifampin, triazolam, ergot derivatives, St. John's wort, lovastatin, simvastatin, pimozide, lurasidone, and sildenafil (for pulmonary hypertension)	• N/D • Hyperlipidemia • Hyperglycemia • Fat redistribution • Hepatotoxicity	• LFTs • Lipids • Blood glucose	• CYP3A4 and CYP2C19 substrate • CYP3A4 inhibitor	• May disperse tabs in water • Take with food
Ritonavir • Norvir • 600 mg PO BID to boost other PIs • Caps, powder, solution, tabs	Concurrent use with alfuzosin, amiodarone, dronedarone, colchicine, flecainide, propafenone, quinidine, voriconazole (with ritonavir doses ≥800 mg/day), triazolam, ergot derivatives, St. John's wort, lovastatin, simvastatin, pimozide, lurasidone, ranolazine, and sildenafil (for pulmonary hypertension)	• Hyperlipidemia • Hepatotoxicity • N/V/D • Hyperglycemia • Fat redistribution • Paresthesia • Taste distur-bance	• LFTs • Lipids • Blood glucose • ECG	• CYP3A4 and CYP2D6 substrate and inhibitor • CYP1A2, CYP2C9, and CYP2C19 inducer	• Only used for boosting • Oral solution contains alcohol • Take with food • Do NOT refrigerate oral solution

Protease Inhibitors (PIs) *(cont'd)*

Generic • Brand • Dose/Dosage Forms	Contraindications	Primary Side Effects	Key Monitoring	Pertinent Drug Interactions	Med Pearl
Saquinavir • Invirase • 1,000 mg PO BID + ritonavir 100 mg PO BID • Caps, tabs	• QT interval prolongation or concurrent use with other drugs that prolong QT interval • Complete atrioventricular block (in absence of pacemaker) • Severe hepatic impairment • Concurrent use with alfuzosin, amiodarone, atazanavir, cobicistat, dofetilide, lidocaine, flecainide, propafenone, quinidine, disopyramide, quinine, trazodone, rifampin, triazolam, clarithromycin, erythromycin, pentamidine, ergot derivatives, St. John's wort, lovastatin, simvastatin, pimozide, lurasidone, clozapine, haloperidol, ziprasidone, phenothiazines, rilpivirine, tacrolimus, dasatinib, sunatinib, and sildenafil (for pulmonary hypertension)	• PR interval prolongation • QT interval prolongation • Hyperlipidemia • Hepatotoxicity • N/V/D • Headache • Hyperglycemia • Fat redistribution	• LFTs • Lipids • Blood glucose • ECG	CYP3A4 substrate and inhibitor	Take with food
Tipranavir • Aptivus • Therapy experienced: 500 mg PO BID + ritonavir 200 mg PO BID • Caps, solution	• Moderate or severe hepatic impairment • Concurrent use with alfuzosin, amiodarone, flecainide, propafenone, quinidine, rifampin, triazolam, ergot derivatives, St. John's wort, lovastatin, simvastatin, pimozide, lurasidone, and sildenafil (for pulmonary hypertension)	• Hepatotoxicity • Intracranial hemorrhage • Rash • N/V/D • Hyperlipidemia • Hyperglycemia • Fat redistribution	• LFTs • Lipids • Blood glucose	• CYP3A4 substrate • CYP2D6 inhibitor • CYP1A2, CYP2C19, and CYP3A4 inducer • Antiplatelets, anticoagulants, and vitamin E ↑ risk of bleeding	• Not for therapy naïve patients • Use with caution in patients with sulfa allergy • Take with food if used with ritonavir tabs • Oral solution contains propylene glycol • Do NOT refrigerate oral solution

Integrase Inhibitors

Generic • Brand • Dose/Dosage Forms	Contraindications	Primary Side Effects	Key Monitoring	Pertinent Drug Interactions	Med Pearl
Mechanism of action – inhibit integration of proviral DNA into host CD4 T-cell genome					
Bictegravir • Only available in combination products	Concurrent use with dofetilide or rifampin	• N/D • Headache	• None	• CYP3A4 substrate • ↑ dofetilide and metformin levels • Carbamazepine, oxcarbazepine, phenytoin, phenobarbital, St. John's wort, rifabutin, and rifampin ↓ levels • Absorption ↓ with antacids and products containing iron, magnesium, aluminum, calcium, or zinc (give bictegravir 2 hr before these medications)	None
Dolutegravir • Tivicay • Therapy naïve or therapy experienced, integrase inhibitor naïve or virologically suppressed switching to dolutegravir + rilpivirine: 50 mg PO daily • Integrase inhibitor experienced with certain integrase inhibitor associated resistance substitutions: 50 mg PO BID • Tabs	Concurrent use with dofetilide	• Hypersensitivity reaction • Insomnia • Headache • Hepatotoxicity • Depression or suicidal thoughts (primarily in patients with pre-existing psychiatric conditions)	• LFTs	• ↑ dofetilide and metformin levels • Etravirine, efavirenz, nevirapine, fosamprenavir/ritonavir, and tipranavir/ritonavir ↓ levels • Carbamazepine, oxcarbazepine, phenytoin, phenobarbital, St. John's wort, and rifampin ↓ levels • Absorption ↓ with antacids and products containing iron, magnesium, aluminum, calcium, or zinc (give dolutegravir 2 hr before or 6 hr after these medications)	• ↑ dose to 50 mg PO BID when used with carbamazepine, efavirenz, fosamprenavir/ritonavir, tipranavir/ritonavir, or rifampin • Use with caution in pregnancy (has been associated with neural tube defects)

Integrase Inhibitors *(cont'd)*

Generic • Brand • Dose/Dosage Forms	Contraindications	Primary Side Effects	Key Monitoring	Pertinent Drug Interactions	Med Pearl
Elvitegravir • Only available in combination products	None	• N/D • Depression or suicidal thoughts (primarily in patients with pre-existing psychiatric conditions)	None	• CYP3A4 substrate • Atazanavir, lopinavir/ritonavir, ketoconazole ↑ levels • Carbamazepine, efavirenz, didanosine, bosentan, oxcarbazepine, phenytoin, phenobarbital, rifampin, rifabutin, dexamethasone, and St. John's wort ↓ levels • Absorption ↓ with antacids and products containing iron, magnesium, aluminum, calcium, or zinc (space administration by ≥2 hr) • May ↑ ketoconazole, rifabutin, bosentan, and buprenorphine levels • May ↓ naloxone and methadone levels	Take with food
Raltegravir • Isentress • Therapy naïve or patients who are virologically suppressed on initial regimen of 400 mg PO BID: 1,200 mg PO daily • Therapy experienced: 400 mg PO BID • Chewable tabs, powder for suspension, tabs	None	• N/D • Headache • Rash • ↑ creatinine kinase • Muscle weakness • Insomnia • Depression or suicidal thoughts (primarily in patients with pre-existing psychiatric conditions)	None	• Rifampin ↓ levels • Absorption ↓ with antacids containing aluminum or magnesium (space administration)	• ↑ dose to 800 mg PO BID when used with rifampin • Chewable tabs and suspension for children

Cytochrome P450 Inhibitor

Generic • Brand • Dose/Dosage Forms	Contraindications	Primary Side Effects	Key Monitoring	Pertinent Drug Interactions	Med Pearl
Mechanism of action – CYP3A inhibitor used to ↑ systemic exposure to the CYP3A substrates, atazanavir and darunavir					
Cobicistat • Tybost • Therapy naïve or experienced: 150 mg PO daily + atazanavir 300 mg PO daily **OR** 150 mg PO daily + darunavir 800 mg PO daily • Tabs	Concurrent use with alfuzosin, dronedarone, irinotecan, rifampin, triazolam, ergot derivatives, St. John's wort, lovastatin, simvastatin, pimozide, lurasidone, sildenafil (for pulmonary hypertension), nevirapine, indinavir, carbamazepine, phenytoin, phenobarbital, ranolazine, colchicine, and drospirenone/ethinyl estradiol	• ↑ SCr/↓ CrCl (monitor closely if SCr ↑ by >0.4 mg/dL) • Jaundice • Nausea	SCr/CrCl	• CYP2D6 and CYP3A substrate and inhibitor • ↑ risk of renal impairment when used with tenofovir (do not use combination if CrCl <70 mL/min)	• ↑ SCr by inhibiting renal tubular secretion • Take with food

CCR5 Inhibitor

Generic • Brand • Dose/Dosage Forms	Contraindications	Primary Side Effects	Key Monitoring	Pertinent Drug Interactions	Med Pearl
Mechanism of action – acts as an antagonist for the CCR5 receptor, a chemokine coreceptor that can facilitate HIV entry into CD4 T-cells					
Maraviroc • Selzentry • Use with strong CYP3A4 inhibitors (including PIs [except tipranavir/ritonavir] and elvitegravir/ritonavir): 150 mg PO BID • Use with strong CYP3A4 inducers (including efavirenz, etravirine, rifampin, phenytoin, phenobarbital, and carbamazepine): 600 mg PO BID • Use with other medications (including tipranavir/ritonavir, nevirapine, raltegravir, NRTIs and enfuvirtide): 300 mg PO BID • Solution, tabs	CrCl <30 mL/min with concurrent use of strong CYP3A4 inhibitors or inducers	• Abdominal pain • Cough • Dizziness • Joint/muscle pain • Rash • Hepatotoxicity • Orthostatic hypotension	• Tropism testing • LFTs • Blood pressure	CYP3A4 substrate	• Only for patients with CCR5-tropic HIV • Hepatotoxicity may be preceded by systemic hypersensitivity reaction (rash, eosinophilia) • Adjust dose in renal impairment

Fusion Inhibitor

Generic • Brand • Dose	Contraindications	Primary Side Effects	Key Monitoring	Pertinent Drug Interactions	Med Pearl
Mechanism of action – blocks conformational changes in gp41 on the surface of HIV that are required for HIV fusion with CD4 cell membranes					
Enfuvirtide • Fuzeon • 90 mg subcut BID • Injection	None	• Local injection site reactions (pain, erythema, induration, nodules and cysts, pruritus, ecchymosis) • Pneumonia • Hypersensitivity reactions	Injection sites	None	Only HIV medication available as subcut injection

Combination Products: See individual drug components for important points.		
Brand	**Components**	**Dosing**
Atripla	Efavirenz, tenofovir disoproxil fumarate, emtricitabine	1 tablet PO daily
Biktarvy	Bictegravir, emtricitabine, tenofovir alafenamide	1 tablet PO daily
Cimduo	Lamivudine, tenofovir disoproxil fumarate	1 tablet PO daily
Combivir	Lamivudine, zidovudine	1 tablet PO BID
Complera	Rilpivirine, tenofovir disoproxil fumarate, emtricitabine	1 tablet PO daily
Descovy	Emtricitabine, tenofovir alafenamide	1 table PO daily
Epzicom	Abacavir, lamivudine	1 tablet PO daily
Evotaz	Atazanavir, cobicistat	1 tablet PO daily
Genvoya	Elvitegravir, cobicistat, emtricitabine, tenofovir alafenamide	1 tablet PO daily
Juluca	Dolutegravir, rilpivirine	1 tablet PO daily
Odefsey	Emtricitabine, rilpivirine, tenofovir alafenamide	1 tablet PO daily
Prezcobix	Darunavir, cobicistat	1 tablet PO daily
Stribild	Elvitegravir, cobicistat, emtricitabine, tenofovir disoproxil fumarate	1 tablet PO daily
Symfi/Symfi Lo	Efavirenz, lamivudine, tenofovir disoproxil fumarate	1 tablet PO daily
Triumeq	Dolutegravir, abacavir, lamivudine	1 tablet PO daily
Trizivir	Abacavir, lamivudine, zidovudine	1 tablet PO BID
Truvada	Emtricitabine, tenofovir disoproxil fumarate	1 tablet PO daily

TUBERCULOSIS

Guidelines Summary

The overall goals for treatment of TB are: (1) To cure the individual patient and (2) to minimize the transmission of *Mycobacterium tuberculosis* to other persons.

- Risk factors
    - Location of birth (New York, New Jersey, California, Florida, and Texas account for 92% of cases)
    - Close contact (>40 hours per week) with TB patients
    - Increase in age
    - Race and ethnicity: Hispanics, African Americans, and Asian Pacific Islanders
- Successful treatment of TB has benefits for both the individual patient and the community in which the patient resides.
- Prescribing physician responsibility for treatment completion is a fundamental principle in TB control.
- Treatment of patients with TB is most successful within a comprehensive framework that addresses both clinical and social issues of relevance to the patient.
- It is strongly recommended that patient-centered care be the initial management strategy, regardless of the source of supervision. This strategy should always include an adherence plan that emphasizes directly observed therapy (DOT).
- Patients with TB caused by drug-susceptible organisms usually are treated initially with a four-drug regimen (rifampin, isoniazid, pyrazinamide, and ethambutol [RIPE]) followed by a two-drug continuation phase (rifampin and isoniazid).

Antitubercular Drugs

Generic • Brand • Dose/Dosage Forms	Contraindications	Primary Side Effects	Key Monitoring	Pertinent Drug Interactions	Med Pearl
Mechanism of action – inhibits mycolic acid synthesis resulting in disruption of the bacterial cell wall					
Isoniazid • Only available generically • Latent: 5 mg/day (max = 300 mg) PO daily × 6–9 mo **OR** 15 mg/kg (max = 900 mg) PO weekly × 6–9 mo • Active: multiple scenarios • Injection, syrup, tabs	• Hepatic impairment • Previous severe reactions (drug fever, chills, arthritis)	• Depression • Flushing • Jaundice	• LFTs • Sputum cultures	CYP2C19 and CYP2D6 inhibitor	• Severe and sometimes fatal hepatitis may occur within 3 mo of treatment • Drinking alcohol not recommended during treatment • Pyridoxine should be administered to prevent peripheral neuropathy
Mechanism of action – inhibits bacterial RNA synthesis by binding to the beta subunit of DNA-dependent RNA polymerase, blocking RNA transcription					
Rifampin • Rifadin • 10 mg/kg/day PO/IV (max = 600 mg/day) • Caps, injection	Concurrent use with PIs	• Numbness • Flu-like syndrome • Rash • Red discoloration of bodily fluids and teeth • Neutropenia/leukopenia	• LFTs • CBC • Sputum cultures • Chest x-ray	CYP1A2, CYP2C9, CYP2C19, and CYP3A4 inducer	None
Mechanism of action – kills mycobacteria replicating in macrophages; exact mechanism is not known					
Pyrazinamide • Only available generically • 40–55 kg: 1,000 mg/day PO • 56–75 kg: 1,500 mg/day PO • 76–90 kg: 2,000 mg/day PO (max dose) • Tabs	• Acute gout • Hepatic impairment	• Malaise • Anorexia • Hepatotoxicity	• LFTs • Uric acid levels • Sputum cultures • Chest x-ray	None	Typically used for the first 2 mo of therapy
Mechanism of action – suppresses mycobacteria multiplication by interfering with RNA synthesis					
Ethambutol • Myambutol • 15–25 mg/kg/day (max = 1,600 mg/day) • Tabs	Optic neuritis	• Myocarditis • Headache • Gout • Hepatotoxicity	• Baseline and periodic (monthly) visual testing • LFTs	Aluminum hydroxide ↓ absorption (separate by 4 hr)	Optic neuritis manifests as ↓ red-green color perception, ↓ visual field

Pulmonary Disorders

3

This chapter covers the following diseases:

- **Asthma**
- **Chronic obstructive pulmonary disease**

ASTHMA

Assessment and Monitoring

Once asthma is diagnosed, accurate classification of severity (prior to treatment initiation) and control (for patients on treatment) is essential. Classification is based upon considerations of both impairment and risk, including frequency of symptoms, night-time awakenings, interference with normal activity, use of a short-acting β_2 agonist (for those on treatment), lung function (spirometry or peak flow), and exacerbations. Assessment varies based upon age (0–4 years, 5–11 years, and 12 years and older). Tables follow for classification of asthma severity and asthma control in patients age 12 years and older.

Classification of Asthma Severity (12 Years and Older)

	Intermittent	Persistent		
		Mild	**Moderate**	**Severe**
Symptoms	≤2 days/week	>2 days /week but not daily	Daily	Throughout the day
Nighttime awakenings	≤2 × /month	3–4 × /month	>1 × /week but not nightly	Often 7 × /week
Short-acting β_2-agonist use for symptom control	≤2 days/week	>2 days/week but not daily	Daily	Several times per day
Interference with normal activity	None	Minor limitation	Some limitation	Extreme limitation

Classification of Asthma Severity (12 Years and Older)   *(cont'd)*

	Intermittent	Persistent		
		Mild	**Moderate**	**Severe**
Lung function	• Normal FEV1 between exacerbations • FEV1 >80% predicted • FEV1/FVC normal	• FEV1 ≥80% predicted **OR** • FEV1/FVC normal	• FEV1 60–79% predicted **OR** • FEV1/FVC reduced 5%	• FEV1 <60% predicted **OR** • FEV1/FVC reduced >5%
Exacerbations (requiring oral corticosteroids)	0–1/year (see note)	≥2/year (see note)		
	Consider severity and interval since last exacerbation. Frequency and severity may fluctuate over time for patients in any severity category.			
	Relative annual risk of exacerbations may be related to FEV1.			

Adapted from National Heart, Lung and Blood Institute, National Asthma Education and Prevention Program, Expert Panel Report 3: Guidelines for the Diagnosis and Management of Asthma—Full Report, 2007. www.nhlbi.nih.gov/files/docs/guidelines/asthgdln.pdf.

Classification of Asthma Control (12 Years and Older)

	Well Controlled	**Not Well Controlled**	**Very Poorly Controlled**
Symptoms	≤2 days/week	>2 days/week	Throughout the day
Nighttime awakenings	≤2 × /month	1–3 × /week	≥4 × /week
Interference with normal activity	None	Some limitation	Extreme limitation
Short-acting β$_2$-agonist use for symptom control	≤2 days/ week	>2 days/week	Several times per day
FEV1 or peak flow	>80% predicted/ personal best	60–80% predicted/ personal best	<60% predicted/ personal best
Validated questionnaires ATQ ACQ ACT	0 ≤0.75 ≥20	1–2 ≥1.5 16–19	3–4 N/A ≤15
Exacerbations	0–1/year	≥2/year	
	Consider severity and interval since last exacerbation.		
Progressive loss of lung function	Evaluation requires long-term follow-up care.		
Treatment-related adverse effects	Medication side effects can vary in intensity from none to very troublesome and worrisome. The level of intensity does not correlate to specific levels of control but should be considered in the overall assessment of risk.		

Adapted from National Heart, Lung and Blood Institute, National Asthma Education and Prevention Program, Expert Panel Report 3: Guidelines for the Diagnosis and Management of Asthma—Full Report, 2007. www.nhlbi.nih.gov/files/docs/guidelines/asthgdln.pdf.

Guidelines Summary

General Principles of Asthma Management

Long-term goals:

- Minimize exacerbations
- Maintain good control of daily symptoms
- Limit fixed airflow limitation
- Minimize side effects of treatment
- Patient's own self-identified goals

Medication categories:

- Controller therapy: Used for maintenance treatment. Decreases airway inflammation, controls symptoms, and decreases risk of exacerbation and declining lung function.
- Rescue therapy: Used as needed for relief of breakthrough symptoms.
- Add-on therapy: Used in severe asthma to address persistent symptoms despite high-dose inhaled corticosteroids (ICS) and long-acting beta agonist (LABA) therapy.

Control-based management:

- Continuous cycle of assessment, treatment, monitoring.
- Stepwise therapy based upon severity and level of control.
- Inhaled corticosteroids are the mainstay of therapy for all persistent asthma.

Asthma Treatment Summary

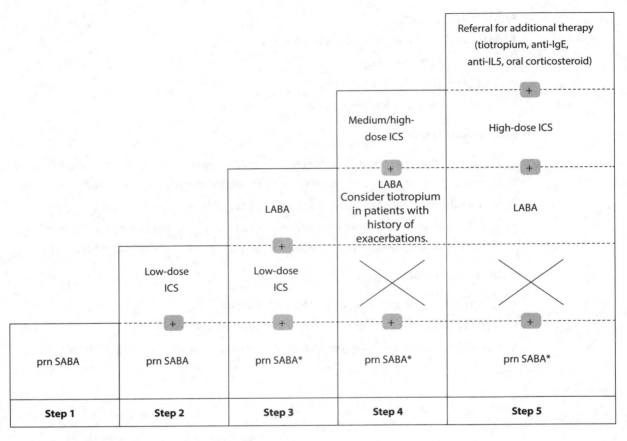

Asthma Stepwise Therapy

Step 6 per NAEPP is addition of daily oral corticosteroids.

Abbreviations: ICS = inhaled corticosteroid; LABA = long-acting β-2 agonist; prn = as needed;
SABA = short-acting β-2 agonist
* Low-dose ICS/formoterol is reliever therapy for those taking low-dose ICS/formoterol or low-dose beclametasone/formoterol
controller therapies.
Adapted from GINA 2017 guidelines

Inhaled Corticosteroids

Generic • Brand • Dose/Dosage Forms	Contraindications	Primary Side Effects	Key Monitoring	Pertinent Drug Interactions	Med Pearl
Mechanism of action – glucocorticoid receptor agonist with an affinity for the receptor resulting in anti-inflammatory and immunosuppressive properties, and antiproliferative actions					
Fluticasone • Flovent Diskus, Flovent HFA • 88–440 mcg BID	Primary treatment of acute bronchospasm	• Throat irritation • Cough • Oral candidiasis • Upper respiratory tract infection • Sinusitis	• FEV1 • Peak flow • Other PFTs • Hypothalamic-pituitary-adrenal axis suppression	• CYP3A4 substrate • Cobicistat (component of Stribild) and ritonavir may ↑ levels	• HFA formulation for Flovent • Most potent corticosteroid
Fluticasone furoate ☆ • Arnuity Ellipta • 100–200 mcg daily					
Fluticasone propionate • Armonair RespiClick • 55–232 mcg BID					
Budesonide ☆ • Pulmicort Flexhaler, Pulmicort Respules • Flexhaler: 180–720 mcg BID • Respules: 0.25–1 mg/day					Respules are the only nebulized corticosteroid
Mometasone • Asmanex HFA, Asmanex Twisthaler • HFA: 100–200 mcg BID • Twisthaler: 110–880 mcg/day					Twisthaler is true once daily
Beclomethasone ☆ • QVAR Redihaler • 40–320 mcg BID					HFA formulation
Flunisolide • Aerospan • 160–320 mcg BID					HFA formulation
Ciclesonide • Alvesco • 80 mcg BID (max = 640 mcg/day)					Drug is a solution aerosol so no shaking is required

Short-Acting β₂ Agonists

Generic • Brand • Dose/Dosage Forms	Contraindications	Primary Side Effects	Key Monitoring	Pertinent Drug Interactions	Med Pearl
Mechanism of action – relaxes bronchial smooth muscle by acting on β₂ receptors in the lungs					
Albuterol ☆ • Ventolin HFA, Proventil HFA, ProAir HFA, ProAir Respiclick • Metered-dose inhaler (MDI): 2 inhalations every 4–6 hr prn (90 mcg/inhalation) • Neb: 2.5 mg 3–4 × /day prn	Hypersensitivity	• Dose-dependent • Angina • Arrhythmias • Chest discomfort • Cough • Tremor	• FEV1 • Peak flow • Blood pressure • HR	Nonselective β-blockers ↓ effects	• Excessive use can ↑ risk of death • Nebulizer is compatible with budesonide, cromolyn, ipratropium
Levalbuterol ☆ • Xopenex, Xopenex HFA • MDI: 2 inhalations every 4–6 hr prn (45 mcg/inhalation) • Neb: 0.63 mg TID	Hypersensitivity	• Tremor • Rhinitis • Tachycardia			Fewer cardiac side effects than albuterol

Long-Acting β₂ Agonists

Generic • Brand • Dose/Dosage Forms	Contraindications	Primary Side Effects	Key Monitoring	Pertinent Drug Interactions	Med Pearl
Mechanism of action – long-acting β2 agonists; relaxes bronchial smooth muscle					
Salmeterol • Serevent Diskus • 50 mcg/inhalation • 1 inhalation BID (max = 2 puffs/day)	• Primary treatment of acute bronchospasm • Presence of tachyarrhythmias • Monotherapy	• Headache • Hypertension • Dizziness • Chest pain • Throat irritation	• FEV1 • Peak flow	• CYP3A4 substrate • Cobicistat (component of Stribild) and ritonavir may ↑ levels	LABAs may ↑ the risk of asthma-related deaths; should be used only in adjunct therapy with inhaled corticosteroids
Formoterol • Only available in combination products in US (for asthma)	• Hypersensitivity • Monotherapy	• Headache • Hypertension • Dizziness • Chest pain • Throat irritation	• FEV1 • Peak flow	Nonselective β-blockers ↓ effects	

Immunomodulators

Generic • Brand • Dose/Dosage Forms	Contraindications	Primary Side Effects	Key Monitoring	Pertinent Drug Interactions	Med Pearl
Mechanism of action – IgG monoclonal antibody which inhibits IgE receptor on mast cells and basophils					
Omalizumab • Xolair • 150–375 mg subcut every 2–4 wk, based on weight and serum IgE	Primary treatment of acute bronchospasm	• Pain and bruising of injection sites • Anaphylaxis • Neuromuscular pain	Be prepared for anaphylaxis	None	Do not administer >150 mg per injection site
Mechanism of action – interleukin-5 antagonist which ↓ production and survival of eosinophils; however, the mechanism of action in asthma has not been definitively established					
Mepolizumab • Nucala • 100 mg subcut every 4 wk	Hypersensitivity	• Anaphylaxis • Injection site reaction • Antibody development • Herpes zoster activation	• FEV1 • Other PFTs	None	• Add-on therapy for severe asthma with eosinophilic phenotype • Zoster vaccination recommended prior to use
Reslizumab • Cinqair • 3 mg/kg IV every 4 wk	Hypersensitivity	• Anaphylaxis • ↑ creatine kinase • Antibody development	• FEV1 • Other PFTs	None	• Add-on therapy for severe asthma with eosinophilic phenotype • Store in refrigerator
Benralizumab • Fasenra • 30 mg subcut every 4 wk for 3 doses, then every 8 wk		• Antibody development • Headache • Pharyngitis			

Leukotriene Receptor Antagonists

Generic • Brand • Dose/Dosage Forms	Contraindications	Primary Side Effects	Key Monitoring	Pertinent Drug Interactions	Med Pearl
Mechanism of action – selective leukotriene receptor antagonist of leukotrienes D4 and E4					
Montelukast ☆ • Singulair • 4–10 mg PO HS • Tabs, chewable tabs, and granules	Hypersensitivity	• Behavioral changes (agitation, hostility, anxiety, depression, hallucinations, insomnia, irritability, suicidal thoughts) • Headache • Churg-Strauss syndrome (rare)	Behavioral changes	None	Approved for adults and children ≥1 yr
Zafirlukast • Accolate • 10–20 mg PO BID		• ↑ liver function tests (LFTs) • Headache • Insomnia • Depression	LFTs	• CYP2C9 substrate • CYP2C9 and CYP3A4 inhibitor • May ↑ effects of warfarin • CYP2C9 inhibitors may ↑ effects • CYP2C9 inducers may ↓ effects	Must be taken on empty stomach

Other Asthma Medications

Generic • Brand • Dose/Dosage Forms	Contraindications	Primary Side Effects	Key Monitoring	Pertinent Drug Interactions	Med Pearl
Mechanism of action – prevents the mast cells from releasing histamine and leukotrienes					
Cromolyn • Only available generically • 60–80 mg/day • Nebulization solution	Primary treatment of acute bronchospasm	• Cough and irritation • Unpleasant taste • ↑ sneezing	PFTs	None	• Safety is the primary advantage of this drug • May take 4–6 wk for full benefit • Approved for adults and children > 2 yr
Mechanism of action – 5-lipoxygenase inhibitor limits neutrophil and monocyte aggregation					
Zileuton • Zyflo, Zyflo CR • IR: 600 mg PO 4 × /day • CR: 1,200 mg PO BID	Acute liver disease	• ↑ LFTs • Headache	• LFTs at baseline, then every 4 wk × 3 mo, then every 2–3 mo for the rest of the yr, then periodically • Peak flow	• CYP1A2, CYP2C9, and CYP3A4 substrate • CYP1A2 inhibitor • May ↑ effects/toxicity of theophylline and warfarin	• 4 × /day dose is disadvantage for IR • CR should be taken with food
Mechanism of action – methylxanthine causes bronchodilation by ↑ tissue concentrations of cyclic adenine monophosphate					
Theophylline ☆ • Theo-24, Theocron, Elixophyllin • 10 mg/kg/day PO up to 600 mg/day • Liquid, sustained-release tabs, and caps	Allergy to corn-derived dextrose	• Tachycardia • Nausea/vomiting • Central nervous system (CNS) stimulation • Theophylline toxicity (persistent, repetitive vomiting)	• Theophylline concentrations (10–20 mcg/mL) • Heart rate • CNS effects	• CYP1A2 substrate • CYP1A2 inhibitors may ↑ effects/toxicity • CYP1A2 inducers may ↓ effects	Dosage adjustments should be in small increments (maximum: 25%); ↓ dose by 25% in older adult patients
Aminophylline • Only available generically • Dose is diagnosis- and age-dependent • Injection	Hypersensitivity to theophylline				Theophylline dose is 80% of aminophylline dose

Combination Products: See individual drug components for important points.		
Brand	**Components**	**Dosing**
Advair Diskus, Advair HFA, Airduo Respiclick	Fluticasone + Salmeterol	Diskus: 1 inhalation BID HFA: 2 inhalations BID Respiclick: 1 inhalation BID
Breo Ellipta	Fluticasone + Vilanterol	1 inhalation daily
Dulera	Mometasone + Formoterol	2 inhalations BID
Symbicort	Formoterol + Budesonide	2 inhalations BID

CHRONIC OBSTRUCTIVE PULMONARY DISEASE

Classification of Airflow Severity

- GOLD I: mild COPD: FEV1 ≥80% predicted
- GOLD II: moderate COPD: 50% ≤FEV1 <80% predicted
- GOLD III: severe COPD: 30% ≤FEV1 <50% predicted
- GOLD IV: very severe COPD: FEV1 <30% predicted

Classification of COPD Exacerbation Risk

- Group A: low risk of exacerbation (0–1 moderate/severe exacerbation history, no hospitalization) + low symptom burden (mMRC 0–1 or CAT score <10)
- Group B: low risk of exacerbation (0–1 moderate/severe exacerbation history, no hospitalization) + with more symptoms than group A (mMRC ≥2 or CAT ≥10)
- Group C: high risk of exacerbation (≥2 moderate/severe exacerbation history OR ≥1 leading to hospitalization) + low symptom burden (mMRC 0–1 or CAT score <10)
- Group D: high risk of exacerbation (≥2 moderate/severe exacerbation history OR ≥1 leading to hospitalization) with more symptoms than group C (mMRC ≥2 or CAT ≥10)

Guidelines Summary

Treatment is based on the **G**lobal Initiative for Chronic **O**bstructive **L**ung **D**isease (GOLD).

- Goals of therapy:
  - Reduce symptoms
  - Reduce frequency and severity of exacerbations
  - Improve health status and exercise tolerance
- Treatment approach to stable COPD:
  - Influenza and pneumococcal (PPSV 23) vaccination should be offered for all patients who smoke and all patients with diagnosed COPD.
  - Pneumococcal (PCV 13) is indicated for all patients ≥65 years of age.
  - Smoking cessation should be encouraged for all patients who smoke.
  - Effectiveness and safety of e-cigarettes is uncertain.
  - Short-acting or long-acting inhaled bronchodilators, including β_2 agonists and anticholinergics, can be used as needed in patients in Group A.
  - Long-acting inhaled bronchodilators, including LABAs and long-acting antimuscarinic antagonists (LAMAs), are first-line pharmacological therapy for patients in Groups B, C, and D.

- Long-acting inhaled bronchodilators may be combined (LABA/LAMA) for enhanced efficacy if monotherapy is insufficient.
- ICS are recommended as an addition to long-acting bronchodilator therapy for Groups C and D after LABA/LAMA.
- Roflumilast may reduce exacerbations for patients with severe or very severe COPD (Group D) with FEV1 <50% predicted, chronic bronchitis, and at least one exacerbation in the past year.
- Macrolide antibiotics (azithromycin) may be considered in Group D patients who are former smokers and are uncontrolled on combination bronchodilator therapy.
- Group D patients with persistent exacerbations on LABA/LAMA/ICS therapy may have ICS withdrawn.
- Theophylline should be reserved for patients unable to access or afford long-acting inhaled bronchodilators.

- Treatment approach to exacerbations:
  - Exacerbation diagnosis is based on clinical presentation of significant change in daily symptoms and sputum production.
  - Goal of therapy is to minimize impact of the current exacerbation and prevent future exacerbations.
  - Use of short-acting bronchodilators and systemic corticosteroids (prednisone 40 mg daily for 5 days) can shorten recovery time.

COPD Treatment Summary

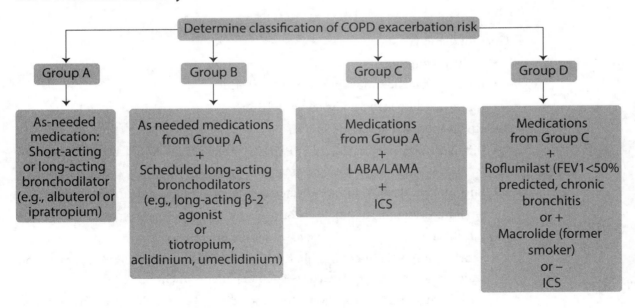

Medications for COPD

(See Asthma section for additional drug tables including ICS, short-acting bronchodilators, and methylxanthines.)

Long-Acting Bronchodilators

Generic • Brand • Dose	Contraindications	Primary Side Effects	Key Monitoring	Pertinent Drug Interactions	Med Pearl
Mechanism of action – long-acting β_2-adrenergic agonist; relaxes bronchial smooth muscle					
Indacaterol • Arcapta Neohaler • 75 mcg daily	Monotherapy in the treatment of asthma	• Cough • Chest pain • Headache • Nasopharyngitis	• PFTs • HR	Nonselective β-blockers	• Indacaterol, arformoterol, formoterol, and olodaterol not approved for the treatment of asthma • Arformoterol and formoterol available as nebulizer solution
Arformoterol • Brovana • 15 mcg BID					
Formoterol • Perforomist • 20 mcg BID					
Salmeterol • Serevent Diskus • 50 mcg/ inhalation • 1 inhalation BID					
Olodaterol • Striverdi Respimat • 2 inhalations daily					

Long-Acting Bronchodilators *(cont'd)*

Generic • Brand • Dose	Contraindications	Primary Side Effects	Key Monitoring	Pertinent Drug Interactions	Med Pearl
Mechanism of action – blocks acetylcholine at the parasympathetic sites in bronchial smooth muscle, causing bronchodilation					
Ipratropium ☆ • Atrovent HFA • MDI: 2 inhalations 4 × /day (max = 12 puffs/24 hrs) • Nebulizer: 500 mcg every 6–8 hr	• Hypersensitivity • Peanut allergy (due to soya lecithin) • Does not apply to Atrovent HFA	• Upper respiratory tract infection • Palpitation • Xerostomia • Pharyngeal irritation	• FEV1 • Peak flow • Other PFTs	Avoid use with other anticholinergic inhalers	• Not recommended for initial treatment of acute episode of bronchospasm • Anticholinergic side effects are possible. Be careful in BPH, narrow-angle glaucoma, and myasthenia gravis
Tiotropium ☆ • Spiriva Handihaler, Spiriva Respimat • Handihaler: 1 cap (18 mcg) via inhalation daily • Respimat: 2 inhalations daily	Contains lactose				
Aclidinium • Tudorza Pressair • 1 inhalation BID	Hypersensitivity to milk protein				
Umeclidinium • Incruse Ellipta • 1 inhalation daily	Hypersensitivity to milk protein				
Glycopyrrolate • Seebri Neohaler • 1 cap (15.6 mcg) by inhalation BID • Lonhala Magnair by nebulizer 25 mcg BID	Hypersensitivity	• Upper respiratory tract infection • Nasopharyngitis			

Phosphodiesterase-4 Inhibitor

Generic • Brand • Dose	Contraindications	Primary Side Effects	Key Monitoring	Pertinent Drug Interactions	Med Pearl
Mechanism of action – inhibits phosphodiesterase-4 leading to an accumulation of cyclic AMP					
Roflumilast • Daliresp • 500 mcg daily	Hepatic impairment (Child-Pugh class B or C)	• Diarrhea • Weight loss • Nausea • Gynecomastia	• Weight • LFTs	• CYP1A2 and CYP3A4 substrate • CYP1A2 and CYP3A4 inhibitors may ↑ effects • CYP1A2 and CYP3A4 inducers may ↓ effects	Not indicated for relieving acute bronchospasms or for use as monotherapy of COPD

Combination Products: See individual drug components for important points.		
Brand	**Components**	**Dosing**
Advair Diskus	Fluticasone + Salmeterol	1 inhalation BID
Anoro Ellipta	Umeclidinium + Vilanterol	1 inhalation daily
Bevespi Aerosphere	Glycopyrrolate + Formoterol	2 inhalations BID
Breo Ellipta	Fluticasone + Vilanterol	1 inhalation daily
Combivent Respimat	Ipratropium + Albuterol	1 inhalation 4×/day
Stiolto Respimat	Tiotropium + Olodaterol	2 inhalations daily
Symbicort	Budesonide + Formoterol	2 inhalations BID
Trelegy Ellipta	Fluticasone + Umeclidinium + Vilanterol	1 inhalation daily
Utibron Neohaler	Glycopyrrolate + Indacaterol	1 cap inhaled BID

Endocrine Disorders

4

This chapter covers the following diseases:

- **Diabetes mellitus**
- **Hypothyroidism**
- **Hyperthyroidism**
- **Polycystic ovary syndrome**

DIABETES MELLITUS

Guidelines Summary

- American Diabetes Association (ADA) Guideline Treatment Targets
  - Preprandial glucose 80–130 mg/dL
  - Postprandial glucose <180 mg/dL
  - A1c <7%
  - Blood pressure <140/90 mmHg
  - Goals should be individualized.

Patient education is integral to successful management of diabetes. Diabetes education should be conducted through an interprofessional approach.

Dietary education should focus on medical nutrition therapy provided by a registered dietitian.

Exercise should include 150 min/week of moderate-intensity aerobic activity or 75 min/week of vigorous aerobic activity.

- Insulin replacement is necessary in type 1 DM and is generally initiated at 0.5–1 units/kg/day.
  - Analog-based basal bolus regimen (50% basal, 50% bolus [divided into 3 meals]) **OR**
  - Human insulin–based split-mixed regimen (70% A.M.; 30% P.M. [each dose $\frac{2}{3}$ NPH to $\frac{1}{3}$ regular])
- Insulin regimens are adjusted based upon patient response (self-monitored blood glucose [SMBG]).
- Metformin is first-line therapy for patients with type 2 DM unless contraindicated.
- Second-line options include insulin, sulfonylureas, dipeptidyl-peptidase 4 (DPP-4) inhibitors, glucagon-like peptide-1 (GLP-1) agonists, sodium-glucose cotransporter 2 (SGLT-2) inhibitors, and thiazolidinediones (TZD).
- Second-line selection is made based upon patient-specific considerations of presence of atherosclerotic cardiovascular disease (ASCVD), efficacy needed, risk of hypoglycemia/weight gain, other side effects, and cost.
- Cardiovascular outcomes trials (CVOT) support ASCVD risk reduction with the use of empagliflozin and liraglutide in patients with ASCVD.

Treatment Algorithm

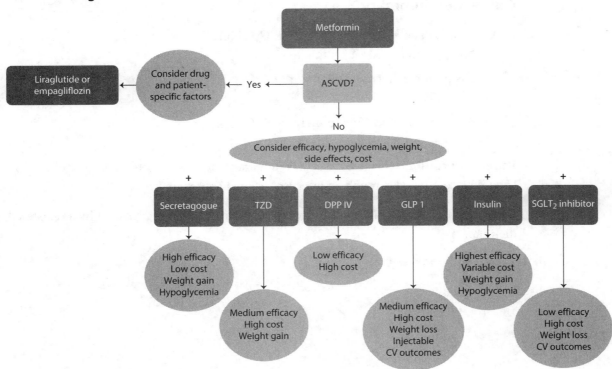

Insulin

Generic • Brand	Onset	Peak	Duration	Comments
Rapid-acting				• Hypoglycemia is the most common side effect. It is defined as blood sugar <70 mg/dL and must be treated as soon as recognized.
Aspart ☆ • NovoLog • Fiasp	5–15 min	30–90 min	<5 hr	
Lispro U-100 ☆ Lispro U-200 • Humalog • Admelog	5–15 min	30–90 min	<5 hr	• Insulin dosage is individually based due to sensitivity; 0.5–1.0 units/kg/day for the average nonobese patient.
Glulisine • Apidra	5–15 min	30–90 min	<5 hr	• Duration of action is prolonged in renal failure.
Short-acting				
Regular ☆ • Humulin R (OTC)	30–60 min	2–3 hr	5–8 hr	
Inhaled, regular • Afrezza	30–60 min	2–3 hr	5–8 hr	
Intermediate, basal				
NPH (Neutral Protamine Hagedorn) ☆ • Humulin N (OTC)	2–4 hr	4–10 hr	10–16 hr	
Long-acting, basal				
Glargine U-100 ☆ • Basaglar, Lantus	2–4 hr	No peak	20–24 hr	
Detemir ☆ • Levemir	3–8 hr	No peak	6–24 hr	
Glargine U-300 • Toujeo	2–4 hr	No peak	22–24 hr	
Degludec • Tresiba	1–3 hr	No peak	42 hr	

Insulin   *(cont'd)*

Generic • Brand	Onset	Peak	Duration	Comments
Premixed				[Same as above]
75% Lispro protamine/ 25% lispro • Humalog Mix 75/25	5–15 min	Dual	10–16 hr	
50% Lispro protamine/ 50% lispro • Humalog Mix 50/50	5–15 min	Dual	10–16 hr	
50% Aspart protamine/ 50% aspart • NovoLog Mix 50/50	5–15 min	Dual	10–16 hr	
70% Aspart protamine/ 30% aspart • NovoLog Mix 70/30	5–15 min	Dual	10–16 hr	
70% Degludec/30% aspart • Ryzodeg	5–15 min	Dual	<5 hr (aspart); 42 hr (degludec)	
70% NPH/30% regular • 70/30 (OTC)	30–60 min	Dual	10–16 hr	
• OTC insulin is available without a prescription. • Rapid-acting insulin should be given at time of meal ingestion, no more than 15 minutes from eating. • Regular insulin should be given 30 minutes prior to meal due to delayed onset of action.				

Sulfonylureas

Generic • Brand • Dose & Max	Contraindications	Primary Side Effects	Key Monitoring	Pertinent Drug Interactions	Med Pearl
Sulfonylureas, first generation — stimulate insulin release from the pancreatic beta cells					
Tolbutamide • Only available generically • 250 mg–3 g daily Tolazamide • Only available generically • 100 mg–1 g daily Chlorpropamide • Diabinese • 100–500 mg daily	• Type 1 DM • Sulfa allergy • Creatinine clearance (CrCl) <50 mL/min (chlorpropamide)	• Hypoglycemia • Weight gain	• Fasting plasma glucose (FPG) • A1c every 3 mo • S/S hypoglycemia	• Tolbutamide = CYP2C9 substrate and inhibitor • Chlorpropamide = CYP2C9 substrate • Chronic ethanol ingestion may ↓ hypoglycemic effect	Response plateaus after half maximum dose

Sulfonylureas   *(cont'd)*

Generic • Brand • Dose & Max	Contraindications	Primary Side Effects	Key Monitoring	Pertinent Drug Interactions	Med Pearl
Sulfonylureas, second generation – stimulate insulin release from the pancreatic beta cells					
Glyburide☆ • DiaBeta, Glynase • 1.25–20 mg/day (given daily BID) • Micronized: 0.75–12 mg/day (given daily BID)	• Type 1 DM • Sulfa allergy	• Hypoglycemia • Weight gain	• FPG • A1c every 3 mo • S/S hypoglycemia	• CYP2C9 substrates • CYP2C9 inhibitors may ↑ effects • CYP2C9 inducers may ↓ effects • Chronic ethanol ingestion may ↓ hypoglycemic effect	• Response plateaus after half maximum dose • Administer with meals
Glipizide☆ • Glucotrol, Glucotrol XR • 2.5–40 mg/day					
Glimepiride☆ • Amaryl • 1–8 mg daily					

Meglitinides

Generic • Brand • Dose & Max	Contraindications	Primary Side Effects	Key Monitoring	Pertinent Drug Interactions	Med Pearl
Mechanism of action – in presence of glucose, stimulate insulin release from the pancreatic beta cells					
Repaglinide • Prandin • 0.5–16 mg/day (taken BID–4 × /day)	• Type 1 DM • Concurrent use of gemfibrozil	• Hypoglycemia • Weight gain	• Postprandial plasma glucose • A1c every 3 mo • S/S hypoglycemia	• CYP2C8 and CYP3A4 substrate • CYP2C8 and CYP3A4 inhibitors may ↑ effects • CYP2C8 and CYP3A4 inducers may ↓ effects	• Faster acting and shorter duration than sulfonylureas • Recommended for postprandial hyperglycemia • Administer each dose 15–30 min before meals
Nateglinide • Starlix • 60–120 mg TID	Type 1 DM			• CYP2C9 and CYP3A4 substrate • CYP2C9 and CYP3A4 inhibitors may ↑ effects • CYP2C9 and CYP3A4 inducers may ↓ effects	

Biguanide

Generic • Brand • Dose & Max	Contraindications	Primary Side Effects	Key Monitoring	Pertinent Drug Interactions	Med Pearl
Mechanism of action – ↓ hepatic glucose production, ↓ intestinal absorption of glucose, and improves insulin sensitivity					
Metformin☆ • Glucophage, Glucophage XR • IR: 500–2,550 mg/day (in 2–3 divided doses) • XR: 500–2,000 mg daily	• CrCl <30 mL/min • Lactic acidosis • Severe heart failure • Radiocontrast dyes (discontinue 48 hr before and after procedure)	• Diarrhea • Flatulence • Lactic acidosis • Vitamin B$_{12}$ deficiency	• Serum creatinine (SCr) • Hemoglobin/hematocrit • Vitamin B12 concentrations • FPG • A1c every 3 mo	Cimetidine may ↑ effects	• Black box warning: lactic acidosis • Maximum daily dose for IR is 2,550 mg

Alpha-Glucosidase Inhibitors

Generic • Brand • Dose & Max	Contraindications	Primary Side Effects	Key Monitoring	Pertinent Drug Interactions	Med Pearl
Mechanism of action – inhibit pancreatic alpha-amylase and alpha-glucosidases, block carbohydrate hydrolysis to glucose; ↓ postprandial blood glucose					
Acarbose • Precose • 25–100 mg TID	• Cirrhosis • Inflammatory bowel disease • Intestinal obstruction	• Abdominal pain • Diarrhea • Flatulence	• Liver function tests (LFTs) every 3 mo × 1 yr • Postprandial plasma glucose • A1c every 3 mo	• Sulfonylureas and insulin ↑ risk of hypoglycemia	• Must treat hypoglycemia with simple carbohydrate such as glucose • Administer with food
Miglitol • Glyset • 25–100 mg TID			• Postprandial plasma glucose • A1c every 3 mo		

Thiazolidinediones

Generic • Brand • Dose & Max	Contraindications	Primary Side Effects	Key Monitoring	Pertinent Drug Interactions	Med Pearl
Mechanism of action – PPAR-gamma activator, which improves insulin sensitivity					
Rosiglitazone • Avandia • 2–8 mg daily	• Liver disease • Unstable heart failure • Previous myocardial infarction • Osteopenia or osteoporosis • History of bladder cancer	• Edema • Hepatotoxicity	• LFTs at baseline and periodically • FPG • A1c every 3 mo	• CYP2C8 substrates • CYP2C8 inhibitors may ↑ effects • CYP2C8 inducers may ↓ effects	Potential link to ↑ risk of cardiovascular events; controversial
Pioglitazone ☆ • Actos • 15–45 mg daily					Thought to have better lipid profile than rosiglitazone

Amylinomimetic

Generic • Brand • Dose & Max	Contraindications	Primary Side Effects	Key Monitoring	Pertinent Drug Interactions	Med Pearl
Mechanism of action – amylin cosecreted with insulin ↓ postprandial blood sugars, prolonging gastric emptying, ↓ postprandial glucagon secretion, and caloric intake through centrally mediated appetite suppression					
Pramlintide • Symlin • 15–120 mcg subcut daily	• Gastroparesis • Hypoglycemia unawareness	• Nausea • Severe hypoglycemia	• Blood sugars (before and after meals and HS) • A1c every 3 mo • S/S hypoglycemia	• May delay absorption of other drugs due to ↑ gastric emptying time (administer other medications 1 hr prior to pramlintide) • Sulfonylureas and insulin ↑ risk of hypoglycemia (↓ dose of mealtime insulin by 50% when starting pramlintide)	Adjunctive treatment *with* mealtime insulin

GLP-1 Receptor Agonists

Generic • Brand • Dose & Max	Contraindications	Primary Side Effects	Key Monitoring	Pertinent Drug Interactions	Med Pearl
Mechanism of action – analogs of GLP-1, which ↑ insulin secretion, ↑ B-cell growth/replication, slow gastric emptying, and ↓ food intake					
Exenatide ☆ • Byetta (IR) • 5–10 mcg subcut BID • Bydureon (ER) and Bydureon B-cise • 2 mg subcut once weekly	• CrCl <30 mL/min • Family history of medullary thyroid carcinoma (ER) • Multiple endocrine neoplasia syndrome type 2 (ER)	• Nausea • Hypoglycemia • ↓ appetite • Weight loss • Pancreatitis • Thyroid tumors	• FPG • A1c every 3 mo • S/S pancreatitis • S/S hypoglycemia • Thyroid tumors	• May delay absorption of other drugs due to ↑ gastric emptying time (administer other medications 1 hour prior) • Sulfonylureas and insulin ↑ risk of hypoglycemia	• IR: Administer within 60 min before main meals of day • ER: Reconstitute prior to injection, must be injected immediately after reconstitution; administer without regard to meals; administer missed dose within 3 days
Liraglutide • Victoza • 0.6–1.8 mg subcut **daily**	• Family history of medullary thyroid carcinoma • Multiple endocrine neoplasia syndrome type 2				• Administer without regard to meals • Saxenda used for chronic weight management
Semaglutide • Ozempic • 0.25–1 mg subcut once weekly					
Albiglutide • Tanzeum • 30–50 mg subcut once weekly					• Reconstitute prior to injection, must be injected within 8 hours of reconstitution • Administer without regard to meals • Administer missed dose within 3 days
Lixisenatide • Adlyxin • 10 mcg subcut daily × 14 days then 20 mcg subcut daily					Administer within 1 hr of 1st meal of day
Dulaglutide • Trulicity • 0.75–1.5 mg subcut once weekly		• Nausea • Hypoglycemia • ↓ appetite • Weight loss • Pancreatitis • Thyroid tumors • Tachycardia • PR interval prolongation • Atrioventricular block	• FPG • A1c every 3 mo • S/S pancreatitis • S/S hypoglycemia • Thyroid tumors • Heart rate • Electrocardiogram		• Administer without regard to meals • Administer missed dose within 3 days

DPP-4 Inhibitors

Generic • Brand • Dose & Max	Contraindications	Primary Side Effects	Key Monitoring	Pertinent Drug Interactions	Med Pearl
Mechanism of action – prolong the active incretin levels of GLP-1 and glucose-dependent insulinotropic polypeptide (GIP)					
Sitagliptin ☆ • Januvia • 25–100 mg daily	None	• Hypoglycemia • Arthralgias • Pancreatitis	• Blood urea nitrogen (BUN)/SCr • FPG • A1c every 3 mo • S/S pancreatitis • S/S hypoglycemia	• Sulfonylureas and insulin ↑ risk of hypoglycemia • May ↑ digoxin concentrations	• 100-mg dose is preferred unless patient has renal impairment • Adjust dose in renal impairment
Saxagliptin • Onglyza • 2.5–5 mg daily		• Hypoglycemia • Arthralgias • Pancreatitis • Heart failure	• BUN/SCr • FPG • A1c every 3 mo • S/S pancreatitis • S/S hypoglycemia • S/S heart failure	• CYP3A4 substrate • CYP3A4 inhibitors may ↑ effects; ↓ dose to 2.5 mg daily when used with strong CYP3A4 inhibitors • CYP3A4 inducers may ↓ effects • Sulfonylureas and insulin ↑ risk of hypoglycemia	Adjust dose in renal impairment
Linagliptin • Tradjenta • 5 mg daily		• Hypoglycemia • Arthralgias • Pancreatitis	• FPG • A1c every 3 mo • S/S pancreatitis • S/S hypoglycemia	• CYP3A4 and P-glycoprotein (P-gp) substrate • CYP3A4 or P-gp inhibitors may ↑ effects • CYP3A4 or P-gp inducers may ↓ effects • Sulfonylureas and insulin ↑ risk of hypoglycemia	No renal dose adjustment
Alogliptin • Nesina • 25 mg daily		• Hypoglycemia • Arthralgias • Pancreatitis • Heart failure	• BUN/SCr • FPG • A1c every 3 mo • S/S pancreatitis • S/S hypoglycemia • S/S heart failure • LFTs (at baseline)	• Sulfonylureas and insulin ↑ risk of hypoglycemia	Adjust dose in renal and hepatic impairment

SGLT2 Inhibitors

Generic • Brand • Dose & Max	Contraindications	Primary Side Effects	Key Monitoring	Pertinent Drug Interactions	Med Pearl
Mechanism of action – ↓ reabsorption of filtered glucose from tubular lumen, ↑ glucosuria					
Canagliflozin • Invokana • 100–300 mg daily	• Hypersensitivity • CrCl <30 mL/min	• Genitourinary infections (especially in females) • Dehydration • Hyperkalemia • Hypotension • DKA • Fractures • Acute kidney injury • Urosepsis/ pyelonephritis • Hypoglycemia • ↑ low-density lipoprotein cholesterol (LDL-C)	• BUN/SCr • FPG • A1c every 3 mo • S/S hypoglycemia • Blood pressure • Serum potassium (K+) • LDL-C • S/S heart failure • LFTs (at baseline) • S/S genital fungal infections or urinary tract infections	• Rifampin, phenytoin, phenobarbital, and ritonavir may ↓ effects • May ↑ digoxin concentrations • Diuretics may ↑ risk of volume depletion and hypotension • Sulfonylureas and insulin ↑ risk of hypoglycemia • Diuretics may ↑ risk of volume depletion and hypotension • Sulfonylureas and insulin ↑ risk of hypoglycemia	Administer before first meal of the day
Dapagliflozin • Farxiga • 5–10 mg daily					
Ertugliflozin • Steglatro • 5–15 mg daily					
Empagliflozin • Jardiance • 10–25 mg daily	• Hypersensitivity • CrCl <45 mL/min				• Administer in A.M. • Administer without regard to meals

Combination Products

See individual drug components for important points.		
Brand	**Components**	**Maximum Daily Dose**
Actoplus Met, Actoplus Met XR	Actoplus Met = Pioglitazone + Metformin Actoplus Met XR = Pioglitazone + Metformin ER	Actoplus Met: Pioglitazone 45 mg/metformin 2,550 mg Actoplus Met XR: Pioglitazone 45 mg/metformin ER 2,000 mg
Avandamet	Rosiglitazone + Metformin	Rosiglitazone 8 mg/metformin 2,000 mg
Avandaryl (only available generically)	Rosiglitazone + Glimepiride	Rosiglitazone 8 mg/glimepiride 4 mg
Duetact	Pioglitazone + Glimepiride	Pioglitazone 45 mg/glimepiride 8 mg
Glucovance	Glyburide + Metformin	Glyburide 20 mg/metformin 2,000 mg
Glyxambi	Empagliflozin + Linagliptin	Empagliflozin 25 mg/linagliptin 5 mg
Invokamet	Canagliflozin + Metformin	Cangliflozin 300 mg/metformin 2,000 mg
Janumet, Janumet XR	Janumet = Sitagliptin + Metformin Janumet XR = Sitagliptin + Metformin ER	Janumet: Sitagliptin 100 mg/metformin 2,000 mg Janumet XR: Sitagliptin 100 mg/metformin ER 2,000 mg

Combination Products *(cont'd)*

Brand	Components	Maximum Daily Dose
Jentadueto, Jentadueto XR	Jentadueto = Linagliptin + Metformin Jentadueto XR = Linagliptin + Metformin ER	Jentadueto: Linagliptin 5 mg/metformin 2,000 mg Jentadueto XR: Linagliptin 5 mg/metformin ER 2,000 mg
Kazano	Alogliptin + Metformin	Alogliptin 25 mg/metformin 2,000 mg
Kombiglyze XR	Saxagliptin + Metformin ER	Saxagliptin 5 mg/metformin ER 2,000 mg
Metaglip (only available generically)	Glipizide + Metformin	Glipizide 20 mg/metformin 2,000 mg
Oseni	Alogliptin + Pioglitazone	Alogliptin 25 mg/pioglitazone 45 mg
Qtern	Dapagliflozin + Saxagliptin	Dapagliflozin 10 mg/saxagliptin 5 mg
Prandimet	Repaglinide + Metformin	Repaglinide 10 mg/metformin 2,500 mg
Segluromet	Ertugliflozin + Metformin	Ertugliflozin 15 mg/metformin 2,000 mg
Soliqua	Insulin Glargine + Lixisenatide	Insulin glargine 60 units/lixisenatide 20 mcg
Steglujan	Ertugliflozin + Sitagliptin	Ertugliflozin 15 mg/sitagliptin 100 mg
Synjardy and Synjardy XR	Synjardy = Empagliflozin + Metformin Synjardy XR = Empagliflozin + Metformin ER	Synjardy: Empagliflozin 25 mg/metformin 2,000 mg Synjardy XR: Empagliflozin 25 mg/metformin ER 2,000 mg
Xigduo XR	Dapagliflozin + Metformin ER	Dapagliflozin 10 mg/metformin ER 2,000 mg
Xultophy	Insulin Degludec + Lixisenatide	Insulin degludec 50 units/lixisenatide 1.8 mg

HYPOTHYROIDISM

Guidelines Summary

The treatment and management of chronic thyroiditis and clinical hypothyroidism must be tailored to the individual patient. Levothyroxine is the treatment of choice, with three primary treatment goals: (1) resolution of signs and symptom, (2) achieving normal serum thyrotropin (TSH 0.4–4 mIU/L), and (3) avoiding overtreatment.

- TSH is the primary marker for medication monitoring. Because thyroid hormone functions on a negative feedback loop, elevated levels indicate hypothyroid state and low levels indicate hyperthyroid state.
- Typical initial dose of levothyroxine is 1.6 mcg/kg/day based upon actual body weight. Dose adjustments are made in 10–25 mcg/day increments based upon clinical response. Half-life of levothyroxine is approximately 1 week. TSH monitoring and dose adjustments occur at 4–8 week intervals.

Medications for Hypothyroidism

Generic • Brand • Dose	Contraindications	Primary Side Effects	Key Monitoring	Pertinent Drug Interactions	Med Pearl
Mechanism of action – T4 is converted to T3 and exerts many metabolic effects through control of DNA transcription and protein synthesis					
Levothyroxine ☆ (T4) • Synthroid, Levoxyl, Tirosint, Tirosint-Sol, Unithroid • 25–300 mcg daily • Caps, injection, solution, tabs Liothyronine (T3) • Cytomel, Triostat • 5–100 mcg daily • Injection, tabs	• Recent myocardial infarction or thyrotoxicosis • Uncorrected adrenal insufficiency	• Angina • Anxiety • Alopecia • ↑ LFTs • Tachycardia	• TSH • T3 • T4 • Free T4 • Heart rate • Blood pressure • Weight	Absorption may be ↓ by: cholestyramine, aluminum-containing medications, sucralfate, sodium polystyrene sulfonate, phenytoin, carbamazepine, rifampin	• T4: not the active compound; must be converted to T3 to become active • Thyroid treatment may also be used to augment depression treatment • Narrow therapeutic index drug • Often involved in medication errors
Desiccated thyroid ☆ T4 (80%) T3 (20%) • Armour, Thyroid • 15–120 mg daily • Tabs	• Hypersensitivity to beef or pork • Recent myocardial infarction or thyrotoxicosis • Uncorrected adrenal insufficiency				• Same as above • Origin: hog, cow, sheep • 80% T4 and 20% T3 is to mimic natural physiologic production
Liotrix • Thyrolar • Levothyroxine 12.5–100 mcg/liothyronine 3.1–25 mcg daily • Tabs	• Uncorrected adrenal cortical insufficiency • Untreated thyrotoxicosis				Liotrix is LT4/LT3 which is T4:T3 ratio; this ratio is 4:1

HYPERTHYROIDISM

Guidelines Summary

Symptomatic Management

Therapy targeting symptoms of hyperthyroidism (primarily tachycardia) is recommended in elderly patients, those with resting heart rate >90 beats per minute, and patients with preexisting cardiovascular disease. Oral β-blockers are the mainstay of therapy; see Cardiovascular Disorders chapter for details on this drug class.

Antithyroid Therapy

Three treatment modalities are available for Graves' disease: surgical intervention, antithyroid drugs, and radioactive iodine.

- In the United States, radioactive iodine is currently the treatment of choice for Graves' disease. Many clinical endocrinologists prefer an ablative dose of radioactive iodine, but some prefer use of a smaller dose in an attempt to render the patient euthyroid. Ablative therapy with radioactive iodine yields quicker resolution of the hyperthyroidism than does small-dose therapy, and thereby minimizes potential hyperthyroid-related morbidity.

- Although thyroidectomy for Graves' disease was frequently used in the past, it is now uncommonly performed in the United States unless coexistent thyroid cancer is suspected.

- Antithyroid medications, methimazole and propylthiouracil, have been used since the 1940s and are prescribed in an attempt to achieve a remission. The remission rates are variable, and relapses are frequent. Patients in whom remission is most likely to be achieved are those with mild hyperthyroidism and small goiters. Antithyroid drug treatment is not without the risk of adverse reactions, including minor rashes and, in rare instances, agranulocytosis and hepatitis.

Medications for Hyperthyroidism

Generic • Brand • Dose	Contraindications	Primary Side Effects	Key Monitoring	Pertinent Drug Interactions	Med Pearl
Mechanism of action – inhibits synthesis of thyroid hormones by blocking the oxidation of iodine in the thyroid gland					
Propylthiouracil • Only available generically • Initial: 300–600 mg/day in 3–4 divided doses • Maintenance: 50–300 mg/day in 2–3 divided doses	Hypersensitivity	• Benign transient leukopenia (white blood cell [WBC] count <4,000/mm³) • Pruritic maculo-papular rash • Arthralgias • Fever • Hepatotoxicity • Lupus-like syndrome	• WBC with differential • LFTs • TSH • T3 • T4	May ↑ effects of warfarin	• Clinical improvement approx. 4–8 weeks • Side effects with propylthiouracil more common with higher doses and in children • Rash may be treated with antihistamine • Severe side effects may require discontinuation of therapy • "PTU" is an error-prone abbreviation; avoid use • Tapering doses may start once clinical improvement seen • Correction of hyperthyroidism may alter disposition of β-blockers, digoxin, and theophylline • Propylthiouracil preferred in pregnancy
Methimazole • Tapazole • Initial: 15–60 mg/day in 3 divided doses • Maintenance: 5–30 mg/day	Hypersensitivity				

POLYCYSTIC OVARY SYNDROME

Guidelines Summary

Treatment is based on a symptoms approach for anovulation, amenorrhea, ovulation induction, and hirsutism.

Anovulation and Amenorrhea

- Hormonal contraceptives (oral, patch, or vaginal ring) are first-line therapy to regulate or restore irregular or absent menses. The agents also improve symptoms of hirsutism and acne.
- Weight-reduction through a combination of calorie restriction and exercise are important; they affect and improve insulin resistance.
- Progestin, including medroxyprogesterone acetate, is often used to induce menses.
- Insulin-sensitizing agents, including metformin, pioglitazone, and rosiglitazone, are used to ↓ insulin resistance primarily in patients with type 2 DM or in those with IFG.

Ovulation Induction

- Lifestyle modifications, especially weight loss, will assist with ovulation induction.
- Clomiphene citrate is used to induce ovulation for up to 6 months.
- Ovarian drilling with laser or diathermy can be considered but is not recommended.
- Insulin-sensitizing agents, such as metformin and thiazolidinediones, can induce ovulation.

Hirsutism

- Oral contraceptives can reduce hair growth.
- Antiandrogens, including spironolactone, flutamide, insulin-sensitizing agents, and eflornithine can be used to ↓ hair growth.
- Mechanical hair removal, such as shaving, plucking, waxing, depilatory creams, electrolysis, and laser vaporization, can also be used.

Medications for Polycystic Ovary Syndrome

Generic • Brand • Dose	Contraindications	Primary Side Effects	Key Monitoring	Pertinent Drug Interactions	Med Pearl
Mechanism of action – inhibits secretion of pituitary gonadotropins, which prevents follicular maturation and ovulation; causes endometrial thinning					
Medroxyprogesterone ☆ • Provera • Amenorrhea: 5–10 mg daily × 10 days	• History of deep venous thrombosis or pulmonary embolism • Pregnancy	• Headache • Weight changes • Edema • Menstrual irregularities	• Pregnancy should be ruled out • Symptoms of migraine	CPY3A4 substrate	Long-term use can lead to ↓ bone mineral density
Mechanism of action – Enclomiphene is less potent in inducing ovulation; however, it is rapidly absorbed and metabolized, allowing for the more potent zuclomiphene to act. Zuclomiphene inhibits normal estrogen negative feedback, which results in release of luteinizing hormone and follicle stimulating hormone; more potent than enclomiphene					
Clomiphene citrate (38% zuclomiphene; 62% enclomiphene) • Clomid • 50–100 mg daily × 5 days	• Liver disease • Abnormal uterine bleeding • Ovarian cysts • Uncontrolled thyroid or adrenal dysfunction • Pregnancy	• Ovarian enlargement • Hot flashes • Breast discomfort • Nausea • Bloating	• Pregnancy test • Menstrual cycle	May ↑ effects of ospemifene	Dosages ≥150 mg do not improve symptoms for PCOS
Mechanism of action – competes with aldosterone receptor sites in the distal tubules					
Spironolactone ☆ • Aldactone • 50–200 mg daily	• Acute renal failure • Hyperkalemia • Pregnancy	• Gynecomastia • Hyperkalemia • Nausea • Cramping	• Blood pressure • Renal function • K+	Use with angiotensin-converting enzyme inhibitors, angiotensin receptor blockers, K+ supplements, or nonsteroidal anti-inflammatory drugs may ↑ risk of hyperkalemia	Adjust dose in renal impairment
Mechanism of action – nonsteroidal antiandrogen that inhibits androgen uptake or inhibits binding to androgen in target tissue					
Flutamide • Only available generically • 125–250 mg BID-TID	• Severe hepatic impairment • Pregnancy	• Gynecomastia • Hot flashes • Breast tenderness • Galactorrhea • ↓ libido	LFTs monthly for 4 mo, then periodically	CYP1A2 substrate	Most cases of liver failure occur within first 3 months of therapy

Medications for Polycystic Ovary Syndrome *(cont'd)*

Generic • Brand • Dose	Contraindications	Primary Side Effects	Key Monitoring	Pertinent Drug Interactions	Med Pearl
Mechanism of action – inhibitor of 5-alpha reductase which results in the inhibition of conversion of testosterone to dihydrotestosterone					
Finasteride ☆ • Proscar, Propecia • 2.5–5 mg daily	• Pregnancy	• Impotence • Ejaculation disturbances • ↓ libido • Orthostatic hypotension	Absolute need for dual forms of birth control	None	Women should avoid contact with crushed or broken tablets and the semen from a male partner exposed to finasteride (teratogen)
Mechanism of action – inhibits ornithine decarboxylase, the rate-limiting enzyme in biosynthesis of putrescine, spermin, and spermidine (rapid dividing cell most susceptible)					
Eflornithine • Vaniqa • Apply BID	Hypersensitivity	• Acne • Pruritus • Alopecia • Stinging	None	None	• Used to ↓ unwanted facial hair • Do not wash affected area for 8 hr following application • Onset of action 4–8 wk

Neurological Disorders

5

This chapter covers the following disease states:

- **Multiple sclerosis**
- **Epilepsy**
- **Parkinson's disease**
- **Migraine headache**
- **Alzheimer's disease**

MULTIPLE SCLEROSIS

Guidelines Summary

The clinical management of MS should include disease-modifying therapy (DMT), alleviation of symptoms, and treatment of acute exacerbations.

Acute exacerbations: The cornerstone of therapy for acute exacerbations is IV corticosteroids. Methylprednisolone is most commonly used at 1,000 mg IV daily for 3–5 days. Oral prednisone may also be considered, but there is not strong evidence for using oral corticosteroids. Although corticosteroids have been shown to be very effective in the treatment of acute exacerbations, they do not alter the disease process.

Altering disease process: DMDs are the therapy of choice in altering the MS disease process. The currently approved DMDs include: interferon-β1a (Avonex and Rebif), interferon-β1b (Betaseron and Extavia), peginterferon β1a (Plegridy), glatiramer acetate (Copaxone), natalizumab (Tysabri), mitoxantrone (Novantrone), dimethyl fumarate (Tecfidera), teriflunomide (Aubagio), fingolimod (Gilenya), and alemtuzumab (Lemtrada).

- The interferon agents glatiramer acetate, teriflunomide, dimethyl fumarate, and fingolimod are considered first-line DMDs.
- Natalizumab, alemtuzumab, mitoxantrone, and ocrelizumab may be considered if a patient cannot tolerate or has a poor response to another MS medication.

- Mitoxantrone is approved to treat worsening relapsing-remitting MS and secondary progressive MS.

- Ocrelizumab is indicated for primary progressive or relapsing MS.

- Patients are generally treated with one DMT at a time, but worsening disease can be treated with combination DMT.

Symptom management: Dalfampridine (Ampyra) is used to improve walking in patients with MS.

Medications for Multiple Sclerosis

Generic • Brand • Dose & Max	Contraindications	Primary Side Effects	Key Monitoring Parameters	Pertinent Drug Interactions	Med Pearls
Disease-Modifying Drugs					
Mechanism of action – anti-inflammatory and immunomodulatory effects are exerted through binding of interferon to human cell-surface receptors and subsequent ↓ T-cell production of pro-inflammatory cytokines, ↓ production of pro-inflammatory lymphocytes, and ↑ production of anti-inflammatory lymphocytes					
Interferon-β1a • Avonex, Rebif • Avonex: 30 mcg IM weekly • Rebif: 4.4–8.8 mcg subcut 3 times weekly × 2 wk, then 11–22 mcg subcut 3 times weekly × 2 wk, then 22–44 mcg 3 times weekly Interferon-β1b • Betaseron, Extavia • 0.0625 mg subcut every other day; ↑ dose by 0.0625 mg every 2 wk to target dose of 0.25 mg subcut every other day Peginterferon-β1a • Plegridy • 63 mcg subcut on day 1, then 94 mcg subcut on day 15, then 125 mcg subcut every 2 wk starting on day 29	• Hypersensitivity to interferon-β or human albumin • Allergy to other interferons	• Flu-like symptoms (fever, chills, fatigue, muscle aches) • Injection site reactions • Anemia • Thrombocytopenia • Hepatotoxicity • Depression	• Liver function tests (LFTs) • Complete blood count (CBC)	None	• Acetaminophen or nonsteroidal anti-inflammatory drugs (NSAIDs) can ↓ flu-like symptoms • Neutralizing antibodies may develop, rendering the drug less efficacious

Medications for Multiple Sclerosis (cont'd)

Generic • Brand • Dose & Max	Contraindications	Primary Side Effects	Key Monitoring Parameters	Pertinent Drug Interactions	Med Pearls
Mechanism of action – influences immature CD4 cells to become less inflammatory, thereby suppressing demyelination and preventing nerve fiber damage					
Glatiramer acetate • Copaxone, Glatopa • 20 mg subcut daily or 40 mg subcut 3 times/week	Hypersensitivity to the drug or to mannitol	• Injection site reactions • Postinjection reactions (chest pain, palpitations)	Injection reactions	• Avoid use of live vaccines	Does not produce neutralizing antibodies
Mechanism of action – ↓ central inflammation by binding to sphingosine 1-phosphate receptors					
Fingolimod • Gilenya • 0.5 mg PO daily	• Myocardial infarction • Unstable angina • Transient ischemic attack/cerebrovascular accident • New York Heart Association class III/IV or decompensated heart failure (HF) • Atrioventricular (AV) block/sick sinus syndrome • QTc interval ≥500 msec • Concurrent use with class Ia or III antiarrhythmic	• Bradycardia • AV block • Hypertension • Infection • Macular edema • Dyspnea • ↑ LFTs • Diarrhea • Headache • Flu-like syndrome • HF • QT interval prolongation • Hypersensitivity reactions • Posterior reversible encephalopathy syndrome (PRES) • Progressive multifocal leukoencephalopathy (PML)	• Heart rate (HR) • Blood pressure (BP) • CBC • Electrocardiogram (ECG) • Ophthalmologic exam • LFTs • S/S of HF • S/S of PRES or PML • S/S of infection	• Class Ia and class III anti-arrhythmics may ↑ risk of bradycardia and AV block • Avoid use of live vaccines • Use with QT-interval prolonging agents may ↑ risk of torsades de pointes (TdP)	Give live attenuated zoster vaccination prior to administration, if needed
Mechanism of action – monoclonal antibody inhibits pro-inflammatory interactions within vascular endothelial cells and parenchymal brain cells					
Natalizumab • Tysabri • 300 mg IV infusion every 4 wk	• Hypersensitivity • Current or history of PML	• Infusion reactions (rash, drowsiness, fever, chills, hypotension, nausea, shortness of breath) • ↑ LFTs • Infection • Headache • Fatigue • Arthralgia • PML	• MRI (baseline, and repeated if PML suspected) • LFTs • Infusion reactions • S/S of infection • JC antibody test	Other DMDs ↑ risk of PML	• Reserved for patients who have not responded to other DMDs • Should be used as monotherapy only • Available only through a restrictive prescribing program (MS-TOUCH) • Also indicated for Crohn's disease

Medications for Multiple Sclerosis   *(cont'd)*

Generic • Brand • Dose & Max	Contraindications	Primary Side Effects	Key Monitoring Parameters	Pertinent Drug Interactions	Med Pearls
Mechanism of action – ↓ migration of T cells into the CNS by arresting the cell cycle and interfering with DNA repair and RNA synthesis					
Mitoxantrone • Only available generically • 12 mg/m² IV infusion every 3 mo; max cumulative dose = 140 mg/m²	Hypersensitivity	• HF • Nausea • Neutropenia • Alopecia • Menstrual irregularities • Infection	• Echocardio-gram (left ventricular ejection fraction [LVEF] at baseline and prior to each IV infusion) • CBC with differential • LFTs • S/S of infection	Avoid use of live vaccines	Discontinue therapy if LVEF <50% or clinically significant decline in LVEF
Mechanism of action – activates nuclear factor–like 2 pathway, ↓ inflammatory response to oxidative stress					
Dimethyl fumarate • Tecfidera • 120 mg PO BID × 7 days, then 240 mg PO BID	Hypersensitivity	• Dermatitis • Flushing • ↑ LFTs • Lymphopenia • Nausea/vomiting/diarrhea (N/V/D) • Hypersensitivity reaction • PML • Infection	• CBC with differential (baseline, 6 mo, then every 6–12 mo) • S/S of PML • S/S of infection • LFTs	May ↓ effectiveness and ↑ toxicity of live vaccines	May give with food or give aspirin 325 mg 30 min before to ↓ flushing
Mechanism of action – inhibits pyrimidine synthesis, ↓ proliferation and inflammation					
Teriflunomide • Aubagio • 7–14 mg PO daily	• Hypersensitivity • Severe hepatic impairment • Pregnancy • Women of reproductive potential without adequate contraception	• Hepatotoxicity • Rash • Hypersensitivity reaction • Hypertension • Infection • Interstitial lung disease • Peripheral neuropathy • Neutropenia • Headache • Alopecia • N/D	• CBC with differential • LFTs (monthly for first 6 months) • BP • Renal function • PPD (prior to initiation) • Pregnancy test (prior to initiation) • S/S of infection	• CYP2C8 inhibitor • CYP1A2 inducer • May ↓ effects of warfarin • Avoid use of live vaccines	• Counsel males and females on appropriate use of contraception during therapy (teratogenic) • Screen for tuberculosis (TB) prior to initiating therapy

Medications for Multiple Sclerosis *(cont'd)*

Generic • Brand • Dose & Max	Contraindications	Primary Side Effects	Key Monitoring Parameters	Pertinent Drug Interactions	Med Pearls
Mechanism of action – monoclonal antibody to CD52 receptors, which causes the depletion of lymphocytes to CD52 receptors, which causes the depletion of lymphocytes					
Alemtuzumab • Lemtrada • 12 mg IV daily × 5 days, then 12 mg daily × 3 days 12 months later	HIV infection	• Autoimmune conditions • Bone marrow suppression • Infection • Infusion reactions • Pulmonary fibrosis • PML • Thyroid disease • Malignancy (melanoma)	• CBC with differential • S/S of infection • Thyroid stimulating hormone • S/S of infusion reactions • S/S of PML • Malignancy • S/S of pulmonary fibrosis • Renal function • Urinalysis • Skin exam	Avoid use of live vaccines	• REMS program • Premedicate with corticosteroids for first 3 days of each treatment course • Initiate antiviral therapy (to prevent herpes infection) on 1st day of therapy and continue for 2 mo or until CD4+ cell count >200/m³
Symptom Management					
Mechanism of action – potassium channel blocker; ↑ action potential in demyelinated axon					
Dalfampridine • Ampyra • 10 mg PO every 12 hr	• History of seizures • Moderate–severe renal impairment (creatinine clearance ≤50 mL/min) • Hypersensitivity	• Seizures • Anaphylaxis • Urinary tract infection • Dizziness • Insomnia • Headache • Nausea • Balance disturbance	• Renal function • Walking ability	None	• Indicated to improve walking in patients with MS • Seizure risk is dose-dependent

EPILEPSY

Guidelines Summary

- Goals of treatment include a lack of seizure activity, minimal medication side effects of treatment, and improved quality of life.

- Treatment with antiepileptic drugs (AEDs) is warranted for patients that experience multiple seizures or have significantly affected quality of life. AED choice is based on the specific seizure type, the patient's age, comorbidities, ability to adhere to the regimen, and insurance coverage.

- AED monotherapy is preferred, but some patients may require combination therapy.

- First-line AEDs for focal seizures include carbamazepine, phenytoin, lamotrigine, valproic acid, levetiracetam, and oxcarbazepine.

- First-line AEDs for generalized absence seizures include valproic acid and ethosuximide.

- First-line AEDs for tonic-clonic seizures include phenytoin, carbamazepine, and valproic acid.

- Alternative AEDs include gabapentin, topiramate, zonisamide, tiagabine, primidone, felbamate, lamotrigine, phenobarbital, lacosamide, vigabatrin, and perampanel.

- The Food and Drug Administration (FDA) issued an alert regarding the relationship between the use of AEDs and suicidality (including suicidal behavior or ideation). Pooled analyses completed by the FDA indicated a significant ↑ of suicidality for patients treated with AEDs when compared to those given placebo. All AEDs appear to ↑ the risk similarly. Manufacturers of all AEDs are now required to include a boxed warning in their prescribing information and to include a medication guide for patients in their product labeling regarding the risk of suicide.

- Abrupt discontinuation of antiepileptic medications should be avoided as this may cause seizure occurrence or precipitate status epilepticus.

Antiepileptic Drugs

Generic • Brand • Dose/Dosage Forms	Contraindications	Primary Side Effects	Key Monitoring Parameters	Med Pearls
Mechanism of action – block voltage-sensitive sodium channels, resulting in stabilization of hyperexcitable neuronal membranes				
Carbamazepine • Carbatrol, Epitol, Equetro, Tegretol, Tegretol-XR • 400–1,600 mg/day in 2–4 divided doses	• Bone marrow suppression • Concomitant use with an MAOI or NNRTI	• Diplopia • Dizziness • Drowsiness/lethargy • Ataxia • N/V • Rash (Stevens-Johnson syndrome possible) • Hyponatremia • Metabolic bone disease • Aplastic anemia • Agranulocytosis	• Seizure occurrence • Serum drug concentrations (4–12 mcg/mL) • Na+ levels • CBC with differential • Suicidal ideation • Renal function • LFTs • Rash	↑ risk of Stevens-Johnson syndrome in patients with HLA-B*1502 allele
Oxcarbazepine • Oxtellar XR, Trileptal • IR: 300–1,200 mg/day BID • ER: 600–2,400 mg daily • XR tabs, suspension, tabs	Hypersensitivity	• Ataxia • Dizziness • Sedation • Nausea • Hyponatremia • Rash (Stevens-Johnson syndrome possible)	• Seizure occurrence • Suicidal ideation • Na+ levels • Rash	• 25–30% cross sensitivity in patients allergic to carbamazepine • ↑ risk of Stevens-Johnson syndrome in patients with HLA-B*1502 allele • Adjust dose in renal impairment
Phenytoin • Dilantin, Dilantin Infatabs, Phenytek • 100–600 mg/day; doses >400 mg dosed BID	Hypersensitivity	• Ataxia • Nystagmus • Fatigue/sedation • Behavior changes • Dizziness • Headache • Cognitive impairment • Gingival hyperplasia • Acne • Hirsutism • Folate deficiency • Metabolic bone disease • Rash (Stevens-Johnson syndrome possible) • Blood dyscrasias	• Serum drug concentrations (10–20 mcg/mL) • Seizure occurrence • Suicidal ideation • Rash	• 7–10 days to reach steady state • Serum drug concentrations must be corrected for hypoalbuminemia (serum albumin <4 g/dL): corrected phenytoin concentration = measured total concentration/ ([0.2 × albumin] + 0.1) • ↑ risk of Stevens-Johnson syndrome in patients with HLA-B*1502 allele
Lacosamide • Vimpat • 50–200 mg BID • IV, oral solution, tabs	Hypersensitivity	• Ataxia • N/V • Dizziness • Vertigo • Diplopia • PR interval prolongation • Headache • ↑ LFTs	• Seizure occurrence • Suicidal ideation • LFTs • ECG	• Schedule V controlled substance • Adjust dose in renal and hepatic impairment

Antiepileptic Drugs   *(cont'd)*

Generic • Brand • Dose/Dosage Forms	Contraindications	Primary Side Effects	Key Monitoring Parameters	Med Pearls
Eslicarbazepine • Aptiom • 400–1,600 mg daily • Tabs	Hypersensitivity to eslicarbazepine or oxcarbazepine	• Dizziness • Drowsiness • Somnolence • N/V • Headache • Diplopia • Fatigue • Vertigo • Blurred vision • Hyponatremia • Rash (Stevens-Johnson syndrome possible)	• Seizure occurrence • Suicidal ideation • Rash • LFTs • Na^+ levels	Adjust dose in renal impairment
Rufinamide • Banzel • 400–3,200 mg in 2 equally divided doses	• Hypersensitivity • Familial short QT syndrome	• N/V • Dizziness • Headache • Leukopenia • Somnolence • Shortened QT interval • Multiorgan sensitivity	• Seizure occurrence • Suicidal ideation • Rash • ECG	May cause status epilepticus
Mechanism of action – inhibits voltage-gated sodium channels and inhibits the release of glutamate				
Lamotrigine • Lamictal, Lamictal XR, Lamictal ODT • IR: 25–700 mg/day in 1–2 divided doses • 25–600 mg daily • Tabs, ODTs, XR tabs, chewable tabs	Hypersensitivity	• Rash (Stevens-Johnson syndrome possible) • Blood dyscrasias • Diplopia • Dizziness • Headache • Unsteadiness • Nausea	• Seizure occurrence • Suicidal ideation • LFTs • Renal function • Rash	• ↑ risk of rash when combined with valproate or initiated at high doses • Slow dosage titration used to reduce risk of rash • Adjust dose in hepatic impairment
Mechanism of action – inhibits calcium channels and facilitates GABA transmission				
Levetiracetam • Keppra, Keppra XR, Roweepra, Roweepra XR, Spritam • IR: 500–1,500 mg BID • XR: 1,000–3,000 mg daily • IV, oral solution, tabs, ODTs, XR tabs	Hypersensitivity	• Dizziness • Sedation • Behavioral disturbances • Fatigue • Rash (Stevens-Johnson syndrome possible) • Psychosis • ↑ BP in children	• Seizure occurrence • Suicidal ideation • CNS depression • BP in children • CBC • Renal function	• Adjust dose in renal impairment • Less CYP450 mediated drug interactions compared to other AEDs

Antiepileptic Drugs   *(cont'd)*

Generic • Brand • Dose/Dosage Forms	Contraindications	Primary Side Effects	Key Monitoring Parameters	Med Pearls
Mechanism of action – not well understood but may be attributed to selective affinity for synaptic vesicle protein 2A (SV2A)				
Brivaracetam • Briviact • 50–100 mg BID • IV, oral solution, tabs	Hypersensitivity	• Somnolence • Fatigue • Dizziness • Gait disturbance • Behavioral disturbances • Ataxia • Psychotic symptoms • N/V	• Seizure occurrence • Suicidal ideation • CBC with differential • LFTs • Renal function	• Schedule V controlled substance • Adjust dose in hepatic impairment
Mechanism of action – increases gamma-aminobutyric acid (GABA) in the brain				
Valproic acid (divalproex sodium) • Depakote, Depakote ER, Depakote Sprinkles, Depacon, Depakene • 10–60 mg/kg/day • Caps, DR caps/tabs, IV, oral solution, ER tabs	• Hypersensitivity • Hepatic impairment • Urea cycle disorders • Known porphyria • Known mitochondrial disorders • Use in pregnant women for migraine prevention	• Hepatotoxicity • Thrombocytopenia • Hyperammonemia • Weight gain • Pancreatitis • Headache • Somnolence • Dizziness • Alopecia • GI upset • Polycystic ovary-like syndrome	• Seizure occurrence • Suicidal ideation • Serum drug concentration (50–100 mcg/mL) • LFTs • CBC with platelets • Serum ammonia levels	• Highly teratogenic • Also indicated for the treatment of mania and migraine prophylaxis • ER product has 85% bioavailability of valproic acid
Mechanism of action – increase levels of GABA, bind to the α2δ subunit of calcium channels				
Gabapentin • Neurontin, Gralise, Fanatrex, Neuraptine • 300–3,600 mg daily in 2–3 divided doses • Caps, cream, oral solution, oral suspension, tabs	Hypersensitivity	• Dizziness • Fatigue • Somnolence • Ataxia • Weight gain • Behavioral disturbances • Edema • Nystagmus	• Seizure occurrence • Suicidal ideation • Renal function	• Adjust dose in renal impairment • Less CYP450 mediated drug interactions compared to other AEDs • Also used for neuropathic pain
Pregabalin • Lyrica, Lyrica CR • IR: 75–300 mg BID • CR: 165–330 mg daily • Caps, ER tab, oral solution	Hypersensitivity	• Dizziness • Dry mouth • Somnolence • Peripheral edema • Weight gain • Blurred vision • Ataxia	• Seizure occurrence • Suicidal ideation • Edema • Weight	• Schedule V controlled substance • Adjust dose in renal failure • Also indicated for fibromyalgia, neuropathic pain, post-herpetic neuralgia

Antiepileptic Drugs   *(cont'd)*

Generic • Brand • Dose/Dosage Forms	Contraindications	Primary Side Effects	Key Monitoring Parameters	Med Pearls
Mechanism of action – inhibits calcium channels				
Ethosuximide • Zarontin • 250–750 mg BID • Caps, oral solution	Hypersensitivity	• Ataxia • Drowsiness • N/V/D • Rash (Stevens-Johnson syndrome possible)	• Seizure occurrence • Suicidal ideation • CBC • Serum drug concentration (40–100 mcg/mL) • Platelets • LFTs • Rash	Used only for absence seizures
Mechanism of action – blocks voltage-dependent sodium channels, augments GABA activity, antagonizes glutamate receptors				
Topiramate • Topamax, Topamax, Trokendi XR, Qudexy XR • IR: 20–200 mg BID • ER: 50–400 mg daily • ER caps, sprinkle caps, tabs	• Hypersensitivity • Trokendi XR: use of alcohol within 6 hr prior or after • Qudexy XR: metabolic acidosis in patients taking metformin	• Difficulty concentrating • Confusion • Memory impairment • Speech problems • Dizziness • Headache • Depression • Somnolence • Kidney stones • Anorexia • Weight loss • Oligohydrosis • Metabolic acidosis • Acute-angle glaucoma • Paresthesia • Hyperammonemia • Hyperthermia	• Seizure occurrence • Suicidal ideation • Serum ammonia levels • Intraocular pressure	• Adjust dose in renal impairment • Slow titration necessary to minimize side effects • Also indicated for migraine prophylaxis • May be used for weight loss
Mechanism of action – prolong the opening of the GABA receptor chloride complex, resulting in potentiation of GABA on GABA$_A$ receptors; inhibit glutamate release				
Phenobarbital • Only available as generic • 60–200 mg/day in 2–3 divided doses • Elixir, oral solution, injection, tabs	• Hypersensitivity • Severe liver impairment • Porphyria • Dyspnea or airway obstruction	• Sedation • Nystagmus • Ataxia • Agitation • Hyperactivity • Headache • Nausea • Sedation • Agranulocytosis • Behavioral changes • Intellectual blunting • Respiratory depression (IV) • Rash (Stevens-Johnson syndrome possible)	• Seizure occurrence • Suicidal ideation • Serum concentrations (10–40 mg/L) • CBC with differential • LFTs	• Schedule IV controlled substance • Titrate dose slowly to minimize side effects • Takes 3–4 wk to reach steady state • Frequency of side effects limits it use
Primidone • Mysoline • 100–1,500 mg in 2–3 divided doses • Tabs			• Seizure occurrence • Suicidal ideation • Serum concentrations (5–12 mcg/mL) • CBC with differential • LFTs	Metabolized to phenobarbital

Antiepileptic Drugs *(cont'd)*

Generic • Brand • Dose/Dosage Forms	Contraindications	Primary Side Effects	Key Monitoring Parameters	Med Pearls
Mechanism of action – inhibits NMDA receptors				
Felbamate • Felbatol • 1,200–3,600 mg/day in 3–4 divided doses • Tabs, oral suspension	• Hypersensitivity • Blood dyscrasias • Hepatic impairment	• Aplastic anemia • Acute liver failure • Anorexia • Weight loss • N/V • Insomnia • Headache	• Seizure occurrence • Suicidal ideation • CBC • LFTs	• Requires signed patient consent for use • Reserved for refractory cases • Discontinue use if AST or ALT >2 × ULN
Mechanism of action – inhibits GABA transporter type 1 (GAT1) and decreases clearance of GABA from synaptic cleft				
Tiagabine • Gabatril • 4–56 mg/day	Hypersensitivity	• Dizziness • Fatigue • Difficulty concentrating • Blurred vision • Nervousness • Tremor • Depression • Weakness	• Seizure occurrence • Suicidal ideation • LFTs	Take with food
Mechanism of action – inhibits GABA transaminase (GABA-T), resulting in increased levels of GABA				
Vigabatrin • Sabril • 500–1,500 mg BID • Packet for oral solution, tabs	Hypersensitivity	• Permanent vision loss • Fatigue • Anemia • Somnolence • Weight gain • Tremor • Peripheral neuropathy • Confusion	• Seizure occurrence • Suicidal ideation • CBC • Ophthalmologic exam	• Adjust dose in renal impairment • Black box warning due to vision loss • Available only through REMS program
Mechanism of action – inhibits voltage-dependent sodium and calcium channels				
Zonisamide • Zonegran • 100–600 mg/day	Hypersensitivity to zonisamide or sulfonamides	• Sedation • Dizziness • Rash (Stevens-Johnson syndrome possible) • Kidney stones • Weight loss • Metabolic acidosis • Oligohydrosis • Hyperthermia • Cognitive impairment • Nausea	• Seizure occurrence • Suicidal ideation • Rash • Renal function • Serum bicarbonate	• Adjust dose in renal impairment • Takes up to 2 wk to achieve steady state

Antiepileptic Drugs *(cont'd)*

Generic • Brand • Dose/Dosage Forms	Contraindications	Primary Side Effects	Key Monitoring Parameters	Med Pearls
Mechanism of action – noncompetitive AMPA-type glutamate receptor antagonist				
Perampanel	Hypersensitivity	• Ataxia • Falls • Behavioral changes • Somnolence • Dizziness • Gait disturbance • Depression • Weight gain • Rash (Stevens-Johnson syndrome possible)	• Seizure occurrence • Suicidal ideation • Weight • Rash	• Schedule III controlled substance • Adjust dose in renal impairment
Mechanism of action – binds to benzodiazepine receptor on the $GABA_A$ receptor				
Clobazam • Onfi • Tabs, oral suspension	• Hypersensitivity • Myasthenia gravis • Narrow-angle glaucoma • Severe hepatic or respiratory disease • Sleep apnea • Use in 1st trimester of pregnancy • Breastfeeding	• Sedation • Somnolence • Ataxia • Fever • Aggressive behavior	• Seizure occurrence • Suicidal ideation • Respiratory status	• Schedule IV controlled substance • Adjust dose in hepatic impairment

Selected AED Drug Interactions

AED	Interacting Medication	Effect
Carbamazepine • 3A4 substrate • Strong CYP1A2, CYP2C19, CYP2C8, CYP2C9, and CYP3A4 inducer	Abiraterone	↓ Abiraterone
	Apixaban	↓ Apixaban
	Bortezomib	↓ Bortezomib
	Cimetidine	↑ Carbamazepine
	Clozapine	↓ Clozapine
	Dabigatran	↓ Dabigatran
	Dolutegravir	↓ Dolutegravir
	Doxycycline	↓ Doxycycline
	Dronedarone	↓ Dronedarone
	Erythromycin	↑ Carbamazepine
	Everolimus	↓ Everolimus
	Fluoxetine	↑ Carbamazepine
	Ibrutinib	↓ Ibrutinib
	Isoniazid	↑ Carbamazepine
	Itraconazole	↓ Itraconazole
	Oral contraceptives	↓ Contraceptives
	Perampanel	↓ Perampanel
	Phenobarbital	↓ Carbamazepine, ↓ phenobarbital
	Phenytoin	↓ Carbamazepine, ↓ phenytoin
	Rivaroxaban	↓ Rivaroxaban
	Theophylline	↓ Theophylline
	Warfarin	↓ Warfarin
Valproic acid	Carbamazepine	↓ Valproic acid, ↑ carbamazepine
	Lamotrigine	↑ Lamotrigine
	Phenobarbital	↓ Valproic acid, ↑ phenobarbital
	Phenytoin	↓ Valproic acid, ↓ phenytoin
	Primidone	↓ Valproic acid, ↑ phenobarbital
Phenytoin • CYP2C19 and CYP2C9 substrate • Strong CYP2C19, CYP2C8, CYP2C9, and CYP3A4 inducer	Abiraterone	↓ Abiraterone
	Antacids	↓ Phenytoin
	Apixaban	↓ Apixaban
	Carbamazepine	↓ Phenytoin
	Cimetidine	↑ Phenytoin
	Clozapine	↓ Clozapine
	Dabigatran	↓ Dabigatran
	Dolutegravir	↓ Dolutegravir
	Dronederone	↓ Dronederone
	Fluconazole	↑ Phenytoin
	Isoniazid	↑ Phenytoin
	Oral contraceptives	↓ Contraceptives
	Perampanel	↓ Perampanel
	Phenobarbital	↑ or ↓ Phenytoin
	Rivaroxaban	↓ Rivaroxaban
	Ticagrelor	↓ Ticagrelor
	Warfarin	↑ Phenytoin, ↑ anticoagulant effect

Selected AED Drug Interactions (cont'd)

AED	Interacting Medication	Effect
Ethosuximide • CYP3A4 substrate	Phenytoin Valproic acid	↑ Phenytoin ↑ or ↓ Ethosuximide
Oxcarbazepine • CYP3A4 inducer	Cobicistat Dolutegravir Elvitegravir Ledipasvir Oral contraceptives Perampanel Phenobarbital Phenytoin Sofosbuvir	↓ Cobicistat ↓ Dolutegravir ↓ Elvitegravir ↓ Ledipasvir ↓ Contraceptives ↓ Perampanel, ↑ oxcarbazepine ↓ Oxcarbazepine ↓ Oxcarbazepine ↓ Sofosbuvir
Felbamate • CYP3A4 substrate	Carbamazepine Phenobarbital Phenytoin Valproic acid	↓ Carbamazepine, ↓ felbamate ↑ Phenobarbital, ↓ felbamate ↑ Phenytoin, ↓ felbamate ↑ Valproic acid
Perampanel • CYP3A4 substrate	Buprenorphine Carbamazepine Oxcarbazepine Phenytoin Progestins	↑ CNS depressant effect ↓ Perampanel ↓ Perampanel ↓ Perampanel ↓ Progestins
Lacosamide • CYP2C19, CYP2C9, and CYP3A4 substrate	Carbamazepine Phenobarbital Phenytoin	↓ Lacosamide ↓ Lacosamide ↓ Lacosamide
Lamotrigine	Carbamazepine Phenobarbital Phenytoin Primidone Valproic acid	↓ Lamotrigine ↓ Lamotrigine ↓ Lamotrigine ↓ Lamotrigine ↑ Lamotrigine
Topiramate	Carbamazepine Oral contraceptives Phenytoin Simeprevir Valproic acid	↓ Topiramate ↓ Contraceptives ↓ Topiramate ↓ Simeprevir ↓ Valproic acid
Phenobarbital • CYP2C19 substrate • Strong CYP1A2, CYP2C8, CYP2C9, and CYP3A4 inducer	Apixaban Dronederone Felbamate Oral contraceptives Phenytoin Rivaroxaban Simeprevir Valproic acid	↓ Apixaban ↓ Dronederone ↑ Phenobarbital ↓ Contraceptives ↑ Phenobarbital ↓ Rivaroxaban ↓ Simeprevir ↑ Phenobarbital

Selected AED Drug Interactions *(cont'd)*

AED	Interacting Medication	Effect
Primidone • Strong CYP1A2, CYP2C8, CYP2C9, and CYP3A4 inducer	Carbamazepine Corticosteroids Phenytoin Valproic acid	↓ Primidone, ↑ phenobarbital ↓ Corticosteroids ↓ Primidone, ↑ phenobarbital ↑ Primidone, ↓ phenobarbital
Tiagabine • CYP3A4 substrate	Carbamazepine Phenytoin	↓ Tiagabine ↓ Tiagabine
Vigabatrin	Clonazepam Phenytoin	↑ Clonazepam ↓ Phenytoin
Zonisamide • CYP3A4 substrate	Carbamazepine Phenobarbital Phenytoin	↓ Zonisamide ↓ Zonisamide ↓ Zonisamide
Brivaracetam • CYP2C19 substrate	Phenytoin	↓ Brivaracetam

PARKINSON'S DISEASE

Summary of Treatment Recommendations

- Initial therapy generally consists of either a dopamine agonist or carbidopa/levodopa.
  - Patients ≥65 years of age or those with significant disability due to their PD should receive carbidopa/levodopa as initial therapy.
  - Patients <65 years of age may receive a dopamine agonist as initial therapy.
  - Inadequate response to maximum tolerable doses of initial therapy with a dopamine agonist or carbidopa/levodopa should result in the addition of the alternate medication.
  - Subsequently, COMT inhibitors may be added to ongoing carbidopa/levodopa therapy, and adjunctive therapies such as amantadine or anticholinergics may also be utilized.
  - Anticholinergic agents are primarily useful for the treatment of tremor-predominant PD but should be used with caution in elderly patients and avoided in patients with pre-existing cognitive impairment.
  - Because dopamine agonists and carbidopa/levodopa are aimed at increasing the available dopamine in the CNS, side effects such as hallucinations and delusions are possible. If psychiatric side effects occur, lowering the dose or slowing the titration of dopamine therapy may help. However, if lowering the dose is not helpful, PD-related psychiatric comorbidities may be treated with the antipsychotic medication quetiapine.

Medications for Parkinson's Disease

Generic • Brand • Dose/Dosage Forms	Contraindications	Primary Side Effects	Key Monitoring Parameters	Pertinent Drug Interactions	Med Pearls
Mechanism of action – unknown, thought to enhance dopamine release and inhibit dopamine reuptake, also acts as an NMDA receptor antagonist					
Amantadine • Gocovri • IR: 100–400 mg/day • ER: 129–322 mg/day • Caps, ER cap, oral syrup, tabs	• Hypersensitivity • End-stage renal disease	• Confusion • Nightmares • Hallucinations • Insomnia • Nervousness • Irritability	• Renal function • Response to therapy • Mental status • BP	Alcohol use with ER product	Adjust dose in renal impairment
Mechanism of action – monoamine-oxidase (MAO) B inhibitors: inhibit the catabolism of dopamine by selectively inhibiting the monoamine oxidase B enzyme					
Selegiline • Eldepryl, Zelapar • Cap/tab: 5 mg BID • ODT: 1.25–2.5 mg daily • Caps, ODTs, tabs	• Hypersensitivity • Concurrent use with meperidine, methadone, dextromethorphan, tramadol, or MAOIs	• Nausea • Hallucinations • Insomnia • Depression • Orthostasis • Impulse control disorders • Hypertensive crisis (if high-tyramine foods are ingested)	• BP • Response to therapy • Presence of anxiety or agitation • Suicidal ideation • S/S of serotonin syndrome	Use with meperidine, other opioid analgesics, dextromethorphan, tramadol, selective serotonin reuptake inhibitors (SSRIs), serotonin-norepinephrine reuptake inhibitors (SNRIs), tricyclic antidepressants (TCAs), cyclobenzaprine, triptans, or St. John's wort may ↑ risk of serotonin syndrome	• Avoid tyramine-containing foods • Should not be abruptly discontinued • Discontinue 14 days prior to surgery if possible; should not be taken with general anesthesia • Transdermal patch (Emsam) used for depression
Rasagiline • Azilect • 0.5–1 mg daily • Tabs	• Hypersensitivity • Concurrent use with meperidine, methadone, tramadol, MAOIs, cyclobenzaprine, dextromethorphan, or St. John's wort	• Hypertension • Nausea • Orthostasis • Somnolence • Hallucinations • Impulse control disorders • Hypertensive crisis (if high-tyramine foods are ingested)	• Response to therapy • BP • S/S of serotonin syndrome	• CYP1A2 substrate • CYP1A2 inhibitors may ↑ effects • CYP1A2 inducers may ↓ effects • Use with meperidine, other opioid analgesics, dextromethorphan, tramadol, SSRIs, SNRIs, TCAs, cyclobenzaprine, triptans, or St. John's wort may ↑ risk of serotonin syndrome	• Avoid tyramine-containing foods > 150 mg • Should not be abruptly discontinued • Adjust dose in hepatic impairment
Xadago • Safinamide • 50–100 mg daily • Tabs	• Hypersensitivity • Concurrent use with meperidine, methadone, tramadol, MAOIs, cyclobenzaprine, dextromethorphan, or St. John's wort	• Dyskinesia • Hypertension • Orthostatic hypotension • Falls • Nausea • ↑ LFTs	• Response to therapy • BP • S/S of serotonin syndrome	Use with meperidine, other opioid analgesics, dextromethorphan, tramadol, SSRIs, SNRIs, TCAs, cyclobenzaprine, triptans, or St. John's wort may ↑ risk of serotonin syndrome	Avoid tyramine-containing foods >150 mg

Medications for Parkinson's Disease *(cont'd)*

Generic • Brand • Dose/Dosage Forms	Contraindications	Primary Side Effects	Key Monitoring Parameters	Pertinent Drug Interactions	Med Pearls
Mechanism of action – levodopa is a direct precursor to dopamine and is converted to dopamine once it crosses the blood-brain barrier; carbidopa is a dopa decarboxylase inhibitor; it is necessary to combine carbidopa with levodopa in order to prevent the peripheral degradation of levodopa prior to entry into the blood-brain barrier					
Carbidopa/levodopa ☆ • Duopa, Rytary, Sinemet, Sinemet CR • Carbidopa 75–300 mg/day in 3–4 divided doses (75 mg required, side effects if >300 mg/day) • Levodopa 100–2,000 mg/day in 3–4 divided doses • Enteral suspension, CR caps, ER tabs, ODTs, tabs	• Hypersensitivity • Narrow-angle glaucoma • Concurrent use with MAOIs	• N/V • Orthostasis • Confusion • Hallucinations • Wearing-off fluctuations • Dyskinesias • Somnolence • Impulse control disorders	• Response to therapy • Presence of side effects • BP	• Nonselective MAOIs may cause hypertensive crisis • Pyridoxine (vitamin B6) ↓ effectiveness of levodopa	• IR tabs and CR caps/tabs often used simultaneously • CR is less bioavailable (~30% less) than IR • Duopa is indicated for PEG-J tube administration
Mechanism of action – dopamine agonists: directly stimulate striatal dopamine receptors					
Bromocriptine (ergot derivative) • Parlodel • 1.25–50 mg BID • Caps, tabs	• Uncontrolled hypertension • Sensitivity to ergot alkaloids • Pregnancy • Postpartum with history of coronary artery disease	• Valvular fibrosis • Nausea • Hallucinations • Dizziness • Drowsiness • Orthostasis • Impulse control disorders	• Response to therapy • Presence of side effects • BP • Impulse control	• ↓ levodopa dose by 20–30% when initiating • Metoclopramide and antipsychotics ↓ effects	Cardiac side effects ↓ clinical use; nonergot derivatives used much more commonly
Pramipexole ☆ (nonergot derivative) • Mirapex, Mirapex ER • IR: 0.125–1.5 mg TID • ER: 0.375–4.5 mg daily • ER tabs, tabs	None	• N/V • Constipation • Orthostasis • Hallucinations • Somnolence • Syncope • Impulse control disorders	• Response to therapy • Presence of side effects • BP • Impulse control	• ↓ levodopa dose by 20–30% when initiating • Metoclopramide and antipsychotics ↓ effects	• Adjust dose in renal impairment • Titrate dose slowly and taper upon discontinuation • Also indicated for restless leg syndrome
Ropinirole ☆ (nonergot derivative) • Requip, Requip XL • IR: 0.25–8 mg TID • ER: 2–24 mg daily • ER tabs, tabs	Hypersensitivity				• Titrate dose slowly and taper upon discontinuation • Also indicated for restless leg syndrome

Medications for Parkinson's Disease   *(cont'd)*

Generic • Brand • Dose/Dosage Forms	Contraindications	Primary Side Effects	Key Monitoring Parameters	Pertinent Drug Interactions	Med Pearls
Rotigotine • Neupro • 2–8 mg daily • Transdermal patch	Hypersensitivity	• Application site reactions • N/V • Orthostasis • Hallucinations • Somnolence • Syncope • Impulse control disorders • Hypertension • Tachycardia • Edema	• Response to therapy • Presence of side effects • BP • HR	Metoclopramide and antipsychotics ↓ effects	• Apply daily • Titrate dose slowly and taper upon discontinuation • Also indicated for restless leg syndrome
Mechanism of action – COMT inhibitors: inhibit the degradation of dopamine through inhibition of the catechol-O-methyltransferase enzyme					
Tolcapone • Tasmar • 100–200 mg TID • Tabs	• Hypersensitivity • Hepatic impairment • History of nontraumatic rhabdomyolysis or hyperpyrexia and confusion due to medication	• Hepatic failure • Dyskinesias • N/V/D • Orthostasis • Hallucinations • Somnolence • Syncope • Impulse control disorders • Rhabdomyolysis	• Frequent LFTs • Response to therapy • Presence of side effects • BP	• May ↑ effects of MAOIs (avoid concurrent use of nonselective MAOIs) • ↑ activity of drugs known to be metabolized by COMT (dopamine, dobutamine, isoproterenol, methyldopa)	• Reserved for third-line therapy in patients that do not respond adequately to carbidopa/levodopa and dopamine agonists • Administer with carbidopa/ levodopa
Entacapone • Comtan • 200–1,600 mg daily (divided up to 8 × daily; administered with each dose of carbidopa/ levodopa) • Tabs	Hypersensitivity	• Dyskinesias • N/V/D • Hallucinations • Urine discoloration (brown-orange) • Orthostasis • Hallucinations • Somnolence • Syncope • Impulse control disorder	• Response to therapy • Presence of side effects • BP	• May ↑ effects of MAOIs (avoid concurrent use of nonselective MAOIs) • ↑ activity of drugs known to be metabolized by COMT (dopamine, dobutamine, isoproterenol, methyldopa)	• Reserved for third-line therapy in patients that do not respond adequately to carbidopa/levodopa and dopamine agonists • Preferred over tolcapone, as no fatal liver injury has been reported with this agent • Administer with carbidopa/ levodopa
Combination product: Levodopa/carbidopa/entacapone (Stalevo)					

Medications for Parkinson's Disease *(cont'd)*

Generic • Brand • Dose/Dosage Forms	Contraindications	Primary Side Effects	Key Monitoring Parameters	Pertinent Drug Interactions	Med Pearls
Mechanism of action – anticholinergics: through diminished activity of acetylcholine, help to ↓ the relative ↑ in activity compared to dopamine, thereby ↓ tremor					
Benztropine ☆ • Cogentin • 0.5–6 mg/day in 2–4 divided doses • Injection, tabs	Hypersensitivity	• Dry mouth • Blurred vision • Constipation • Urinary retention • Confusion • Memory impairment • Hallucinations	• Response to therapy • Presence of side effects	Additive anticholinergic side effects when co-administered with other anticholinergic medications	• Use with caution in elderly patients who are at risk for mental status changes with anticholinergic medications • Primarily used for tremor and/or drooling
Trihexyphenidyl • Only available as generic • 1–15 mg/day in 3–4 divided doses • Solution, tabs	None				
Mechanism of action – second-generation atypical antipsychotic; inverse agonist and antagonist activity at 5-HT2A and 5-HT2C receptors					
Pimavanserin • Nuplazid • 17–34 mg daily • Tabs	None	• Edema • Confusion • Hallucination • Gait disturbance • QT interval prolongation	• ECG • Response to therapy	• CYP3A4 substrate • CYP3A4 inhibitors may ↑ toxicity/effect (↓ pimavanserin dose to 17 mg/day) • CYP3A4 inducers may ↓ effect • Use with QT-interval prolonging agents may ↑ risk of TdP	Indicated to treat hallucinations and delusions associated with PD psychosis

MIGRAINE HEADACHE

Summary of Treatment Recommendations

- Migraine treatment is divided into abortive treatment, rescue treatment, and prophylactic treatment. Most patients will respond to abortive treatment and can be controlled without the addition of rescue or prophylactic therapy.

- Abortive treatment options include analgesics (over-the-counter [OTC] and prescription), NSAIDs (detailed in bone and joint chapter), ergotamine and dihydroergotamine, serotonin agonists, and butorphanol. Over-the-counter analgesics, prescription non-opioid analgesics, and NSAIDs are reserved for patients with mild symptoms.

- The serotonin agonists are the mainstay of abortive therapy options for patients with moderate to severe symptoms. Various dosage forms are available and there is only slight variability between the efficacy and safety of available agents. Patients may respond to one agent in this class and not to another; therefore, trial and error is often the approach taken.

- For patients who have >2 headaches/week or >8 headaches/month, or who do not have an adequate response to abortive therapy, prophylactic therapy may be warranted.

- Available prophylactic agents include antihypertensive medications such as propranolol, atenolol, and metoprolol (detailed in cardiovascular chapter); antidepressant medications such as amitriptyline, paroxetine, fluoxetine, and sertraline (detailed in psychiatric disorders chapter); and anticonvulsant medications such valproic acid, gabapentin, tiagabine, and topiramate (detailed earlier in this chapter). In general, migraine prophylactic doses are low compared to normal doses of these medications.

Medications for Migraine

Generic • Brand • Dose/Dosage Forms	Contraindications	Primary Side Effects	Key Monitoring Parameters	Pertinent Drug Interactions	Med Pearls
Analgesics					
Acetaminophen, aspirin, caffeine • Excedrin Migraine, Anacin • 2 tabs at onset, then every 6 hr PRN • Tabs	• Hypersensitivity to any component • Pregnancy	Minimal	• Response to therapy • Presence of side effects	Other acetaminophen-containing meds (do not exceed 4 g/day)	Available OTC
Aspirin or acetaminophen with butalbital and caffeine☆ • Fiorinal, Fioricet • 1–2 tabs every 4–6 hrs PRN (max = 6 doses/day)	• Hypersensitivity to any component • Pregnancy	• Tachycardia • Dizziness • Drowsiness • Insomnia • Orthostatic hypotension	• Response to therapy • Presence of side effects	Alcohol ↑ CNS depression with butalbital	• Limit to 4 tabs/day and use max of 2 days/wk • Dependence may develop with continued use
Isometheptene/dichloral-phenazone/APAP • Nodolor • 2 caps at onset, then 1 cap every hr PRN (max = 5 capsules/24 hr)	• Glaucoma • Severe renal disease • Hypertension • Cardiovascular disease • Cerebrovascular accident • MAOI use	• Dizziness • Skin rash	• Response to therapy • Presence of side effects	Use with MAOIs may ↑ risk for hyper-tensive crisis	Max 6 caps/day; 20 caps/mo
Mechanism of action – exert serotonergic agonist activity, resulting in vasoconstriction					
Ergotamine tartrate • Ergomar • 2 mg at onset, then 2 mg every 30 min PRN • Not to exceed 6 mg/24 hr or 10 mg/wk • SL tabs	• Hypersensitivity • Peripheral arterial disease • Coronary artery disease • Hypertension • Hepatic or renal impair-ment • Concurrent use of strong 3A4 inhibitors • Pregnancy	• Chest pain • Myocardial infarction • Hyperten-sion • Tachycardia • Nausea • Valvular fibrosis	• Response to therapy • Presence of side effects • BP • HR	• CYP3A4 substrate • CYP3A4 inhibitors may ↑ effects/toxicity • CYP3A4 inducers may ↓ effects	Potential for dependence with long-term use
Dihydroergotamine • DHE 45, Migranal • IV, IM, or subcut: 1 mg at onset, repeated at 1-hr intervals (max = 2 mg/day IV or 3 mg/day subcut or IM or 6 mg/wk) • Nasal: 1 spray (0.5 mg) in each nostril; repeat in 15 min with spray in each nostril (max = 3 mg/day or 8 sprays/wk)	• Hypersensitivity • Peripheral arterial disease • Coronary artery disease • Hypertension • Hepatic or renal impairment • Concurrent use of strong 3A4 inhibitors • Pregnancy • Within 24 hr of triptan product • Within 2 wk of MAOI				

Medications for Migraine   *(cont'd)*

Mechanism of action – serotonin agonists (triptans): serotonin 5HT1 receptor agonists, resulting in vasoconstriction in the cerebral vasculature

Generic • Brand • Dose/Dosage Forms	Contraindications	Primary Side Effects	Key Monitoring Parameters	Pertinent Drug Interactions	Med Pearls
Sumatriptan ☆ • Imitrex oral tablets • 25–100 mg at onset, may redose at >2 hr (max = 200 mg/day) • Imitrex or Alsuma subcut injection • 4–6 mg subcut; may repeat in 1 hr (max = 2 doses/day) • Imitrex nasal spray • 5–20-mg spray in 1 nostril at onset; may repeat after 2 hr (max = 40 mg/day) • Sumavel Dosepro, needle-free subcut injection • 6 mg subcut; may repeat in 1 hr (max = 12 mg/day) • Zembrace SymTouch subcut injection • 3 mg subcut; may repeat in 1 hr (max = 12 mg/day) • Onzetra Xsail powder for nasal inhalation • 22 mg, delivered by one nosepiece (11 mg in each nostril); may repeat in 2 hr (max = 44 mg/day)	• Coronary artery disease • Wolff-Parkinson-White syndrome • Stroke or transient ischemic attack • Peripheral arterial disease • Ischemic bowel disease • Uncontrolled hypertension • Within 24 hr of an ergot product • Within 2 wk of MAOI • Within 24 hr of strong 3A4 inhibitor (eletriptan) • Severe hepatic impairment (sumatriptan) • Severe renal or hepatic impairment (naratriptan)	• Fatigue • Dizziness • Flushing • Chest/neck/throat pressure • Unpleasant taste • Hypertension	• Response to therapy • Presence of side effects • BP	Use with meperidine, dextromethorphan, tramadol, SSRIs, SNRIs, TCAs, MAOIs, triptans, or St. John's wort may ↑ risk of serotonin syndrome	Onset: 30 min (PO); 15–30 min (intranasal); 10 min (subcut)
Zolmitriptan • Zomig, Zomig ZMT • Tabs: 1.25–2.5 at onset; may repeat in >2 hr if needed (max = 10 mg/day) • ODTs: 2.5 mg at onset; may repeat in >2 hr if needed (max = 10 mg/day) • Nasal spray: 2.5-mg spray in 1 nostril at onset; may repeat in >2 hr if needed (max = 10 mg/day)					Onset: 45 min

Medications for Migraine *(cont'd)*

Generic • Brand • Dose/Dosage Forms	Contraindications	Primary Side Effects	Key Monitoring Parameters	Pertinent Drug Interactions	Med Pearls
Naratriptan • Amerge • Tabs: 1–2.5 mg at onset; may repeat in >4 hr if needed (max = 5 mg/day)	[Same as above]	[Same as above]	[Same as above]	[Same as above]	Onset: 1–2 hr
Rizatriptan ☆ • Maxalt, Maxalt MLT • Tabs, ODTs: 5–10 mg at onset; repeat in >2 hr if needed (max = 30 mg/day)					Onset: Within 2 hr
Almotriptan • Axert • Tabs: 6.25–12.5 mg at onset; repeat in >2 hr if needed (max = 2 doses/day)					Onset: 30 min
Eletriptan • Relpax • Tabs: 20–40 mg at onset; repeat in >2 hr if needed (max = 80 mg/day)					Onset: 30 min
Frovatriptan • Frova • Tabs: 2.5 mg at onset; repeat in >2 hr if needed (max = 7.5 mg/day)					Onset: 3 hr
Combination product: Sumatriptan/naproxen (Treximet)					
Mechanism of action – butorphanol: mixed opioid agonist/antagonist with opioid analgesic properties					
Butorphanol • Only available generically • Nasal spray: 1 mg (1 spray) in 1 nostril at onset; may repeat in >1 hour; may then repeat in 3–4 hr after last dose if needed	• Hypersensitivity • Patients with a history of narcotic dependence	• Somnolence • Dizziness • Nausea • Nasal congestion • Insomnia	• Response to therapy • Presence of adverse effects	Concurrent use of other CNS depressants will have additive adverse effects and should be avoided	• Schedule IV controlled substance • Not routinely used for migraines • High addiction potential
Mechanism of action – calcitonin gene-related peptide receptor antagonist					
Erenumab-aooe • Aimovig • 70–140 mg subQ once monthly • SQ injection	None	• Injection site reaction • Constipation • Antibody development	Response to therapy	Belimumab	Used only for migraine prophylaxis

ALZHEIMER'S DISEASE

Guidelines Summary

- Goals of treatment include preservation of function and symptomatic slowing of cognitive decline. A commonly used benchmark is the change in MMSE within one year. Without therapy, MMSE would be expected to ↓ approximately 2–4 points per year. Therapeutic efficacy is often determined if MMSE ↓ by ≤2 points per year. None of the available therapies has an impact on halting disease progression or reversing pathophysiology.

- Cholinesterase inhibitors are the treatment of choice in mild to moderate AD. Although slight differences exist in the mechanism of action of these agents, there is no evidence to indicate greater efficacy with one agent over another. Agent selection is typically made based upon patient preference, cost, and potential for drug interactions. There is insufficient evidence to support a dose-response relationship within this class. It is currently recommended that patients be started on the lowest dose and titrated slowly to the typical maintenance dose.

- Memantine is the only currently available N-methyl-D-aspartate (NMDA) receptor antagonist and has been studied and approved in moderate to severe AD as either monotherapy or an adjunct to a cholinesterase inhibitor.

- The most widely accepted approach to treatment is to initiate a low dose of a cholinesterase inhibitor at the time of diagnosis with slow titration to a typical maintenance dose. After 6 months to 1 year, efficacy is assessed. If this therapy is not efficacious, the patient can be switched to an alternate cholinesterase inhibitor or memantine can be added (in moderate to severe disease).

Cholinesterase Inhibitors

Generic • Brand • Dose/Dosage Forms	Contraindications	Primary Side Effects	Key Monitoring Parameters	Pertinent Drug Interactions	Med Pearls
Mechanism of action – inhibit the activity of the cholinesterase enzyme, thereby allowing ↑ acetylcholine activity					
Donepezil ☆ • Aricept • 5 mg daily, then ↑ to 10 mg daily after 4–6 wk (max = 23 mg daily in moderate–severe AD) • ODTs, tabs	Hypersensitivity	• N/V/D • Peptic ulcer disease • Weight loss • Urinary incontinence • Dizziness • Headache • Syncope • Salivation • Sweating • Bradycardia • AV block • Rash (Stevens-Johnson syndrome possible)	• Presence of side effects • ECG • HR • MMSE (at 6–12 mo intervals)	• May ↑ neuromuscular blockade with succinylcholine • Anticholinergic drugs ↓ efficacy • Cholinergic drugs ↑ toxicity	Slow titration can ↑ tolerability
Galantamine • Razadyne, Razadyne ER • IR: 4 mg BID × 4 wk, then 8 mg BID × ≥4 wk, then 12 mg BID • ER: 8 mg daily × 4 wk, then 16 mg daily × ≥4 wk, then 24 mg daily • ER caps, solution, tabs					
Rivastigmine • Exelon • Caps: 1.5–6 mg BID • Patch: 4.6–13.3 mg daily • Caps, transdermal patch				• May ↑ neuromuscular blockade with succinylcholine • Anticholinergic drugs ↓ efficacy • Cholinergic drugs ↑ toxicity • Metoclopramide ↑ risk of extrapyramidal symptoms	• Capsules should be administered with meals • Also indicated for Parkinson-related dementia

NMDA Receptor Antagonist

Generic • Brand • Dose/Dosage Forms	Contraindications	Primary Side Effects	Key Monitoring Parameters	Pertinent Drug Interactions	Med Pearls
Mechanism of action – NMDA receptor antagonist, preventing detrimental effects of glutamate					
Memantine ☆ • Namenda, Namenda XR • IR: 5 mg daily × ≥1 wk, then 5 mg BID × ≥1 wk, then 5 mg AM and 10 mg PM × ≥1 wk, then 10 mg BID • ER: 7–28 mg daily • ER caps, solution, tabs	Hypersensitivity	• Confusion • Constipation • Dizziness • Headache • D/V • Hypertension	• Presence of side effects • BP • MMSE at 6–12 month intervals	Carbonic anhydrase inhibitors and sodium bicarbonate may ↑ effects/ toxicity	• Indicated for moderate–severe AD as monotherapy or in combination with cholinesterase inhibitor • Adjust dose in renal impairment
Combination product: Donepezil/memantine (Namzaric)					

Gastrointestinal Disorders

6

This chapter covers the following diseases:

- **Gastroesophageal reflux disease/peptic ulcer disease**
- **Inflammatory bowel disease**

GASTROESOPHAGEAL REFLUX DISEASE/ PEPTIC ULCER DISEASE

Guidelines Summary

Gastroesophageal Reflux Disease

The goals of therapy are to relieve symptoms, promote healing of esophageal mucosa, prevent recurrence, and prevent complications.

- **Lifestyle modifications**
  - Unlikely to control symptoms, when used alone, in most patients
  - Dietary changes: Avoid foods that can worsen symptoms (alcohol, caffeine, chocolate, citrus juices, peppermint/spearmint, coffee, spicy foods, tomatoes, high-fatty meals, garlic, onions); avoid eating before bedtime; remain upright after meals
  - Weight loss
  - Smoking cessation
  - Head elevated off the bed by 6–8 inches
  - No tight-fitting clothes
  - No medications that can worsen symptoms

- **Pharmacological therapy**
  - Step 1: Antacids and over-the-counter (OTC) acid suppressants (H2RAs, omeprazole, lansoprazole, esomeprazole) can be used initially on an as-needed basis for intermittent or mild symptoms. If symptoms persist after 2 weeks, proceed to Step 2.
  - Step 2: PPI or H2RA (can be used at higher prescription doses)
    - » PPIs are considered more effective than H2RAs.
  - A promotility agent (e.g., metoclopramide) can be used as adjunctive therapy, if needed.

Peptic Ulcer Disease

The goals of therapy are to relieve symptoms, promote healing of the ulcer, eradicate *H. pylori* (if present), prevent recurrence, and prevent complications.

- **Lifestyle modifications:** Reduce stress, smoking cessation, discontinue NSAID use, avoid foods that can worsen symptoms.
- **Pharmacological therapy**
  - *H. pylori*-associated ulcers: See treatment algorithm below (duration = 10–14 days, depending on regimen).

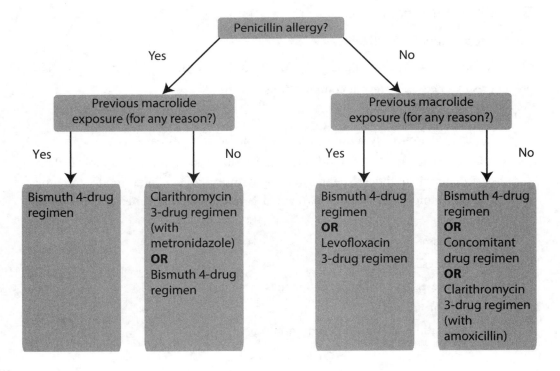

- NSAID-induced ulcers
  - » Treatment
    - First-line therapy: PPI (duration of therapy = 6–8 weeks; may be longer if recurrent symptoms, heavy smoker, or continued NSAID use)
    - Second-line therapies: Misoprostol or H2RA
  - » Primary prevention
    - Recommendations based on whether patient is at low, moderate, or high risk for NSAID GI toxicity (see Definitions) and the patient's risk for CV disease; high CV risk is defined by the patient's need for low-dose aspirin to prevent future CV events

	Low GI Risk	Moderate GI Risk	High GI Risk
Low CV Risk	NSAID alone	NSAID + PPI/misoprostol	Alternative therapy, if possible; or, cyclooxygenase-2 inhibitor + PPI/misoprostol
High CV Risk	Naproxen + PPI/ misoprostol	Naproxen + PPI/misoprostol	Avoid NSAIDs or cyclooxygenase-2 inhibitors; use alternative therapy

Antacids

Generic • Brand • Dose	Contraindications	Primary Side Effects	Key Monitoring	Pertinent Drug Interactions	Med Pearl
Mechanism of action – neutralize stomach acid and ↑ gastric pH					
Magnesium hydroxide/aluminum hydroxide • Mag-Al • 15 mL with meals and at bedtime	None	• Diarrhea (from magnesium [Mg^{2+}]) • Constipation (from aluminum [Al^{3+}] or calcium [Ca^{2+}])	S/S of GERD	• May bind to numerous drugs (separate from other drugs by at least 2 hr) • May ↓ absorption of drugs whose absorption is pH-dependent (e.g., itraconazole, ketoconazole, iron, atazanavir, nelfinavir, rilpivirine, mycophenolate mofetil, and erlotinib)	Use Mg^{2+}- and Al^{3+}- containing products with caution in patients with renal impairment
Calcium carbonate • Tums, Maalox Chewables • 1–2 tabs q2h as needed					

H$_2$ Receptor Antagonists

Generic • Brand • Dose	Dosage Forms	Primary Side Effects	Key Monitoring	Pertinent Drug Interactions	Med Pearl
Mechanism of action – reversibly inhibit histamine (H$_2$) receptors in the gastric parietal cells, which inhibits secretion of gastric acid					
Cimetidine • Tagamet HB • 200–1,600 mg/day	• Rx: Solution, tabs • OTC: Tabs	• Headache • Fatigue • Dizziness • Confusion • Gynecomastia (cimetidine)	S/S of GERD/PUD	• Cimetidine inhibits cytochrome P450 (CYP) enzymes to greater extent than the other drugs (inhibits CYP1A2, CYP2C19, CYP2D6, and CYP3A4) • May ↓ absorption of drugs whose absorption is pH-dependent (e.g., itraconazole, ketoconazole, iron, atazanavir, ledipasvir/ sofosbuvir, nelfinavir, rilpivirine, mycophenolate mofetil, dasatinib, nilotinib, and erlotinib)	Adjust dose of all H2RAs in renal impairment
Famotidine ☆ • Pepcid • 20–80 mg/day	• Rx: Injection, suspension, tabs • OTC: Tabs				
Nizatidine • Only available generically • 150–300 mg/day	Rx: Caps, solution				
Ranitidine ☆ • Zantac • 75–300 mg/day	• Rx: Caps, injection, syrup, tabs • OTC: Tabs				
Combination products: Famotidine/calcium carbonate/magnesium hydroxide (Pepcid Complete) ibuprofen/famotidine (Duexis)					

Proton Pump Inhibitors

Generic • Brand • Dose	Dosage Forms	Primary Side Effects	Key Monitoring	Pertinent Drug Interactions	Med Pearl
Mechanism of action – irreversibly inhibit H^+/K^+-ATPase in gastric parietal cells, which inhibits secretion of gastric acid					
Dexlansoprazole☆ • Dexilant • 30–60 mg/day	Caps	• Diarrhea • Headache	S/S of GERD/PUD	• May ↓ absorption of drugs whose absorption is pH-dependent (e.g., itraconazole, ketoconazole, iron, atazanavir, ledipasvir/ sofosbuvir, nelfinavir, rilpivirine, mycophenolate mofetil, dasatinib, nilotinib, and erlotinib) • May ↓ antiplatelet effects of clopidogrel • May ↑ effects/ toxicity of methotrexate	Long-term therapy may be associated with: • Osteoporosis-related fractures • ↓ Mg^{2+} • *Clostridium difficile* • Vitamin B_{12} deficiency • Acute interstitial nephritis • Cutaneous/ systemic lupus erythematosus • Fundic gland polyps
Esomeprazole ☆ • Nexium, Nexium 24 hr • 20–40 mg/day	• Rx: Caps, granules for suspension, injection • OTC: Caps, tabs				
Lansoprazole☆ • Prevacid • 15–30 mg/day	• Rx: Caps, orally disintegrating tabs (ODTs) • OTC: Caps				
Omeprazole ☆ • Prilosec • 20 mg/day	• Rx: Caps, granules for suspension • OTC: Tabs				
Pantoprazole☆ • Protonix • 20–40 mg/day	Granules for suspension, injection, tabs				
Rabeprazole☆ • Aciphex • 20 mg/day	Sprinkle capsules, tabs				
Combination products: Esomeprazole/naproxen (Vimovo)		Omeprazole/sodium bicarbonate (Zegerid)			Omeprazole/aspirin (Yosprala)

Promotility Drug

Generic • Brand • Dose/Dosage Forms	Contraindications	Primary Side Effects	Key Monitoring	Pertinent Drug Interactions	Med Pearl
Mechanism of action – dopamine antagonist; ↑ LES pressure and accelerates gastric emptying					
Metoclopramide☆ • Reglan, Metozolv ODT • 40–60 mg/day • Injection, ODTs, solution, tabs	Seizures	• Dizziness • Sedation • Diarrhea • Extrapyramidal symptoms (EPS)	• S/S of GERD • EPS	Use with antipsychotic agents may ↑ risk of EPS	• Can also be used for diabetic gastroparesis; erythromycin is an alternative • Adjust dose in renal impairment

Mucosal Protectant Drug

Generic • Brand • Dose/Dosage Forms	Contraindications	Primary Side Effects	Key Monitoring	Pertinent Drug Interactions	Med Pearl
Mechanism of action – nonabsorbable aluminum salt that forms bonds with damaged and normal GI tissue; complex forms protective cover over ulcerated area					
Sucralfate ☆ • Carafate • 4 g/day • Suspension, tabs	None	Constipation	S/S of PUD	May bind to numerous drugs (separate from other drugs by at least 2 hrs)	• Limited value in treatment of GERD; more useful in treatment of PUD • Use cautiously in patients with chronic kidney disease (↑ risk of Al^{3+} toxicity)

Prostaglandin Analog

Generic • Brand • Dose/Dosage Forms	Contraindications	Primary Side Effects	Key Monitoring	Pertinent Drug Interactions	Med Pearl
Mechanism of action – prostaglandin E1 analog; replaces protective prostaglandins inhibited by NSAID therapy					
Misoprostol • Cytotec • 400–800 mcg/day • Tabs	Pregnancy (abortifacient)	Diarrhea	S/S of PUD	None	• Women of reproductive potential should have a pregnancy test before initiating therapy; educate regarding appropriate use of contraception • Can also be used for medical termination of pregnancy
Combination product: Misoprostol/diclofenac (Arthrotec)					

Helicobacter pylori First-Line Treatment Regimens (for PUD)

Proton Pump Inhibitor	Drug #2	Drug #3	Drug #4	Duration of Therapy	Comments
Three-Drug Regimen					
Esomeprazole 40 mg daily **OR** Lansoprazole 30 mg BID **OR** Omeprazole 20 mg BID **OR** Pantoprazole 40 mg BID **OR** Rabeprazole 20 mg BID	Amoxicillin 1,000 mg BID **OR** Metronidazole 500 mg TID (if penicillin allergy)	Clarithromycin 500 mg BID	None	14 days	• Clarithromycin 3-drug regimen • Prevpac is a compliance package that contains individual units of lansoprazole, amoxicillin, and clarithromycin • Omeclamox-Pak is a compliance package that contains individual units of omeprazole, amoxicillin, and clarithromycin
Esomeprazole 40 mg daily **OR** Lansoprazole 30 mg BID **OR** Omeprazole 20 mg BID **OR** Pantoprazole 40 mg BID **OR** Rabeprazole 20 mg BID	Amoxicillin 1,000 mg BID	Levofloxacin 500 mg daily	None	10–14 days	Levofloxacin 3-drug regimen
Four-Drug Regimen					
Esomeprazole 40 mg daily **OR** Lansoprazole 30 mg BID **OR** Omeprazole 20 mg BID **OR** Pantoprazole 40 mg BID **OR** Rabeprazole 20 mg BID	Bismuth subsalicylate 300 mg 4 × daily **OR** Bismuth subcitrate 120–300 mg 4 × daily	Metronidazole 250–500 mg 4 × daily **OR** Metronidazole 500 mg TID	Tetracycline 500 mg 4 × daily	10–14 days	• Bismuth 4-drug regimen • Pylera contains bismuth, metronidazole, and tetracycline in each capsule
Esomeprazole 40 mg daily **OR** Lansoprazole 30 mg BID **OR** Omeprazole 20 mg BID **OR** Pantoprazole 40 mg BID **OR** Rabeprazole 20 mg BID	Amoxicillin 1,000 mg BID	Clarithromycin 500 mg BID	Metronidazole 500 mg BID	10–14 days	Concomitant drug regimen

INFLAMMATORY BOWEL DISEASE

Guidelines Summary

The goals of therapy are to induce and maintain remission, to prevent and resolve complications and systemic symptoms, and to maintain quality of life. There is no pharmacologic cure for these diseases; therefore, treatment focuses on management of symptoms.

- **Nonpharmacologic therapy**
  - Lifestyle changes/diet: Avoid foods that may worsen disease symptoms
  - Possible surgery when complications (e.g., fistulas, strictures, perforation) develop or to manage refractory disease
- **Pharmacologic therapy**
  - Adjunctive therapies: antidiarrheals (e.g., loperamide), antispasmodics (e.g., dicyclomine, propantheline, hyoscyamine)
  - Ulcerative colitis
    » Treatment based upon whether inflammation is distal (below the splenic flexure; topical therapy appropriate) or extensive (proximal to the splenic flexure; requires systemic therapy)
    » Mild/moderate distal disease
      - Active disease: Topical mesalamine (enema or suppository preferred), oral aminosalicylate, or topical corticosteroid
      - Maintenance of remission: Topical mesalamine or oral aminosalicylate
    » Mild/moderate extensive disease
      - Active disease: Oral aminosalicylate (first-line), oral corticosteroids, azathioprine, 6-mercaptopurine, infliximab, adalimumab, golimumab, or vedolizumab
      - Maintenance of remission: Oral aminosalicylate (first-line), azathioprine, 6-mercaptopurine, infliximab, adalimumab, golimumab, or vedolizumab
    » Severe disease
      - Infliximab (if urgent hospitalization not needed), intravenous (IV) corticosteroids (if urgent hospitalization needed), IV cyclosporine
  - Crohn's disease
    » Mild/moderate active disease
      - First-line: Aminosalicylate (sulfasalazine or topical mesalamine), budesonide (disease localized to ileum and/or right colon)
      - Second-line: Metronidazole
    » Moderate/severe disease
      - First-line: Prednisone
      - Second-line: Infliximab, adalimumab, certolizumab pegol, vedolizumab, natalizumab, ustekinumab, methotrexate (IM or subcut)

» Severe/fulminant disease

– First-line: IV corticosteroids

– Second-line: Infliximab

» Maintenance therapy

– First-line: Azathioprine, 6-mercaptopurine, methotrexate, infliximab, adalimumab, certolizumab pegol, vedolizumab, ustekinumab, or natalizumab

Aminosalicylates

Generic • Brand • Dose	Dosage Forms	Contraindications	Primary Side Effects	Key Monitoring	Med Pearl
Mechanism of action – ↓ inflammation in GI tract by inhibiting prostaglandin synthesis and subsequent production of various immune mediators; sulfasalazine is cleaved in colon to mesalamine (responsible for therapeutic effect) + sulfapyridine (causes side effects); olsalazine and balsalazide also contain mesalamine					
Sulfasalazine • Azulfidine, Azulfidine EN • Induction: 3–4 g/day • Maintenance: 2 g/day	Tabs, delayed-release (DR) (enteric-coated) tabs	• Aspirin allergy • Sulfa allergy • Glucose-6-phosphate dehydrogenase (G6PD) deficiency • Pregnancy (near term)	• Stevens-Johnson syndrome • Photosensitivity • N/V • Headache • Folate deficiency • Hemolytic anemia • Agranulocytosis • Hepatitis • Orange discoloration of bodily fluids	• S/S of IBD • Liver function tests (LFTs) (with sulfasalazine) • Complete blood count (CBC) (with sulfasalazine)	• Mesalamine, olsalazine, and balsalazide are not sulfa derivatives; are poorly absorbed from GI tract (better tolerated than sulfasalazine) • Folic acid should be given to patients on sulfasalazine • Sulfasalazine may ↑ effects of warfarin and oral hypoglycemics • All may ↓ absorption of digoxin
Mesalamine • Apriso, Asacol HD, Canasa, Delzicol, Lialda, Pentasa, Rowasa • Oral: *Induction* 2.4–4.8 g/day; *Maintenance,* 1.5–4 g/day • Rectal enema (Rowasa): 4 g at bedtime • Rectal suppository (Canasa): 1 g at bedtime	Extended-release (ER) caps, DR tabs, rectal enema, rectal suppository	• Aspirin allergy • G6PD deficiency	• Nausea • Diarrhea • Headache • Malaise		
Olsalazine • Dipentum • 1–3 g/day	Caps				
Balsalazide • Colazal, Giazo • 1.5–6.75 g/day	Caps, tabs				

Corticosteroids

Generic • Brand • Dose	Dosage Forms	Contraindications	Primary Side Effects	Key Monitoring	Med Pearl
Mechanism of action – quickly ↓ inflammation during acute exacerbations of IBD					
Budesonide • Entocort EC, Uceris • Entocort EC: *Initial*: 9 mg daily for up to 2 mo; *Maintenance*: 6 mg daily for up to 3 mo • Uceris (PO): 9 mg daily for up to 2 mo • Uceris (rectal foam): 1 metered dose (2 mg) BID for 2 wk, then 1 metered dose (2 mg) daily for 4 wk	DR caps, ER tabs, rectal foam	None	• Hyperglycemia • ↑ appetite • Insomnia • Hypertension • Edema • Adrenal suppression • Osteoporosis • Cataracts • Delayed wound healing	• S/S of IBD • Blood glucose • Blood pressure (BP) • Electrolytes	• Methylprednisolone and prednisone should only be used to treat acute exacerbation (4–8 wk) and then tapered • IV therapy given for severe exacerbations for 7–10 days, then switched to PO therapy • Budesonide has localized effect; has minimal systemic side effects • Entocort EC indicated for CD • Uceris indicated for UC
Methylprednisolone☆ • Solu-Medrol • 10–100 mg/day	Injection, tabs				
Prednisone☆ • Sterapred • 20–60 mg/day	Tabs				

Immunomodulators

Generic • Brand • Dose	Contraindications	Primary Side Effects	Key Monitoring	Pertinent Drug Interactions	Med Pearl
Mechanism of action – ↓ production of inflammatory mediators (e.g., interleukins) through various mechanisms					
Azathioprine • Azasan, Imuran • 75–150 mg/day 6-Mercaptopurine • Purixan • 50–100 mg/day	• Pregnancy • Bone marrow suppression • Hepatic impairment	• Pancreatitis • Arthralgias • Nausea • Diarrhea • Rash • Bone marrow suppression • Hepatotoxicity	• Amylase/lipase (if symptoms) • CBC with differential • LFTs • TPMT and NUDT15 deficiency	• Allopurinol and febuxostat may ↑ risk of side effects (↓ azathioprine dose by 75% when used with allopurinol; avoid concomitant use with febuxostat) • Aminosalicylates may ↑ risk of side effects • May ↓ effects of warfarin	• 6-mercaptopurine is active metabolite of azathioprine • Adjust dose in renal impairment • Patients with TMPT or NUDT15 deficiency are at ↑ risk of bone marrow suppression
Cyclosporine • Sandimmune • 4–8 mg/kg/day IV	Renal failure	• Hypertension • Nephrotoxicity • Hypomagnesemia • Infection • Anaphylaxis	• BP • Blood urea nitrogen (BUN)/serum creatinine (SCr) • Electrolytes • S/S of infection • Cyclosporine levels	• CYP3A4 substrate and inhibitor • CYP3A4 inhibitors may ↑ levels/toxicity • CYP3A4 inducers may ↓ effects • May ↑ effects of other CYP3A4 substrates	• Used only for severe disease that has not responded to corticosteroids • Used only for 7–10 days
Methotrexate ☆ • Rheumatrex • 15–25 mg/wk IM or subcut	• Pregnancy • Bone marrow suppression • Severe renal or hepatic impairment	• Hepatotoxicity • Bone marrow suppression • Pneumonitis • Rash • N/V • Diarrhea	• LFTs • CBC with differential • Chest x-ray (if symptoms)	• NSAIDs and salicylates ↑ risk of toxicity • Penicillins, sulfonamides, and tetracyclines may ↑ risk of toxicity	• Only effective for CD (useful for steroid-dependent and steroid-refractory CD) • Adjust dose in renal impairment

Biological Agents

Generic • Brand • Dose	Contraindications	Primary Side Effects	Key Monitoring	Pertinent Drug Interactions	Med Pearl
Mechanism of action – inhibit tumor necrosis factor (TNF)					
Adalimumab • Humira • 160 mg subcut on day 1 or over 2 days, then 80 mg 2 wk later (day 15), then 40 mg every other wk beginning day 29	None	• Headache • Rash • Injection site reactions • Anaphylaxis • Infection (especially tuberculosis [TB], fungal infections and hepatitis B virus [HBV] reactivation) • Malignancy • Heart failure (HF) exacerbation • Bone marrow suppression • Lupus-like syndrome • Demyelinating disorders	• S/S of infection • S/S of HF • CBC with differential	Do not administer live vaccines	• PPD and HBV screening should be done before initiating treatment • Approved for moderately to severely active CD or UC in patients who have not responded despite adequate therapy with a corticosteroid or immunomodulator
Certolizumab pegol • Cimzia • 400 mg subcut at 0, 2, and 4 wks; then 400 mg every 4 wk	None				• PPD and HBV screening should be done before initiating treatment • Only approved for moderately to severely active CD in patients who have not responded despite adequate therapy with a corticosteroid or immunomodulator
Golimumab • Simponi • 200 mg subcut at wk 0, then 100 mg at wk 2, then 100 mg every 4 wk	None				• PPD and HBV screening should be done before initiating treatment • Only approved for moderately to severely active UC in patients who have not responded despite adequate therapy with a corticosteroid or immunomodulator
Infliximab • Inflectra, Remicade, Renflexis • 5 mg/kg IV at 0, 2, and 6 wk; then every 8 wk	New York Heart Association class III or IV HF (for doses >5 mg/kg)	• Infusion reactions (hypotension, dyspnea, urticaria, myocardial infarction, stroke) • Delayed hypersensitivity reactions (fever, rash, myalgia, headache, sore throat, hand/facial edema, dysphagia, arthralgias) • Infection (especially TB, fungal infections, or HBV reactivation) • HF exacerbation • Bone marrow suppression • Malignancy • Hepatotoxicity	• BP • LFTs • S/S of infection • S/S of HF • CBC with differential		• Delayed hypersensitivity reaction may occur as early as after 2nd dose • Premedicate with H_1 antagonist, H2RA, acetaminophen, and/or corticosteroid • PPD and HBV screening should be done before initiating treatment • Approved for moderately to severely active CD or UC in patients who have not responded despite adequate therapy with a corticosteroid or immunomodulator

Biological Agents   *(cont'd)*

Generic • Brand • Dose	Contraindications	Primary Side Effects	Key Monitoring	Pertinent Drug Interactions	Med Pearl
Mechanism of action – interleukin (IL)-12 and IL-23 inhibitor					
Ustekinumab • Stelara • Induction: ≤55 kg: 260 mg IV × 1, 56–85 kg: 390 mg IV × 1, >85 kg: 520 mg IV × 1; Maintenance: 90 mg IV 8 wk after initial dose, then every 8 wk	Hypersensitivity	• Infection (especially TB, fungal infections, or bacterial/viral infections) • Malignancy • Hypersensitivity reactions (anaphylaxis, angioedema) • Reversible posterior leukoencephalopathy syndrome (RPLS)	• S/S of infection • S/S of RPLS • CBC with differential	Do not administer live vaccines	• PPD screening should be done before initiating treatment • Approved only for moderately to severely active CD in patients who have failed or were intolerant to immunomodulators or corticosteroids, but never failed treatment with a TNF inhibitor; or have failed or were intolerant to treatment with a TNF inhibitor
Mechanism of action – ↓ inflammation by binding to α4-subunit of integrins					
Natalizumab • Tysabri • 300 mg IV every 4 wk; discontinue if no response by wk 12	• Progressive multifocal leukoencephalopathy (PML) • Concurrent use of TNF inhibitors or immunosuppressants	• PML (may be fatal) • Headache • Fatigue • Depression • Rash • Nausea • Arthralgia • Hypersensitivity reactions (hypotension, urticaria, fever, rash, rigors, nausea, flushing, dizziness, chest pain) • Anaphylaxis • Infection (especially opportunistic infections, herpes encephalitis meningitis, or herpes acute retinal necrosis) • Hepatotoxicity	• S/S of PML • Brain MRI (at baseline) • S/S of infection • LFTs • Anti-JCV antibody	Do not administer live vaccines	• Patients need to be enrolled in CD-TOUCH program • Must be administered as monotherapy • Only approved for moderate to severely active CD in patients who are refractory to or unable to tolerate conventional therapies and TNF inhibitors
Mechanism of action – ↓ inflammation by binding to α4β7-subunit of integrins					
Vedolizumab • Entyvio • 300 mg IV at 0, 2, and 6 wk; then every 8 wk; discontinue if no response by wk 14	None	• Hypersensitivity reactions • Anaphylaxis • Infusion reactions • Infection (especially TB) • PML • Hepatotoxicity	• S/S of infection • S/S of PML • LFTs	Do not administer live vaccines	• Consider performing PPD before treatment • Approved for moderately to severely active CD or UC in patients who are refractory to or unable to tolerate a TNF inhibitor or immunomodulator; or had an inadequate response to, were intolerant to, or were dependent on corticosteroids

Oncology

9

This chapter covers the following topics:

- **Cancer chemotherapy drugs**
- **Targeted and biologic agents**
- **Supportive care**

Many of the drugs used in chemotherapy are indicated for multiple types of cancer (e.g., lymphoma, leukemia, lung cancer, colorectal cancer, breast cancer, prostate cancer, ovarian cancer). Because cancer therapy is generally protocol-driven, your focus should be mostly on drug toxicities and on certain cases where a specific drug is indicated on the basis of cell-surface markers such as CD20 or HER-2 overexpression. Supportive care (antiemetic agents and colony-stimulating factors) is covered at the end of this chapter.

CANCER CHEMOTHERAPY DRUGS

Alkylating Agents

Generic • Brand • Dosage Forms	Contraindications	Primary Side Effects	Key Monitoring	Pertinent Drug Interactions	Med Pearl
Mechanism of action – alkylate DNA, making it more prone to breakage; most effective against rapidly dividing cells					
Cyclophospha-mide • Only available generically • Caps, injection (IV)	Hypersensitivity to any alkylating agent	• Alopecia • Hemorrhagic cystitis • Infertility • Nausea, vomiting (N/V), mucositis, stomatitis • Bone marrow suppression	• Complete blood count (CBC) with differential • Blood urea nitrogen (BUN)/ serum creatinine (SCr) • Uric acid (UA)	Cytochrome P450 (CYP) 3A4 inducers may ↑ levels of active metabolite (acrolein)	• Maintain adequate hydration to avoid hemorrhagic cystitis; can also use mesna • High emetogenic potential
Chlorambucil • Leukeran • Tabs		• Bone marrow suppression • Infertility • Secondary leukemias • Seizures • Stevens-Johnson syndrome • Hepatotoxicity	• CBC with differential • Liver function tests (LFTs)	None	Take on empty stomach
Carmustine • BiCNU, Gliadel • Injection (IV), intracranial implant		• Bone marrow suppression • Pulmonary fibrosis • Severe N/V • Hypotension (IV) • Secondary leukemias (with long-term use) • Reversible elevation of LFTs	• CBC with differential • Pulmonary function tests • LFTs • Blood pressure (BP) (during IV administration)	IV solution contains ethanol; do not give aldehyde-dehydrogenase inhibitors	Very high emetogenic potential

Platinum-Based Agents

Generic • Brand • Dosage Forms	Contraindications	Primary Side Effects	Key Monitoring	Pertinent Drug Interactions	Med Pearl
Mechanism of action – crosslink DNA, causing it to break					
Cisplatin • Only available generically • Injection (IV)	• Hypersensitivity to any platinum-containing compounds • Renal impairment • Pre-existing hearing impairment (cisplatin)	• Anaphylaxis • Dose-related myelosuppression • N/V • Ototoxicity (cisplatin) • Nephrotoxicity with cumulative doses (esp. cisplatin) • Peripheral neuropathy • QT interval prolongation (oxaliplatin) • Rhabdomyolysis (oxaliplatin)	• BUN/SCr • Electrolytes • Neurologic exam • CBC with differential • Urine output	Administration with taxane derivatives may ↑ myelosuppression and ↓ efficacy of platinum agents	• Do not administer doses exceeding 100 mg/m^2 every 3 wk • High emetogenic potential
Carboplatin • Only available generically • Injection (IV)					• Moderate emetogenic potential • Dose often calculated by target AUC using Calvert formula (total dose [mg] = Target AUC × [GFR + 25]) • Adjust dose in renal impairment
Oxaliplatin • Eloxatin • Injection (IV)					• Moderate emetogenic potential • Warn patients to wear a scarf if being treated during cold weather • Adjust dose in renal impairment

Enzyme Inhibitors

Generic • Brand • Dosage Forms	Contraindications	Primary Side Effects	Key Monitoring	Pertinent Drug Interactions	Med Pearl
Mechanism of action – target enzymes responsible for DNA replication and repair					
Irinotecan • Camptosar • Injection (IV)	Concurrent therapy with strong CYP3A4 inhibitors	• Bone marrow suppression • Severe, life-threatening diarrhea	• CBC with differential • Electrolytes (esp. if diarrhea)	CYP3A4 substrate	• Diarrhea may be early or late onset • Moderate emetogenic potential • Atropine can be used to treat early-onset diarrhea; loperamide for late-onset diarrhea
Irinotecan liposomal • Onivyde • Injection (IV)	None	• Bone marrow suppression • Severe, life-threatening diarrhea • Interstitial lung disease (ILD) • Hypersensitivity reactions	• CBC with differential • Electrolytes (esp. if diarrhea) • S/S of ILD	CYP3A4 substrate	• Diarrhea may be early or late onset • Atropine can be used to treat early-onset diarrhea; loperamide for late-onset diarrhea

Enzyme Inhibitors *(cont'd)*

Generic • Brand • Dosage Forms	Contraindications	Primary Side Effects	Key Monitoring	Pertinent Drug Interactions	Med Pearl
Etoposide • Only available generically • Caps, injection (IV)	None	• Bone marrow suppression • Hypersensitivity reactions	• CBC with differential • LFTs • BUN/SCr	CYP3A4 substrate	• Do NOT give IV push (may cause hypotension) • Do NOT give IM (necrosis) • Adjust dose in renal impairment

Antimitotic Agents

Generic • Brand • Dosage Forms	Contraindications	Primary Side Effects	Key Monitoring	Pertinent Drug Interactions	Med Pearl
Mechanism of action – spindle poisons; interfere with mitotic spindle; prevent chromosome segregation and lead to cell death					
Vincristine • Only available generically • Injection (IV)	None	• Peripheral neuropathy (dose-limiting) • Constipation • Paralytic ileus (secondary to neurologic toxicity)	• Neurologic exam • Change in frequency of bowel movements	CYP3A4 substrate	• Do NOT give intra-thecally (IT) (fatal) • All patients should be on a prophylactic bowel management regimen • Avoid extravasation (vesicant) • Should NOT exceed 2 mg/dose
Vincristine liposomal • Marqibo • Injection (IV)	Demyelinating conditions	• Peripheral neuropathy (dose-limiting) • Bone marrow suppression • Constipation • Paralytic ileus (secondary to neurologic toxicity) • Hepatotoxicity	• Neurologic exam • Change in frequency of bowel movements • LFTs	CYP3A4 substrate	• NOT interchange-able with vincristine • Associated with less neurotoxicity than vincristine • Do NOT give IT (fatal) • Avoid extravasation (vesicant)
Vinblastine • Only available generically • Injection (IV)	None	• Peripheral neuropathy • Bone marrow suppression (dose-limiting)	• CBC with differential • Neurologic exam	CYP3A4 substrate	• Do not give IT (fatal) • Avoid extravasation (vesicant)

Antimitotic Agents   (cont'd)

Generic • Brand • Dosage Forms	Contraindications	Primary Side Effects	Key Monitoring	Pertinent Drug Interactions	Med Pearl
Paclitaxel • Taxol • Injection (IV)	• Hypersensitivity to Cremophor • Baseline neutrophils <1,500/mm³ (ovarian, lung, or breast cancer) • ANC <1,000/mm³ (Kaposi's sarcoma)	• Bone marrow suppression (dose-limiting) • Hypersensitivity reactions • Peripheral neuropathy • Cardiac rhythm abnormalities • Mucositis, stomatitis (severe)	• CBC with differential • Electrocardiogram (ECG) • Neurologic exam	• CYP2C8 and CYP3A4 substrate • Administer prior to platinum derivatives to limit myelosuppression and enhance efficacy	• Premedicate with dexamethasone, diphenhydramine, and H₂-receptor antagonist • Adjust dose in hepatic impairment
Paclitaxel protein-bound particles • Abraxane • Injection (IV)	Baseline neutrophils <1,500/mm³				• No need for premedication • Adjust dose in hepatic impairment
Docetaxel • Taxotere • Injection (IV)	• Hypersensitivity to polysorbate 80 • Baseline neutrophils <1,500/mm³ • Severe hepatic impairment	• Significant, dose-dependent fluid retention • Bone marrow suppression • Hypersensitivity reactions • Erythema (with edema) • Peripheral-neuropathy	• CBC with differential • LFTs • Weight, signs of edema	CYP3A4 substrate	• Avoid doses >100 mg/m² • Premedicate with corticosteroids for 3 days (starting 1 day before docetaxel administration) to prevent fluid retention and hypersensitivity reactions • Contains ethanol • Adjust dose in hepatic impairment

Antimetabolites

Generic • Brand • Dosage Forms	Contraindications	Primary Side Effects	Key Monitoring	Pertinent Drug Interactions	Med Pearl
Mechanism of action – nucleoside analogs					
Cytarabine • Only available generically • Injection (IV)	None	• Severe bone marrow suppression • Cytarabine syndrome: myalgia, bone pain, rash, conjunctivitis, and fever • Sudden respiratory distress syndrome • Tumor lysis syndrome	• CBC with differential • BUN/SCr • Uric acid	None	• Premedicate with corticosteroid; may prevent cytarabine syndrome • May be administered IV, IT, or subcut • Moderate emetogenic potential • Premedicate with antihyperuricemics and hydration in patients at ↑ risk for tumor lysis syndrome

Antimetabolites *(cont'd)*

Generic • Brand • Dosage Forms	Contraindications	Primary Side Effects	Key Monitoring	Pertinent Drug Interactions	Med Pearl
Cytarabine liposomal • DepoCyt • Injection (IT)	Active meningeal infection	• Chemical arachnoiditis (N/V, headache, and fever) • Neurotoxicity	Monitor closely for signs of immediate reactions and neurotoxicity	None	• Coadminister dexamethasone to lessen chemical arachnoiditis • Moderate emetogenic potential
5-Fluorouracil • Only available generically • Injection (IV)	Dihydropyrimidine dehydrogenase (DPD) deficiency	• Hand-and-foot syndrome • N/V/D • Mucositis • Stomatitis • Bone marrow suppression	CBC with differential	• CYP2C9 inhibitor • May ↑ risk of bleeding with warfarin	Leucovorin ↑ effectiveness and toxicity; dose of fluorouracil may need to be ↓
Mechanism of action – folic acid antagonist					
Methotrexate ☆ • Trexall (PO), Xatmep (PO) • Injection (IM, IT, IV), solution, tabs	None	• Nephrotoxicity • Bone marrow suppression • Stevens-Johnson syndrome • Severe diarrhea and ulcerative stomatitis • Neurotoxicity • Hepatotoxicity • Pneumonitis • Tumor lysis syndrome	• CBC with differential • BUN/SCr • Uric acid • LFTs • Chest x-ray	Diuretics and nonsteroidal anti-inflammatory drugs may ↑ risk of toxicity	• Give leucovorin rescue 24 hr after dosing to limit toxicity; do not administer concurrently • Premedicate with antihyperuricemics and hydration in patients at ↑ risk for tumor lysis syndrome • Can be given IT for leukemias • Also used subcut or PO as DMARD for rheumatoid arthritis

Anthracyclines

Generic • Brand • Dosage Forms	Contraindications	Primary Side Effects	Key Monitoring	Pertinent Drug Interactions	Med Pearl
Mechanism of action – intercalate DNA and generate reactive oxygen species					
Daunorubicin • Cerubidine • Injection (IV) Doxorubicin • Only available generically • Injection (IV) Doxorubicin liposomal • Doxil • Injection (IV)	• Pre-existing severe myocardial insufficiency or arrhythmia • Baseline neutrophils <1,500/mm^3 • Severe hepatic impairment	• Dose-related cardiotoxicity • Severe bone marrow suppression • Secondary leukemias • Red coloration of body fluids	• CBC with differential • ECG • Left ventricular ejection fraction (LVEF)	↑ risk of cardiotoxiocity with trastuzumab, pertuzumab, cyclophosphamide, and taxane derivatives	• Greatest risk of irreversible myocardial damage at cumulative dose >550 mg/m^2 • Moderate emetogenic potential • Avoid extravasation (vesicant) • Dexrazoxane indicated to prevent doxorubicin-induced cardiotoxicity or to treat anthracycline-induced extravasation • Liposomal doxorubicin indicated for Kaposi's sarcoma, multiple myeloma, and ovarian cancer

Hormonal Agents

Generic • Brand • Dosage Forms	Contraindications	Primary Side Effects	Key Monitoring	Pertinent Drug Interactions	Med Pearl
Mechanism of action – treat cancers in which growth is accelerated by hormones					
Apalutamide • Erleada • Tabs	None	• ↓ bone mineral density • Seizures • N/V/D • Hypertension • Hot flashes/sweats	• Leutinizing hormone (LH) and follicle-stimulating hormone (FSH) levels • Serum testosterone • BP • Bone mineral density	• CYP2C8 and CYP3A4 substrate • CYP2C9, CYP2C19, and CYP3A4 inducer	None

Hormonal Agents *(cont'd)*

Generic • Brand • Dosage Forms	Contraindications	Primary Side Effects	Key Monitoring	Pertinent Drug Interactions	Med Pearl
Leuprolide • Eligard, Lupron Depot • Injection (subcut, IM/subcut depot)	• Spinal cord compression • Undiagnosed abnormal vaginal bleeding	• Abnormal menses • Exacerbation of endometriosis • Hot flashes/ sweats • ↓ bone mineral density (if used >6 mo) • Spinal cord compression and urinary tract obstruction in prostate cancer • Tumor flare • Depression, mood disturbances	• LH and FSH levels • Serum testosterone (males), estradiol (females) • Bone mineral density	None	• Subcut injection administered daily • Rotate injection sites • Subcut/IM depot injection administered every 1–6 mo depending on dosage
Tamoxifen ☆ • Soltamox • Solution, tabs	• Concurrent warfarin therapy • History of deep vein thrombosis (DVT) or pulmonary embolism	• Thromboembolic events • ↑ risk of endometrial cancer • Hot flashes • Altered menses • Mood disturbances, depression • ↓ bone mineral density	Annual gynecologic exams	• CYP3A4 substrate • May ↑ risk of bleeding with warfarin • Selective serotonin reuptake inhibitors may ↓ effects	• Bone pain may indicate a good therapeutic response; manage with mild analgesia • Duration of treatment = 5–10 yr (depending on menopausal status)
Anastrozole ☆ • Arimidex • Tabs	None	• ↓ bone mineral density • Hyperlipidemia • Mood disturbances • Hot flashes • Insomnia	• Bone mineral density • Low-density lipoprotein (LDL) and total cholesterol	None	• Aromatase inhibitor • Indicated for postmenopausal women with breast cancer • Duration of treatment = 5 yr
Exemestane • Aromasin • Tabs		• ↓ bone mineral density • Hot flashes • Insomnia	Bone mineral density	CYP3A4 substrate	• Aromatase inhibitor • Indicated for postmenopausal women with breast cancer • Duration of treatment = 5 yr
Letrozole • Femara • Tabs		• ↓ bone mineral density • Hyperlipidemia • Hot flashes	• Bone mineral density • LDL and total cholesterol	None	• Aromatase inhibitor • Indicated for postmenopausal women with breast cancer • Duration of treatment = 5 yr • Adjust dose in hepatic impairment

Chemotherapy Agents: Common Adverse Effects

- Cardiotoxicity
  - Doxorubicin
  - Daunorubicin
  - Idarubicin
  - Lapatinib
  - Mitoxantrone
  - Pertuzumab
  - Trastuzumab
- N/V
  - Cisplatin
  - Carboplatin
  - Cytarabine
  - Doxorubicin
  - Cyclophosphamide
- Mucositis
  - Cytarabine
  - Cyclophosphamide
  - 5-Fluorouracil
  - Methotrexate
- Neuropathy
  - Vincristine
  - Vinblastine
  - Oxaliplatin
  - Paclitaxel
- Renal impairment
  - Cisplatin
  - Cyclophosphamide
  - Ifosfamide
- Pulmonary fibrosis
  - Bleomycin
  - Busulfan
- Infusion reactions
  - Monoclonal antibodies
  - Paclitaxel

TARGETED AND BIOLOGIC AGENTS

Monoclonal Antibodies

Generic • Brand • Dosage Forms	Contraindications	Primary Side Effects	Key Monitoring	Pertinent Drug Interactions	Med Pearl
Mechanism of action – target the CD20 antigen					
Ibritumomab • Zevalin • Injection (IV)	None	• Infusion-related reactions • Myelosuppression (prolonged) • Secondary leukemia • Myelodysplastic syndrome • Rash (can be severe)	• CBC with differential • S/S of infusion reactions • S/S of dermatologic reactions	Do not administer live vaccines	• Indicated for CD20-positive, B-cell NHL • Linked to a radioisotope that targets B cells • Used in combination with rituximab as part of a 2-step process • Premedicate with diphenhydramine and acetaminophen (to prevent infusion reactions)
Obinutuzumab • Gazyva • Injection (IV)		• Infusion-related reactions • Tumor lysis syndrome • Myelosuppression (prolonged) • Infection (esp. bacterial, fungal, or hepatitis B virus [HBV] reactivation) • Progressive multifocal leukoencephalopathy (PML)	• CBC with differential • BUN/SCr • Uric acid • S/S of infusion reactions • S/S of infection • S/S of PML		• Indicated for CLL; obinutuzumab also indicated for follicular lymphoma • HBV screening should be done before initiating treatment • Premedicate with diphenhydramine, acetaminophen, and glucocorticoid (to prevent infusion reactions) • Premedicate with antihyperuricemics and hydration in patients at ↑ risk for tumor lysis syndrome
Ofatumumab • Arzerra • Injection (IV)		• Infusion-related reactions • Tumor lysis syndrome • Myelosuppression (prolonged) • HBV reactivation • PML	• CBC with differential • BUN/SCr • Uric acid • S/S of infusion reactions • S/S of HBV • S/S of PML		
Rituximab • Rituxan • Injection (IV)		• Infusion-related reactions • Tumor lysis syndrome • Rash (can be severe) • PML • Arrhythmias • Infection (esp. bacterial, fungal, or HBV reactivation) • Nephrotoxicity • Bowel obstruction/ perforation	• CBC with differential • S/S of infusion reactions • S/S of infection • S/S of PML • BUN/SCr • Electrolytes • Uric acid • ECG • S/S of abdominal pain • S/S of dermatologic reactions		• Indicated for CD20-positive, B-cell NHL and CD20-positive CLL • Also indicated for rheumatoid arthritis • HBV screening should be done before initiating treatment • Premedicate with diphenhydramine and acetaminophen (to prevent infusion reactions) • Premedicate with antihyperuricemics and hydration in patients at ↑ risk for tumor lysis syndrome

Epidermal Growth Factor Receptor (EGFR) Inhibitors

Generic • Brand • Dosage Forms	Contraindications	Primary Side Effects	Key Monitoring	Pertinent Drug Interactions	Med Pearl
Mechanism of action – prevent tumor growth by inhibiting the various EGFR receptors					
Afatinib • Gilotrif • Tabs	None	• Diarrhea • Rash (can be severe) • ILD • Hepatotoxicity • Keratitis	• EGFR mutation status • LFTs • BUN/SCr • S/S of dermatologic reactions • S/S of dehydration • Electrolytes • S/S of ILD • S/S of eye inflammation/ visual abnormalities	P-glycoprotein (P-gp) substrate	• Indicated for metastatic NSCLC with non-resistant EGFR mutations and metastatic squamous NSCLC • Adjust dose in renal impairment • Take 1 hr before or 2 hr after a meal
Cetuximab • Erbitux • Injection (IV)		• Infusion-related reactions • Rash (can be severe) • ILD • Sudden cardiac death • Electrolyte abnormalities ($\downarrow$ Mg^{2+}, $\downarrow$ K$^+$, $\downarrow$ Ca^{2+})	• EGFR and *K-Ras* status (for colorectal cancer) • S/S of infusion reactions • S/S of dermatologic reactions • S/S of ILD • Electrolytes	None	• Indicated for squamous cell cancer of head and neck and *K-Ras* wild type, EGFR expressing colorectal cancer • Premedicate with diphenhydramine (to prevent infusion reactions)
Erlotinib • Tarceva • Tabs		• Rash (can be severe) • Diarrhea • ILD • Renal failure • Hepatotoxicity • Gastrointestinal (GI) perforation • Myocardial ischemia/ infarction • Stroke • Keratitis	• EGFR mutation status • S/S of dermatologic reactions • S/S of dehydration • S/S of ILD • BUN/SCr • Electrolytes • LFTs • S/S of GI perforation • S/S of eye inflammation/ visual abnormalities	• CYP1A2 and CYP3A4 substrate • CYP3A4 inducers, CYP1A2 inducers, and cigarette smoking $\downarrow$ levels ($\uparrow$ erlotinib dose) • May $\uparrow$ risk of bleeding with warfarin • H$_2$-antagonists, proton pump inhibitors (PPIs), and antacids may $\downarrow$ absorption (avoid use with PPIs; space apart from H$_2$- antagonists or antacids)	Indicated for locally advanced/ metastatic NSCLC with EGFR exon 19 deletions or exon 21 substitution mutations and locally advanced, surgically unresect- able, or metastatic pancreatic cancer
Gefitinib • Iressa • Tabs		• Rash (can be severe) • Diarrhea • ILD • Hepatotoxicity • GI perforation • Keratitis	• EGFR mutation status • S/S of dermatologic reactions • S/S of dehydration • BUN/SCr • Electrolytes • S/S of ILD • LFTs • S/S of GI perforation • S/S of eye inflammation/ visual abnormalities	• CYP3A4 substrate • Strong CYP3A4 inducers $\downarrow$ levels ($\uparrow$ gefitinib dose) • May $\uparrow$ risk of bleeding with warfarin • H$_2$-antagonists, PPIs, and antacids may $\downarrow$ absorption (avoid concomitant use of PPIs; may use H$_2$-antagonists or antacids [need to space administration])	Indicated for metastatic NSCLC with EGFR exon 19 deletions or exon 21 substitution mutations

Epidermal Growth Factor Receptor (EGFR) Inhibitors *(cont'd)*

Generic • Brand • Dosage Forms	Contraindications	Primary Side Effects	Key Monitoring	Pertinent Drug Interactions	Med Pearl
Lapatinib • Tykerb • Tabs	None	• Cardiomyopathy • Diarrhea • Hepatotoxicity • Rash (can be severe) • QT interval prolongation • ILD	• HER2 status • LVEF • S/S of dehydration • Electrolytes • LFTs • S/S of dermatologic reactions • ECG • S/S of ILD	• CYP3A4 and P-gp substrate • CYP2C8, CYP3A4, and P-gp inhibitor • Avoid concomitant use of strong CYP3A4 inhibitors and inducers • May ↑ digoxin levels • ↑ risk of torsade de pointes (TdP) with other drugs that prolong QT interval	• Indicated for HER2-positive metastatic breast cancer • Adjust dose in hepatic imparment
Necitumumab • Portrazza • Injection (IV)		• Cardiopulmonary arrest • ↓ Mg^{2+} • Thromboembolic events • Rash (can be severe) • Infusion-related reactions	• Electrolytes • S/S of thromboembolism • S/S of dermatologic reactions • S/S of infusion reactions	None	• Indicated for metastatic squamous NSCLC • Premedicate if patients experienced previous infusion reaction
Neratinib • Nerlynx • Tabs		• Diarrhea (severe) • Hepatotoxicity	• HER2 status • Electrolytes • LFTs	• CYP3A4 substrate and P-gp inhibitor • Avoid concomitant use of strong CYP3A4 inhibitors and inducers • May ↑ digoxin levels • H_2-antagonists, PPIs, and antacids may ↓ absorption (avoid concomitant use of PPIs; may use H_2-antagonists or antacids [need to space administration])	• Indicated for early stage HER2-overexpressed/amplified breast cancer • Antidiarrheal prophylaxis (with loperamide) recommended for first 2 cycles
Osimertinib • Tagrisso • Tabs		• ILD • QT interval prolongation • Cardiomyopathy • Keratitis	• EGFR mutation status • S/S of ILD • ECG • LVEF	• CYP3A4 substrate and inhibitor • CYP1A2 and CYP3A4 inducer • Avoid concomitant use of strong CYP3A4 inhibitors and inducers • ↑ risk of TdP with other drugs that prolong QT interval	Indicated for metastatic NSCLC with EGFR T790M mutation or EGFR exon 19 deletions or exon 21 L858R mutations

Epidermal Growth Factor Receptor (EGFR) Inhibitors *(cont'd)*

Generic • Brand • Dosage Forms	Contraindications	Primary Side Effects	Key Monitoring	Pertinent Drug Interactions	Med Pearl
Panitumumab • Vectibix • Injection (IV)	None	• Diarrhea • Rash (can be severe) • Infusion-related reactions • ILD • Electrolyte abnormalities ($\downarrow$ Mg^{2+}, $\downarrow$ K$^+$, $\downarrow$ Ca^{2+}) • Keratitis • Photosensitivity	• *K-Ras* status • S/S of dehydration • Electrolytes • S/S of dermatologic reactions • S/S of infusion reactions • S/S of ILD • S/S of eye inflammation/ visual abnormalities	None	• Indicated for wild-type *Ras* metastatic colorectal cancer • Advise patients to wear sunscreen
Pertuzumab • Perjeta • Injection (IV)		• Cardiomyopathy • Infusion-related reactions • Anaphylaxis	• HER2 status • LVEF • S/S of infusion reactions/ anaphylaxis	$\uparrow$ risk of cardiomyopathy with anthracyclines	Indicated for HER2-positive metastatic breast cancer; HER2-positive, locally advanced, inflammatory, or early stage breast cancer; and HER2-positive early breast cancer at high risk of recurrence
Trastuzumab • Herceptin • Injection (IV)		• Cardiomyopathy • Infusion-related reactions • Myelosuppression • ILD	• HER2 status • LVEF • S/S of infusion reactions • CBC with differential • S/S of ILD	$\uparrow$ risk of cardiomyopathy with anthracyclines	Indicated for HER2-positive metastatic breast cancer and gastric cancer
Ado-trastuzumab emtansine • Kadcyla • Injection (IV)		• Hepatotoxicity • Cardiomyopathy • Infusion-related reactions • ILD • Myelosuppression • Peripheral neuropathy • Hemorrhage	• HER2 status • LFTs • LVEF • S/S of infusion reactions • S/S of ILD • CBC with differential • S/S of neuropathy • S/S of bleeding	• CYP3A4 substrate • Avoid concomitant use of strong CYP3A4 inhibitors or inducers • $\uparrow$ risk of cardiomyopathy with anthracyclines	Indicated for HER2-positive metastatic breast cancer

Vascular Endothelial Growth Factor (VEGF) Inhibitors

Generic • Brand • Dosage Forms	Contraindications	Primary Side Effects	Key Monitoring	Pertinent Drug Interactions	Med Pearl
Mechanism of action – block angiogenesis and tumor growth by inhibiting VEGF receptors					
Axitinib • Inlyta • Tabs	None	• Thromboembolic events • Hypertension • Hemorrhage • Heart failure • GI perforation/fistula formation • Hypo-/hyperthyroidism • Proteinuria • ↑ LFTs • Impaired wound healing • Reversible posterior leuko-encephalopathy syndrome (RPLS)	• S/S of thromboembolism • BP • S/S of bleeding • S/S of heart failure • Thyroid function tests (TFTs) • Urinalysis • LFTs • S/S of GI perforation/fistula formation • S/S of RPLS	• CYP3A4 substrate • Avoid concomitant use of strong CYP3A4 inhibitors or inducers	• Indicated for metastatic renal cell carcinoma • Adjust dose in hepatic impairment
Bevacizumab • Avastin • Injection (IV)		• Thromboembolic events • Hypertension • Heart failure • Hemorrhage • GI perforation/fistula formation • Proteinuria • ↑ LFTs • Impaired wound healing • Infusion-related reactions • RPLS	• S/S of thromboembolism • BP • S/S of bleeding • Urinalysis • LFTs • S/S of GI perforation/fistula formation • S/S of infusion reactions • S/S of RPLS	↑ risk of cardiomyopathy with anthracyclines	Indicated for metastatic colorectal cancer; locally advanced, recurrent, or metastatic nonsquamous NSCLC; recurrent glioblastoma; metastatic renal cell carcinoma; persistent, recurrent, or metastatic cervical cancer; and stage III or IV epithelial ovarian, fallopian tube, or primary peritoneal cancer
Cabozantinib • Cabometyx, Cometriq • Caps (Cometriq), tabs (Cabometyx)		• Thromboembolic events • Hypertension • Hemorrhage • GI perforation/fistula formation • Diarrhea • Palmar-plantar erythro-dysesthesia syndrome • RPLS	• S/S of thromboembolism • BP • S/S of bleeding • S/S of GI perforation/fistula formation • S/S of dehydration • Electrolytes • S/S of RPLS	• CYP3A4 substrate • Avoid concomitant use of strong CYP3A4 inhibitors or inducers	• Indicated for advanced renal cell carcinoma (Cabometyx) or metastatic, medullary thyroid cancer (Cometriq) • Adjust dose in hepatic impairment

Vascular Endothelial Growth Factor (VEGF) Inhibitors *(cont'd)*

Generic • Brand • Dosage Forms	Contraindications	Primary Side Effects	Key Monitoring	Pertinent Drug Interactions	Med Pearl
Ramucirumab • Cyramza • Injection (IV)	None	• Thromboembolic events • Hypertension • Hemorrhage • GI perforation • Hypo-/hyperthyroidism • Proteinuria • ↑ LFTs • Impaired wound healing • Infusion-related reactions • RPLS	• S/S of thromboembolism • BP • S/S of bleeding • TFTs • Urinalysis • LFTs • S/S of GI perforation • S/S of infusion reactions • S/S of RPLS	None	• Indicated for advanced gastric adenocarcinoma; metastatic NSCLC; and metastatic colorectal cancer • Premedicate with diphenhydramine
Sorafenib • Nexavar • Tabs		• Myocardial ischemia/ infarction • Hepatotoxicity • Diarrhea • Rash (can be severe) • Hand-foot syndrome • Hypertension • QT interval prolongation • Hemorrhage • Hypo-/hyperthyroidism • Impaired wound healing • GI perforation	• LFTs • S/S of dehydration • Electrolytes • S/S of dermatologic reactions • BP • ECG • S/S of bleeding • TFTs • S/S of GI perforation	• CYP3A4 substrate • Avoid concomitant use of strong CYP3A4 inducers • May ↑ risk of bleeding with warfarin • ↑ risk of TdP with other drugs that prolong QT interval	Indicated for advanced renal cell carcinoma; unresectable hepatocellular carcinoma; and locally recurrent or metastatic, progressive differentiated thyroid cancer
Sunitinib • Sutent • Caps		• Hepatotoxicity • Diarrhea • Stevens-Johnson syndrome, toxic epidermal necrolysis • Hypertension • Heart failure • QT interval prolongation • Hemorrhage • Tumor lysis syndrome • Hypo-/hyperthyroidism • Proteinuria • Hypoglycemia • Impaired wound healing • Osteonecrosis (jaw)	• LFTs • S/S of dehydration • Electrolytes • S/S of dermatologic reactions • BP • LVEF • S/S of heart failure • ECG • S/S of bleeding • TFTs • Urinalysis • Glucose • BUN/SCr • Uric acid	• CYP3A4 substrate • Avoid concomitant use of strong CYP3A4 inhibitors or inducers • ↑ risk of osteonecrosis of the jaw with bisphosphonates	• Indicated for gastrointestinal stromal tumor (GIST); advanced renal cell carcinoma; high risk of recurrent renal cell carcinoma after nephrectomy; and unresectable locally advanced or metastatic pancreatic neuroendocrine tumors • Premedicate with antihyperuricemics and hydration in patients at ↑ risk for tumor lysis syndrome

Tyrosine Kinase Inhibitors

Generic • Brand • Dosage Forms	Contraindications	Primary Side Effects	Key Monitoring	Pertinent Drug Interactions	Med Pearl
Mechanism of action – halt proliferation of tumor cells by inhibiting tyrosine kinase					
Bosutinib • Bosulif • Tabs	None	• N/V/D • Myelosuppression • Hepatotoxicity • Renal impairment • Fluid retention	• S/S of dehydration • Electrolytes • CBC with differential • LFTs • BUN/SCr • S/S of peripheral/pulmonary edema	• CYP3A4 and P-gp substrate • P-gp inhibitor • Avoid concomitant use of strong or moderate CYP3A4 inhibitors or inducers • H_2-antagonists, PPIs, and antacids may ↓ absorption (avoid concomitant use of PPIs; may use H_2-antagonists or antacids [need to space administration])	• Indicated for Philadelphia-positive (Ph+) CML • Adjust dose in hepatic or renal impairment
Dasatinib • Sprycel • Tabs		• Myelosuppression • Hemorrhage • Fluid retention • Pulmonary arterial hypertension • Arrhythmias • Stevens-Johnson syndrome • Tumor lysis syndrome • QT interval prolongation	• CBC with differential • BUN/SCr • Uric acid • S/S of bleeding • S/S of peripheral/pulmonary edema • S/S of pulmonary arterial hypertension • S/S of dermatologic reactions • ECG	• CYP3A4 substrate and inhibitor • Avoid concomitant use of strong 3A4 inhibitors or inducers • H_2-antagonists, PPIs, and antacids may ↓ absorption (avoid concomitant use of H_2-antagonists and PPIs; may use antacids [need to space administration]) • ↑ risk of TdP with other drugs that prolong QT interval	• Indicated for Ph+ CML and Ph+ ALL • Premedicate with antihyperuricemics and hydration in patients at ↑ risk for tumor lysis syndrome
Imatinib • Gleevec • Tabs		• Myelosuppression • Hemorrhage • Fluid retention • Rash (can be severe) • Tumor lysis syndrome • Heart failure • Hepatotoxicity • Hypothyroidism • Renal impairment	• CBC with differential • BUN/SCr • Uric acid • S/S of bleeding • S/S of peripheral/pulmonary edema • S/S of dermatologic reactions • S/S of heart failure • LFTs • TFTs	• CYP3A4 substrate and inhibitor • CYP2D6 inhibitor • Avoid concomitant use of strong CYP3A4 inhibitors or inducers	• Indicated for Ph+ CML, Ph+ ALL, Kit (CD117)-positive GIST, and a variety of other disorders • Adjust dose in hepatic or renal impairment • Premedicate with antihyperuricemics and hydration in patients at ↑ risk for tumor lysis syndrome

Tyrosine Kinase Inhibitors *(cont'd)*

Generic • Brand • Dosage Forms	Contraindications	Primary Side Effects	Key Monitoring	Pertinent Drug Interactions	Med Pearl
Lenvatinib • Lenvima • Caps	None	• Thromboembolic events • Hypertension • Hemorrhage • Heart failure • Hepatotoxicity • Proteinuria • Renal failure • GI perforation/fistula formation • QT interval prolongation • Hypocalcemia • RPLS • Hypothyroidism • Impaired wound healing	• S/S of thromboembolism • BP • S/S of bleeding • LVEF • S/S of heart failure • LFTs • Urinalysis • BUN/SCr • S/S of GI perforation/ fistula formation • ECG • Electrolytes • S/S of RPLS • TFTs	↑ risk of TdP with other drugs that prolong QT interval	• Indicated for locally recurrent or metastatic, progressive radioactive iodine-refractory differentiated thyroid cancer and renal cell carcinoma • Adjust dose in hepatic or renal impairment
Nilotinib • Tasigna • Caps	• Hypokalemia • Hypomagnesemia • Long QT syndrome	• Myelosuppression • Hemorrhage • Fluid retention • QT interval prolongation • Cardiovascular events • Pancreatitis • Hepatotoxicity • Electrolyte abnormalities ($\downarrow PO_4$, $\downarrow$/$\uparrow K^+$, $\downarrow Na^+$) • Tumor lysis syndrome	• CBC with differential • BUN/SCr • Uric acid • S/S of bleeding • S/S of peripheral/ pulmonary edema • ECG • S/S of cardiovascular events • Amylase/lipase • Glucose • LFTs • Electrolytes	• CYP3A4 substrate and inhibitor • CYP2C8, CYP2C9, CYP2D6, and P-gp inhibitor • CYP2C9 inducer • Avoid concomitant use of strong CYP3A4 inhibitors or inducers • H_2-antagonists, PPIs, and antacids may $\downarrow$ absorption (avoid concomitant use of PPIs; may use antacids and H_2-antagonists [need to space administration]) • ↑ risk of TdP with other drugs that prolong QT interval	• Indicated for Ph+ CML • Take on empty stomach • Adjust dose in hepatic impairment • Premedicate with antihyperuricemics and hydration in patients at ↑ risk for tumor lysis syndrome

Anaplastic Lymphoma Kinase (ALK) Inhibitors

Generic • Brand • Dosage Forms	Contraindications	Primary Side Effects	Key Monitoring	Pertinent Drug Interactions	Med Pearl
Mechanism of action – reduce proliferation of tumor cells by inhibiting ALK					
Alectinib • Alecensa • Caps	None	• Hepatotoxicity • ILD • Bradycardia • Myalgias • Renal impairment	• ALK status • S/S of ILD • ECG • Heart rate (HR) • Creatine kinase • BUN/SCr	None	• Indicated for ALK-positive, metastatic NSCLC • Adjust dose in hepatic impairment
Brigatinib • Alunbrig • Tabs		• ILD • Hypertension • Bradycardia • Visual disturbances • Myalgias • Hyperglycemia • Pancreatitis	• ALK status • S/S of ILD • BP • ECG • HR • Creatine kinase • Glucose • Amylase/lipase • Ophthalmologic examination	• CYP3A4 substrate and inducer • Avoid concomitant use of strong 3A4 inhibitors or inducers	Indicated for ALK-positive, metastatic NSCLC
Ceritinib • Zykadia • Caps		• N/V/D • Hepatotoxicity • ILD • QT interval prolongation • Hyperglycemia • Bradycardia • Pancreatitis	• ALK status • S/S of dehydration • Electrolytes • LFTs • S/S of ILD • ECG • Glucose • HR • Amylase/lipase	• CYP3A4 substrate • CYP2C9 and CYP3A4 inhibitor • Avoid concomitant use of strong 3A4 inhibitors or inducers	• Indicated for ALK-positive, metastatic NSCLC • Adjust dose in hepatic impairment
Crizotinib • Xalkori • Caps		• N/V/D • Hepatotoxicity • ILD • QT interval prolongation • Bradycardia • Vision loss	• ALK status • ROS-1 status • S/S of dehydration • Electrolytes • BUN/SCr • LFTs • S/S of ILD • ECG • HR	• CYP3A4 substrate and inhibitor • Avoid concomitant use of strong CYP3A4 inhibitors or inducers • Avoid concomitant use of CYP3A4 substrates with narrow therapeutic range • ↑ risk of TdP with other drugs that prolong QT interval	• Indicated for ALK-positive or ROS-1-positive, metastatic NSCLC • Adjust dose in renal impairment

Platelet-Derived Growth Factor Receptor (PDGFR)-α Blocker

Generic • Brand • Dosage Forms	Contraindications	Primary Side Effects	Key Monitoring	Pertinent Drug Interactions	Med Pearl
Mechanism of action – monoclonal antibody that prevents binding of PDGF-AA, PDGF-BB, and PDGF-CC to PDGFR-α, which subsequently inhibits signaling to reduce cancer cell proliferation and metastasis					
Olaratumab • Lartruvo • Injection (IV)	None	• Infusion-related reactions • Myelosuppression	• CBC with differential • S/S of infusion reactions	None	• Indicated for soft tissue sarcoma • Should be used in combination with doxorubicin (for first 8 cycles) • Premedicate with diphenhydramine and dexamethasone (to prevent infusion reactions)

Poly (ADP-Ribose) Polymerase (PARP) Inhibitors

Generic • Brand • Dosage Forms	Contraindications	Primary Side Effects	Key Monitoring	Pertinent Drug Interactions	Med Pearl
Mechanism of action – inhibit PARP enzymes, resulting in ↑ formation of PARP-DNA complexes and subsequent DNA damage, apoptosis, and cell death					
Niraparib • Zejula • Caps	None	• Myelodysplastic syndrome/AML • Myelosuppression • Hypertension	• CBC with differential • BP	None	Indicated for recurrent epithelial ovarian, fallopian tube, or primary peritoneal cancer
Olaparib • Lynparza • Tabs		• Myelodysplastic syndrome/AML • Pneumonitis	• *BRCA* mutation status • CBC with differential • BUN/SCr • S/S of pneumonitis	• CYP3A4 substrate • Avoid concomitant use of strong or moderate CYP3A4 inhibitors or inducers	• Indicated for deleterious *BRCA*-mutated advanced ovarian cancer and deleterious *BRCA*-mutated HER2-negative metastatic breast cancer • Adjust dose in renal impairment
Rucaparib • Rubraca • Tabs		• Myelodysplastic syndrome/AML • Anemia	• *BRCA* mutation status • CBC with differential	None	Indicated for deleterious *BRCA*-mutated advanced ovarian cancer and recurrent epithelial ovarian, fallopian tube, or primary peritoneal cancer

Programmed Death Receptor-1 (PD-1) Inhibitors

Generic • Brand • Dosage Forms	Contraindications	Primary Side Effects	Key Monitoring	Pertinent Drug Interactions	Med Pearl
Mechanism of action – monoclonal antibody that binds to the PD-1 receptor and prevents binding of PD-L1 and PD-L2, which restores antitumor T-cell function, resulting in ↓ tumor growth					
Nivolumab • Opdivo • Injection (IV)	None	• Infusion-related reactions • ILD • Colitis/diarrhea • Hepatotoxicity • Hypophysitis • Adrenal insufficiency • Hypo-/hyperthyroidism • Type 1 diabetes • Renal impairment • Stevens-Johnson syndrome, toxic epidermal necrolysis • Encephalitis	• S/S of infusion reactions • S/S of ILD • LFTs • TFTs • Glucose • S/S of infection • BUN/SCr • Electrolytes (esp. if diarrhea)	None	Indicated for unresectable or metastatic melanoma; melanoma with involvement of lymph nodes or completely resected metastatic melanoma; metastatic NSCLC; advanced renal cell carcinoma; classical Hodgkin lymphoma; recurrent or metastatic squamous cell carcinoma of head and neck; locally advanced or metstatic urothelial carcinoma; unresectable or metastatic microsatellite instability; high or mismatch repair deficient colorectal cancer; and hepatocellular carcinoma

Programmed Death Receptor-1 (PD-1) Inhibitors   *(cont'd)*

Generic • Brand • Dosage Forms	Contraindications	Primary Side Effects	Key Monitoring	Pertinent Drug Interactions	Med Pearl
Pembrolizumab • Keytruda • Injection (IV)	None	• Infusion-related reactions • ILD • Colitis/diarrhea • Hepatotoxicity • Hypophysitis • Adrenal insufficiency • Hypo-/hyperthyroidism • Type 1 diabetes • Renal impairment • Stevens-Johnson syndrome, toxic epidermal necrolysis	• S/S of infusion reactions • S/S of ILD • LFTs • TFTs • Glucose • BUN/SCr • Electrolytes (esp. if diarrhea)	None	Indicated for unresectable or metastatic melanoma; metastatic NSCLC; advanced renal cell carcinoma; classical Hodgkin lymphoma; metastatic squamous cell carcinoma of head and neck; refractory primary mediastinal large B-cell lymphoma; locally advanced or metastatic urothelial carcinoma; unresectable or metastatic microsatellite instability; high or mismatch repair deficient solid tumors or colorectal cancer; locally advanced or metastatic gastric cancer; and recurrent or metastatic cervical cancer

Programmed Death Ligand-1 (PD-L1) Inhibitors

Generic • Brand • Dosage Forms	Contraindications	Primary Side Effects	Key Monitoring	Pertinent Drug Interactions	Med Pearl
Mechanism of action – monoclonal antibody that prevents binding of PD-L1 to PD-1 and B7.1 receptors on T cells, which restores antitumor T-cell function, resulting in ↓ tumor growth					
Atezolizumab • Tecentriq • Injection (IV)	None	• Infusion-related reactions • ILD • Hepatotoxicity • Colitis/diarrhea • Hypo-/hyperthyroidism • Hypophysitis • Adrenal insufficiency • Type 1 diabetes • Meningitis/encephalitis • Neuropathy • Pancreatitis • Myocarditis • Stevens-Johnson syndrome, toxic epidermal necrolysis • Infection	• S/S of infusion reactions • S/S of ILD • LFTs • TFTs • Glucose • S/S of infection • Electrolytes (esp. if diarrhea)	None	Indicated for locally advanced or metastatic urothelial carcinoma and metastatic NSCLC
Avelumab • Bavencio • Injection (IV)		• Infusion-related reactions • ILD • Hepatotoxicity • Colitis/diarrhea • Hypo-/hyperthyroidism • Adrenal insufficiency • Type 1 diabetes • Renal impairment	• S/S of infusion reactions • S/S of ILD • LFTs • TFTs • Glucose • BUN/SCr • Electrolytes (esp. if diarrhea)		• Indicated for metastatic Merkel cell carcinoma and locally advanced or metastatic urothelial carcinoma • Premedicate with diphenhydramine and acetaminophen before first 4 infusions (to prevent infusion reactions)

Programmed Death Ligand-1 (PD-L1) Inhibitors *(cont'd)*

Generic • Brand • Dosage Forms	Contraindications	Primary Side Effects	Key Monitoring	Pertinent Drug Interactions	Med Pearl
Durvalumab • Imfinzi • Injection (IV)	None	• Infusion-related reactions • ILD • Hepatotoxicity • Colitis/diarrhea • Hypo-/hyperthyroidism • Hypophysitis • Adrenal insufficiency • Type 1 diabetes • Renal impairment • Stevens-Johnson syndrome, toxic epidermal necrolysis • Infection	• S/S of infusion reactions • S/S of ILD • LFTs • TFTs • Glucose • BUN/SCr • S/S of infection • Electrolytes (esp. if diarrhea)	None	Indicated for locally advanced or metastatic urothelial carcinoma and unresectable Stage III NSCLC

B-Cell Lymphoma-2 (BCL-2) Inhibitor

Generic • Brand • Dosage Form	Contraindications	Primary Side Effects	Key Monitoring	Pertinent Drug Interactions	Med Pearl
Mechanism of action – inhibits BCL-2, an anti-apoptotic protein, which subsequently restores the apoptotic process					
Venetoclax • Venclexta • Tabs	Concurrent therapy with strong CYP3A4 inhibitors during the ramp-up period (first 5 weeks)	• Tumor lysis syndrome • Myelosuppression	• 17p deletion status • CBC with differential • BUN/SCr • Uric acid	• CYP3A4 and P-gp substrate • Avoid concomitant use of strong or moderate CYP3A4 inhibitors or inducers or P-gp inhibitors	• Indicated for CLL or small lymphocytic leukemia with/without 17p deletion • Take with a meal • Premedicate with antihyperuricemics and hydration in patients at ↑ risk for tumor lysis syndrome

Cyclin-Dependent Kinase (CDK) Inhibitors

Generic • Brand • Dosage Forms	Contraindications	Primary Side Effects	Key Monitoring	Pertinent Drug Interactions	Med Pearl
Mechanism of action – inhibits CDK 4 and 6, which subsequently reduces cell cycle progression, cellular proliferation, and cell cycle progression					
Abemaciclib • Verzenio • Tabs	None	• Diarrhea • Neutropenia • Hepatotoxicity • Venous thromboembolic events	• Electrolytes • CBC with differential • LFTs • S/S of thromboembolism	• CYP3A4 substrate • Avoid concomitant use of ketoconazole; for other strong CYP3A4 inhibitors, ↓ abemaciclib dose • Avoid concomitant use of strong CYP3A4 inducers	• Indicated for hormone receptor-positive, HER2-negative, advanced or metastatic breast cancer • Adjust dose in hepatic impairment
Palbociclib • Ibrance • Caps		Myelosuppression	CBC with differential	• CYP3A4 substrate and inhibitor • Avoid concomitant use of strong CYP3A4 inhibitors or inducers	• Indicated for hormone-receptor positive, HER2-negative, advanced or metastatic breast cancer • Should be used with aromatase inhibitor (in postmenopausal women) or fulvestrant • Adjust dose in hepatic impairment
Ribociclib • Kisqali • Tabs		• QT interval prolongation • Hepatotoxicity • Myelosuppression	• ECG • Electrolytes • LFTs • CBC with differential	• CYP3A4 substrate and inhibitor • Avoid concomitant use of strong CYP3A4 inhibitors or inducers • ↑ risk of TdP with other drugs that prolong QT interval and tamoxifen	• Indicated for postmenopausal women with hormone receptor-positive, HER2-negative advanced or metastatic breast cancer (with fulvestrant); also for pre-/perimenopausal or postmenopausal women with hormone receptor-positive, HER2-negative advanced or metastatic breast cancer (with aromatase inhibitor) • Adjust dose in hepatic impairment

SUPPORTIVE CARE

Nausea and Vomiting

About 55% of cancer patients experience nausea and vomiting during the first week of chemotherapy. $5HT_3$ antagonists are useful in most cases, but should be used only for prevention of nausea and vomiting. Corticosteroids should be given unless contraindicated, as they are synergistic with the $5HT_3$ antagonists; other drug therapies depend on the type of nausea and vomiting experienced.

- Benzodiazepines: Treatment of choice for anticipatory nausea and vomiting (caused by the sights and smells of the chemotherapy environment)
- Neurokinin-1 (NK-1) antagonist: Useful for delayed nausea and vomiting caused by drugs with high emetic potential (cisplatin, cyclophosphamide, doxorubicin)
- Prochlorperazine or metoclopramide: May be used in less severe cases

Management of Neutropenia and Anemia

Neutropenia and its major complication, neutropenic fever, are major concerns in many types of cancer. The nadir, or lowest, concentration of WBCs in the peripheral blood usually occurs 1–2 weeks following the administration of chemotherapy and is typically proportional to the dose. Subsequent chemotherapy is delayed until the ANC recovers, which explains the 3- to 4-week cycle length of most chemotherapy regimens. Classification of ANC is:

- Normal: 3,000–7,000 neutrophils/mm^3
- Mild neutropenia: 500–1,000/mm^3
- Moderate neutropenia: 100–500/mm^3
- Severe neutropenia: <100/mm^3

Colony-stimulating factors (CSF) such as filgrastim or PEG-filgrastim have been shown to shorten the duration of neutropenia, but they have little effect on mortality and are very expensive. CSFs do decrease hospitalizations, however, and clinical judgment should be used to determine which patients are most likely to benefit. Because infection leads to death in a large percentage of neutropenic patients (possibly up to 30%), anti-infective therapy is frequently needed. Broad-spectrum bactericidal antibiotics are generally used (third- and fourth-generation cephalosporins, carbapenems, or fluoroquinolones with or without aminoglycosides or β-lactams), with antipseudomonal activity being particularly important. If antifungal therapy is needed, amphotericin B is the drug of choice.

Anemia is also common in cancer patients. Treatment of anemia is currently the subject of much controversy; use of erythropoiesis-stimulating agents, including erythropoietin and darbepoetin, is no longer supported in myeloid malignancies (these agents have been associated with increase in mortality compared to patients not receiving erythropoietin). The hypothesis is that the drug may be stimulating cancer growth. These drugs should NOT be used in patients with myeloid malignancies who are receiving chemotherapy when the anticipated outcome is a cure. This finding may not apply to solid tumors; more information is needed. Refer to Chapter 8 for discussion of the erythropoiesis-stimulating agents.

Antiemetic Drugs

Generic • Brand • Dose • Dosage Forms	Contraindications	Primary Side Effects	Key Monitoring	Pertinent Drug Interactions	Med Pearl
Mechanism of action – 5HT$_3$ antagonists; prevent release of serotonin in GI mucosa					
Ondansetron ☆ • Zofran, Zuplenz • 16–24 mg PO or 8–12 mg IV • Films, injection (IV), orally disintegrating tabs, solution, tabs	Current N/V (useful only for prevention)	• Headache • Constipation or diarrhea • Fatigue • Dry mouth • Transient ↑ LFTs • QT interval prolongation	None	• CYP3A4 substrates • Use with serotonergic agents may ↑ risk of serotonin syndrome • ↑ risk of TdP with other drugs that prolong QT interval	• Single dose prior to chemotherapy; repeat doses do not ↑ effect • Palonosetron effective in preventing acute and delayed N/V • Extended-release granisetron subcut injection should NOT be administered more frequently than every 7 days (every 14 days in renal impairment)
Granisetron • Sancuso, Sustol • 2 mg PO, 1 mg IV, or 10 mg subcut • Extended-release injection (subcut), injection (IV), tabs, transdermal patch					
Dolasetron • Anzemet • 100 mg PO • Tabs					
Palonosetron • Aloxi • 0.25 mg IV • Injection (IV)					
Mechanism of action – NK-1 antagonist; block substance P from NK-1 receptor					
Aprepitant • Cinvanti, Emend • PO: 125 mg on day 1, then 80 mg daily on days 2 and 3 • IV: 100-130 mg on day 1 • Caps, injection (IV), suspension	None	• Asthenia • Fatigue • Diarrhea • Hiccups • Dizziness • Dehydration	Monitor levels of chemotherapy agents metabolized by CYP3A4	• CYP3A4 substrate and inhibitor • CYP2C9 inducer	• Use in combination with 5HT$_3$ antagonist and dexamethasone • Prevents acute and delayed N/V
Fosprepitant • Emend IV • 150 mg on day 1 • Injection (IV)					

Antiemetic Drugs   *(cont'd)*

Generic • Brand • Dose • Dosage Forms	Contraindications	Primary Side Effects	Key Monitoring	Pertinent Drug Interactions	Med Pearl
Rolapitant • Varubi • PO: 180 mg on day 1 • IV: 166.5 mg on day 1 • Tabs, injection (IV)	Concurrent therapy with thioridazine	• Neutropenia • Hiccups • Anorexia • Dizziness • Dyspepsia	CBC with differential	• CYP3A4 substrate • CYP2D6 inhibitor	• Used in combination with 5HT$_3$ antagonist and dexamethasone • Prevents delayed N/V
Netupitant (fosnetupitant)/palonosetron • Akynzeo • PO: 1 capsule (300 mg netupitant/0.5 mg palonosetron) on day 1 • IV: 235 mg fosnetupitant/0.25 mg palonosetron on day 1 • Caps, injection (IV)	None	• Dyspepsia • Fatigue • Constipation • Headache • Asthenia	Monitor levels of chemotherapy agents metabolized by CYP3A4	• CYP3A4 substrate and inhibitor • Use with serotonergic agents may ↑ risk of serotonin syndrome	• Netupitant is NK-1 antagonist; palonosetron is 5HT$_3$ antagonist • Used in combination with dexamethasone • Prevents acute and delayed N/V
Mechanism of action – corticosteroids; potentiate antiemetic properties of 5HT$_3$ antagonists					
Dexamethasone • Decadron • 8–40 mg daily PO/IV • Injection, solution, tabs	Systemic fungal infections	• Hyperglycemia • Immunosuppression • Adrenal suppression • Insomnia • Mood changes, anxiety • GI irritation • Weight gain	• Hemoglobin/hematocrit • Serum potassium • Glucose	CYP3A4 substrates	• Synergistic with 5HT$_3$ antagonists • Can use as single agents for mild chemotherapy-induced N/V
Methylprednisolone ☆ • Solu-Medrol • 40–125 mg daily IV • Injection					
Mechanism of action – dopamine-2 antagonist					
Metoclopramide ☆ • Reglan • 10–20 mg PO/IV q4–6h PRN • Injection, solution, tabs	Seizures	• Dizziness • Sedation • Diarrhea • Extrapyramidal symptoms (EPS)	EPS	Antipsychotic agents may ↑ risk of EPS	Should not drive or operate heavy machinery while taking this drug

Colony-Stimulating Factors

Generic • Brand • Dosage	Contraindications	Primary Side Effects	Key Monitoring	Pertinent Drug Interactions	Med Pearl
Mechanism of action – stimulate production of WBCs					
Filgrastim • Granix, Neupogen, Zarxio • 5 mcg/kg subcut daily	Hypersensitivity to *E. coli*	• Bone pain • Hypertension • Swelling • Redness • Hypersensitivity reactions	CBC with differential	Use lithium with caution, as it can potentiate neutrophil release	• Requires daily administration • Neutrophil-specific
Pegfilgrastim • Fulphila, Neulasta • 6 mg subcut with each chemotherapy cycle					• PEG unit ↑ half-life; can give once per chemotherapy cycle • Neutrophil-specific
Sargramostim • Leukine • 250–500 mcg/m^2/day subcut	• Hypersensitivity to yeast • Excessive leukemic myeloid blasts in bone marrow	• Fever, chills • Bone pain • Myalgia • Hypertension • Hypersensitivity reactions			• Requires daily administration • Stimulates formation of all WBCs except lymphocytes

Psychiatric Disorders

10

This chapter covers the following disease states:

- **Depression**
- **Anxiety**
- **Bipolar disorder**
- **Schizophrenia**
- **Sleep disorders**
- **Attention-deficit/hyperactivity disorder (ADHD)**

DEPRESSION

Guidelines Summary

- The primary goal of therapy is remission of symptoms.
- There are various antidepressant medications available. Clinical evidence indicates that, in general, efficacy is similar between classes.
- Initial choice of pharmacotherapy agent is based on anticipated side effects, tolerability of these side effects for an individual patient, comorbid conditions, drug interactions, patient preference, quantity and quality of clinical evidence, and cost.
- First-line options for most patients include selective serotonin reuptake inhibitors (SSRIs), serotonin norepinephrine reuptake inhibitors (SNRIs), bupropion, and mirtazapine. Because of the potential for serious side effects and drug interactions, monoamine oxidase inhibitors (MAOIs) should be reserved for patients who do not respond to other therapies.
- An adequate therapy trial requires at least 4–8 weeks. Dose adjustments or treatment changes are made at 4- to 6-week intervals based upon response but may occur earlier if medications are not tolerated.

- There is significant interpatient variability in response to antidepressants. Patients may respond to classes/agents that have been effective in the past or that have been effective for family members.

- Bupropion has a lower incidence of sexual side effects and may be preferred in patients presenting with this complaint related to therapy.

- In 2005, the Food and Drug Administration required that all product labeling for antidepressants include a boxed warning regarding the potential for ↑ risk of clinical worsening and suicidality in children, adolescents, and young adults (<24 years old) taking these agents.

Antidepressants

Generic • Brand • Dose/Dosage Forms	Contraindications	Primary Side Effects	Key Monitoring Parameters	Pertinent Drug Interactions	Med Pearls
Mechanism of action – SSRIs: inhibit reuptake of serotonin, allowing more serotonin availability in synapses					
Citalopram ☆ • Celexa • 10–40 mg daily • Age >60 yr: max = 20 mg daily • Solution, tabs	• Hypersensitivity • Use of MAOI within 2 wk • Concurrent use of pimozide • Concurrent use of linezolid or methylene blue • Congenital long QT syndrome • Use not recommended in patients with bradycardia, recent myocardial infarction (MI), uncompensated heart failure, hypokalemia, and hypomagnesemia	• Lightheadedness • Syncope • ↑ sweating • N/D • Xerostomia • Confusion • Dizziness • Somnolence • Insomia • Tremor • Ejaculation disorders • Impotence • Fatigue • Female sexual disorder • QT interval prolongation • Serotonin syndrome • Hyponatremia	• Reduction or resolution of symptoms • Withdrawal symptoms from abrupt discontinuation • Abnormal bleeding • Worsening of depression, suicidality, or unusual behavior at initiation of therapy or when changing dose • S/S of serotonin syndrome	• CYP2C19 and CYP3A4 substrate • CYP2C19 or CYP3A4 inhibitors may ↑ effects/toxicity; max dose = 20 mg/day when used with CYP2C19 inhibitors due to risk of QTc interval prolongation • CYP2C19 or CYP3A4 inducers may ↓ effects • ↑ risk of serotonin syndrome with MAOIs, SNRIs, triptans, tricyclic antidepressants (TCAs), amphetamines, fentanyl, lithium, dextromethorphan, meperidine, buspirone, linezolid, methylene blue, St. John's wort, and tramadol • ↑ risk of bleeding when used with aspirin, nonsteroidal anti-inflammatory drugs (NSAIDs), or anticoagulants	• Racemic mixture of R- and S- isomers • QTc interval prolongation, dose dependent risk, highest risk > 40 mg/ day • Max dose of 20 mg/day in severe hepatic impairment
Escitalopram ☆ • Lexapro • 10–20 mg daily • Solution, tabs	• Hypersensitivity • Use of MAOI within 2 wk • Concurrent use of pimozide • Concurrent use of linezolid or methylene blue				• Contains only the S-isomer of citalopram • Adjust dose in hepatic impairment

Antidepressants *(cont'd)*

Generic • Brand • Dose/Dosage Forms	Contraindications	Primary Side Effects	Key Monitoring Parameters	Pertinent Drug Interactions	Med Pearls
Fluoxetine ☆ • Prozac, Prozac Weekly, Sarafem • 20–80 mg daily or 90 mg weekly • Caps, ER caps, solution, tabs	• Hypersensitivity • Use of MAOI within 5 wk • Use of thioridazine within 5 wk • Concurrent use of pimozide • Concurrent use of linezolid or methylene blue	[Same as above]	[Same as above]	• CYP2C9 and CYP2D6 substrate • CYP2D6 inhibitor • CYP2C9 or CYP2D6 inhibitors may ↑ effects/toxicity • CYP2C9 inducers may ↓ effects • May ↑ effects/toxicity of CYP2D6 substrates • ↑ risk of serotonin syndrome with MAOIs, SNRIs, triptans, TCAs, amphetamines, fentanyl, lithium, dextromethorphan, meperidine, buspirone, linezolid, methylene blue, St. John's wort, and tramadol • ↑ risk of bleeding when used with aspirin, NSAIDs, or anticoagulants	• Allow 5 wk washout prior to using MAOI due to long half-life • Does not require taper due to long half-life • Also indicated for premenstrual dysphoric disorder (PMDD)
Fluvoxamine • Luvox • 50–300 mg daily • ER caps, tabs	• Hypersensitivity • Concurrent use of tizanidine, thioridazine, alosetron, or pimozide • Use of MAOI within 2 wk • Concurrent use of linezolid or methylene blue			• CYP1A2 and CYP2D6 substrate • CYP1A2 and CYP2C19 inhibitor • CYP1A2 or CYP2D6 inhibitors may ↑ effects/toxicity • CYP1A2 inducers may ↓ effects • May ↑ effects/toxicity of CYP1A2 or CYP2C19 substrates • ↑ risk of serotonin syndrome with MAOIs, SNRIs, triptans, TCAs, amphetamines, fentanyl, lithium, dextromethorphan, meperidine, buspirone, linezolid, methylene blue, St. John's wort, and tramadol • ↑ risk of bleeding when used with aspirin, NSAIDs, or anticoagulants	Only approved to treat obsessive-compulsive disorder (OCD)

Antidepressants *(cont'd)*

Generic • Brand • Dose/Dosage Forms	Contraindications	Primary Side Effects	Key Monitoring Parameters	Pertinent Drug Interactions	Med Pearls
Paroxetine ☆ • Paxil, Paxil CR, Pexeva • IR: 20–50 mg daily • ER: 25–62.5 mg daily • Suspension, tabs	• Hypersensitivity • Concurrent use of thioridazine or pimozide • Use of MAOI within 2 wk • Concurrent use of linezolid or methylene blue	[Same as above]	[Same as above]	• CYP2D6 substrate and inhibitor • CYP2D6 inhibitors may ↑ effects/toxicity • May ↑ effects/toxicity of CYP2D6 substrates • ↑ risk of serotonin syndrome with MAOIs, SNRIs, triptans, TCAs, amphetamines, fentanyl, lithium, dextromethorphan, meperidine, buspirone, linezolid, methylene blue, St. John's wort, and tramadol • ↑ risk of bleeding when used with aspirin, NSAIDs, or anticoagulants	• Short half-life may ↑ risk for discontinuation syndrome • Associated with more sedation, weight gain, sexual dysfunction, and anticholinergic adverse events compared to other SSRIs • Brisdelle approved to treat vasomotor symptoms of menopause • Paxil CR also approved for PMDD • Adjust dose in renal impairment
Sertraline ☆ • Zoloft • 50–200 mg daily • Solution, tabs	• Hypersensitivity • Use of MAOI within 2 wk • Concurrent use of pimozide • Concurrent use of disulfiram-like products (oral concentrate contains alcohol) • Concurrent use of linezolid or methylene blue			• CYP2C19 and CYP2D6 substrate • CYP2D6 inhibitor • CYP2C19 or CYP2D6 inhibitors may ↑ effects/toxicity • CYP2C19 inducers may ↓ effects • May ↑ effects/toxicity of CYP2D6 substrates • ↑ risk of serotonin syndrome with MAOIs, SNRIs, triptans, TCAs, amphetamines, fentanyl, lithium, dextromethorphan, meperidine, buspirone, linezolid, methylene blue, St. John's wort, and tramadol • ↑ risk of bleeding when used with aspirin, NSAIDs, or anticoagulants	• Associated with high prevalence of nausea and diarrhea • Oral concentrate contains alcohol • Also indicated for PMDD

Antidepressants *(cont'd)*

Generic • Brand • Dose/Dosage Forms	Contraindications	Primary Side Effects	Key Monitoring Parameters	Pertinent Drug Interactions	Med Pearls
Mechanism of action – SSRI, 5-HT1A receptor agonist, 5-HT3 receptor antagonist					
Vortioxetine • Trintellix • 5–20 mg daily • Tabs	• Hypersensitivity • Use of MAOI within 2–3 wk • Concurrent use of linezolid or methylene blue	• N/V/D • Sexual dysfunction • Dizziness • Xerostomia • Constipation • Serotonin syndrome	• Reduction or resolution of symptoms • Withdrawal symptoms from abrupt discontinuation • Abnormal bleeding • Worsening of depression, suicidality, or unusual behavior at initiation of therapy or when changing dose • S/S of serotonin syndrome	• CYP2D6 and 3A4 substrate • CYP2D6 or CYP3A4 inhibitors may ↑ effects/toxicity; ↓ dose by 50% when used with strong CYP2D6 inhibitor • CYP3A4 inducers may ↓ effects • ↑ risk of serotonin syndrome with MAOIs, SNRIs, triptans, TCAs, amphetamines, fentanyl, lithium, dextromethorphan, meperidine, buspirone, linezolid, methylene blue, St. John's wort, and tramadol • ↑ risk of bleeding when used with aspirin, NSAIDs, or anticoagulants	Associated with high prevalence of nausea and diarrhea
Mechanism of action – SSRI, partial 5-HT1A receptor agonist					
Vilazodone • Viibryd • 10–40 mg daily • Tabs	Use of MAOI within 2 wk	• N/D • Xerostomia • Dizziness • Insomnia • Serotonin syndrome	• Reduction or resolution of symptoms • Withdrawal symptoms from abrupt discontinuation • Abnormal bleeding • Worsening of depression, suicidality, or unusual behavior at initiation of therapy or when changing dose • S/S of serotonin syndrome	• CYP3A4 substrate • CYP3A4 inhibitors may ↑ effects/toxicity; max dose = 20 mg/day when used with strong CYP3A4 inhibitors • CYP3A4 inducers may ↓ effects; consider ↑ dose when used with strong CYP3A4 inducers (max dose = 80 mg/day) • ↑ risk of serotonin syndrome with MAOIs, SNRIs, triptans, TCAs, amphetamines, fentanyl, lithium, dextromethorphan, meperidine, buspirone, linezolid, methylene blue, St. John's wort, and tramadol • ↑ risk of bleeding when used with aspirin, NSAIDs, or anticoagulants	• Take with food to enhance absorption • Associated with high prevalence of nausea and diarrhea

Antidepressants *(cont'd)*

Generic • Brand • Dose/Dosage Forms	Contraindications	Primary Side Effects	Key Monitoring Parameters	Pertinent Drug Interactions	Med Pearls
Mechanism of action – TCAs: ↑ synaptic concentration of norepinephrine and serotonin					
Amitriptyline ☆ • Only available as generic • 25–300 mg/day in 1–3 divided doses • Tabs Amoxapine • Only available as generic • 50–600 mg/day in 2–3 divided doses • Tabs	• Hypersensitivity • Use of MAOI within 2 wk • Concurrent use of linezolid or methylene blue • Acute recovery period post-MI	• Anticholinergic symptoms • Weight gain • Bloating • Blurred vision • Xerostomia • Constipation • Dizziness • Somnolence • Headache • Fatigue • Serotonin syndrome	• Reduction or resolution of symptoms • Withdrawal symptoms from abrupt discontinuation • Worsening of depression, suicidality, or unusual behavior at initiation of therapy or when changing dose • Blood pressure (BP) • Electrocardiogram (ECG) (in patients with cardiac disease or hyperthyroidism) • Incidence of seizures due to seizure threshold lowering • S/S of serotonin syndrome • Therapeutic blood concentrations	• CYP2D6 substrate • CYP2D6 inhibitors may ↑ effects/ toxicity • ↑ risk of serotonin syndrome with MAOIs, SSRIs, SNRIs, triptans, fentanyl, lithium, dextromethorphan, meperidine, buspirone, linezolid, methylene blue, St. John's wort, and tramadol	• Dangerous in overdose situations • Avoid in patients with high suicidality • Avoid dispensing large quantities • Also used for sleep disorders and for the treatment of neuropathic pain • Anticholinergic side effects may adversely effect older adults
Clomipramine • Anafranil • 25–250 mg/day in 3 divided doses • Caps					• Dangerous in overdose situations • Avoid in patients with high suicidality • Avoid dispensing large quantities • Indicated only for OCD
Desipramine • Norpramin • 25–300 mg/day in 1–2 divided doses • Tabs					• Dangerous in overdose situations • Avoid in patients with high suicidality • Avoid dispensing large quantities

Antidepressants *(cont'd)*

Generic • **Brand** • **Dose/Dosage Forms**	**Contraindications**	**Primary Side Effects**	**Key Monitoring Parameters**	**Pertinent Drug Interactions**	**Med Pearls**
Doxepin ☆ • Silenor, Zonalon • 25–300 mg/day in 1–3 divided doses • Caps, solution, tabs, topical cream	[Same as above]	[Same as above]	[Same as above]	[Same as above]	• Dangerous in overdose situations • Avoid in patients with high suicidality • Avoid dispensing large quantities • Silenor approved for the treatment of insomnia • Zonalon approved for treatment of pruritus
Imipramine ☆ • Tofranil • 75–300 mg/day in 1–2 divided doses • Caps, tabs					• Dangerous in overdose situations • Avoid in patients with high suicidality • Avoid dispensing large quantities
Nortriptyline ☆ • Pamelor • 75–150 mg/day in 3–4 divided doses • Caps, solution					
Protriptyline • Vivactil • 10–60 mg/day in 3–4 divided doses • Tabs					
Trimipramine • Surmontil • 25–300 mg/day in 1–3 divided doses • Caps				• CYP2C19, CYP2D6, and CYP3A4 substrate • CYP2C19, CYP2D6, or CYP3A4 inhibitors may ↑ effects/toxicity • CYP2C19 or CYP3A4 inducers may ↓ effects • ↑ risk of serotonin syndrome with MAOIs, SSRIs, SNRIs, triptans, fentanyl, lithium, dextromethorphan, meperidine, buspirone, linezolid, methylene blue, St. John's wort, and tramadol	

Antidepressants *(cont'd)*

Generic • Brand • Dose/Dosage Forms	Contraindications	Primary Side Effects	Key Monitoring Parameters	Pertinent Drug Interactions	Med Pearls
Mechanism of action – SNRIs: inhibit the reuptake of serotonin and norepinephrine to allow higher available synaptic concentrations					
Duloxetine ☆ • Cymbalta • 30–120 mg/day in 1–2 divided doses • DR caps	• Hypersensitivity • Use of MAOI within 2 wk • Concurrent use of linezolid or methylene blue • Hepatic impairment • Severe renal impairment (CrCl <30 mL/min)	• Hepatotoxicity • Orthostatic hypotension • Rash (Stevens-Johnson syndrome possible) • Palpitations • ↑ sweating • Constipation • ↓ appetite • N/D • Xerostomia • Asthenia • Dizziness • Insomnia or somnolence • Vertigo • Blurred vision • Polyuria • ↓ libido • Serotonin syndrome	• Liver function tests (LFTs) • BP • Reduction or resolution of symptoms • Withdrawal symptoms from abrupt discontinuation • Abnormal bleeding • Worsening of depression, suicidality, or unusual behavior at initiation of therapy or when changing dose • S/S of serotonin syndrome	• CYP1A2 and CYP2D6 substrate • CYP1A2 or CYP2D6 inhibitors may ↑ effects/toxicity; avoid concomitant use with strong CYP1A2 inhibitors • CYP1A2 inducers may ↓ effects • ↑ risk of serotonin syndrome with MAOIs, SSRIs, triptans, amphetamines, TCAs, fentanyl, lithium, dextromethorphan, meperidine, buspirone, linezolid, methylene blue, St. John's wort, and tramadol • ↑ risk of bleeding when used with aspirin, NSAIDs, or anticoagulants	• Doses >60 mg/day may not provide additional benefit • May also be used to treat neuropathic and musculo-skeletal pain, fibromyalgia, and GAD
Venlafaxine ☆ • Effexor XR • IR: 37.5–225 mg/day in 2–3 divided doses • XR: 37.5–225 mg/day • ER caps/tabs, IR tabs		• Hypertension • ↑ sweating • Weight loss • Constipation • ↓ appetite • Nausea • Xerostomia • Insomnia or somnolence • Erectile dysfunction • Serotonin syndrome	• BP • Reduction or resolution of symptoms • Withdrawal symptoms from abrupt discontinuation • Abnormal bleeding • Worsening of depression, suicidality, or unusual behavior at initiation of therapy or when changing dose • S/S of serotonin syndrome	• CYP2D6 and CYP3A4 substrate • CYP2D6 or CYP3A4 inhibitors may ↑ effects/toxicity • CYP3A4 inducers may ↓ effects • ↑ risk of serotonin syndrome with MAOIs, SSRIs, triptans, amphetamines, TCAs, fentanyl, lithium, dextromethorphan, meperidine, buspirone, linezolid, methylene blue, St. John's wort, and tramadol • ↑ risk of bleeding when used with aspirin, NSAIDs, or anticoagulants	Adjust dose in renal or hepatic impairment

Antidepressants *(cont'd)*

Generic • Brand • Dose/Dosage Forms	Contraindications	Primary Side Effects	Key Monitoring Parameters	Pertinent Drug Interactions	Med Pearls
Levomilnacipran • Fetzima • 20–120 mg daily • ER caps	[Same as above]	• Nausea • Orthostasis • Constipation • ↑ sweating • Tachycardia • Serotonin syndrome • Sexual dysfunction • Hypertension • Urinary retention	• BP • Heart rate • Renal function • Reduction or resolution of symptoms • Withdrawal symptoms from abrupt discontinuation • Abnormal bleeding • Worsening of depression, suicidality, or unusual behavior at initiation of therapy or when changing dose • S/S of serotonin syndrome	• CYP3A4 substrate • CYP3A4 inhibitors may ↑ effects/ toxicity; max dose = 80 mg/day when used with strong CYP3A4 inhibitors • CYP3A4 inducers may ↓ effects • ↑ risk of serotonin syndrome with MAOIs, SSRIs, triptans, amphet- amines, TCAs, fentanyl, lithium, dextromethorphan, meperidine, buspirone, linezolid, methylene blue, St. John's wort, and tramadol • ↑ risk of bleeding when used with aspirin, NSAIDs, or anticoagulants	Adjust dose in renal impairment
Milnacipran • Savella • 12.5–200 mg/day in 2 divided doses • Tabs		• N/V • Headache • Insomnia • Hot flashes • Constipation • Dizziness • Hypertension • Palpitations • ↑ sweating • Sexual dysfunction • Urinary retention		• ↑ risk of serotonin syndrome with MAOIs, SSRIs, triptans, amphet- amines, TCAs, fentanyl, lithium, dextromethorphan, meperidine, buspirone, linezolid, methylene blue, St. John's wort, and tramadol • ↑ risk of bleeding when used with aspirin, NSAIDs, or anticoagulants	Indicated only for fibromyalgia
Desvenlafaxine ☆ • Khedezla, Pristiq • 50 mg daily • ER tabs		• Hypertension • Nausea • Dizziness • Insomnia or somnolence • ↑ sweating • Constipation • ↓ appetite • Anxiety • Sexual dysfunction • Serotonin syndrome	• BP • Reduction or resolution of symptoms • Withdrawal symptoms from abrupt discontinuation • Abnormal bleeding • Worsening of depression, suicidality, or unusual behavior at initiation of therapy or when changing dose • S/S of serotonin syndrome	• ↑ risk of serotonin syndrome with MAOIs, SSRIs, triptans, amphet- amines, TCAs, fentanyl, lithium, dextromethorphan, meperidine, buspirone, linezolid, methylene blue, St. John's wort, and tramadol • ↑ risk of bleeding when used with aspirin, NSAIDs, or anticoagulants	Adjust dose in renal or hepatic impairment

Antidepressants (cont'd)

Generic • Brand • Dose/Dosage Forms	Contraindications	Primary Side Effects	Key Monitoring Parameters	Pertinent Drug Interactions	Med Pearls
Mechanism of action – serotonin reuptake inhibitor/antagonist					
Trazodone • Only available as generic • 25–600 mg/day • Tabs	• Hypersensitivity • Use of MAOI within 14 days • Concurrent use of linezolid or methylene blue	• Sedation • Headache • Dizziness • Fatigue • Constipation • Sexual dysfunction • Blurred vision • Serotonin syndrome	• LFTs • Worsening of depression, suicidality, or unusual behavior at initiation of therapy or when changing dose • S/S of serotonin syndrome	• CYP3A4 substrate • ↑ risk of serotonin syndrome with MAOIs, SSRIs, SNRIs, triptans, amphetamines, fentanyl, lithium, dextromethorphan, meperidine, buspirone, linezolid, methylene blue, St. John's wort, and tramadol • ↑ risk of bleeding when used with aspirin, NSAIDs, or anticoagulants	Mostly used for the treatment of insomnia
Nefazodone • Only available as generic • 100–600 mg/day in 1–2 divided doses • Tabs	• Hypersensitivity • Previous nefazodone-induced hepatic damage • Hepatic impairment • Use of MAOI within 2 wk • Concurrent use with carbamazepine, tri-azolam, or pimozide	• Hepatotoxicity • Lightheaded-ness • Constipation • Nausea • Xerostomia • Urinary retention • Blurred vision • Confusion • Dizziness • Insomnia or somnolence • Sexual dysfunction • Serotonin syndrome	• LFTs • Reduction or resolution of symptoms • Withdrawal symptoms from abrupt discontinuation • Abnormal bleeding • Worsening of depression, suicidality, or unusual behavior at initiation of therapy or when changing dose • S/S of serotonin syndrome	• CYP2D6 and CYP3A4 substrate • CYP2D6 or CYP3A4 inhibitors may ↑ effects/toxicity • CYP3A4 inducers may ↓ effects • ↑ risk of serotonin syndrome with MAOIs, SSRIs, triptans, amphet-amines, TCAs, fentanyl, lithium, dextromethorphan, meperidine, buspirone, linezolid, methylene blue, St. John's wort, and tramadol • ↑ risk of bleeding when used with aspirin, NSAIDs, or anticoagulants	Black box warning for hepatotoxicity

Antidepressants *(cont'd)*

Generic • Brand • Dose/Dosage Forms	Contraindications	Primary Side Effects	Key Monitoring Parameters	Pertinent Drug Interactions	Med Pearls
Mechanism of action – MAOIs: ↑ epinephrine, norepinephrine, dopamine, and serotonin through inhibition of monoamine oxidase					
Isocarboxazid • Marplan • 10–60 mg/day in 2–4 divided doses • Tabs	• Hypersensitivity • Concurrent use of sympathomimetics, SSRIs, SNRIs, TCAs, central nervous system depressants, bupropion, meperidine, buspirone, dextromethorphan, anesthetics, or high-tyramine foods • Cardiovascular disease • Hypertension • Cerebrovascular disease • History of headache • Pheochromocytoma • Hepatic impairment • Severe renal impairment	• Weight gain • Orthostatic hypotension • Constipation • Xerostomia • Dizziness • Headache • Insomnia or somnolence • Blurred vision • Anxiety • Serotonin syndrome	• BP • LFTs • Reduction or resolution of symptoms • Withdrawal symptoms from abrupt discontinuation • Abnormal bleeding • Worsening of depression, suicidality, or unusual behavior at initiation of therapy or when changing dose • S/S of serotonin syndrome	• ↑ risk of serotonin syndrome with SSRIs, SNRIs, triptans, amphetamines, TCAs, fentanyl, lithium, dextromethorphan, meperidine, buspirone, linezolid, methylene blue, St. John's wort, and tramadol • ↑ risk of hypertensive crises with sympathomimetics and high-tyramine foods	Used very infrequently due to poor side effect profile and risk of drug and food interactions
Phenelzine • Nardil • 45–90 mg daily (TID–QID) • Tabs	• Cardiovascular disease • Hypertension • Cerebrovascular disease • Concurrent administration of interacting medications • General anesthesia • History of headache • Hypersensitivity • Pheochromocytoma • Severe renal impairment				
Tranylcypromine • Parnate • 30–60 mg daily (divided doses) • Tabs					
Selegiline • Emsam • 6–12 mg daily transdermal patch (max = 12 mg/ 24 hrs) • Transdermal patch	• Concurrent use of sympathomimetics, SSRIs, SNRIs, TCAs, bupropion, meperidine, tramadol, methadone, buspirone, dextromethorphan, carbamazepine, or high-tyramine foods • <12 yr old • Pheochromocytoma				• Apply patch once daily • Patch indicated for depression, not Parkinson's disease

Antidepressants *(cont'd)*

Generic • Brand • Dose/Dosage Forms	Contraindications	Primary Side Effects	Key Monitoring Parameters	Pertinent Drug Interactions	Med Pearls
Mechanism of action – weak inhibitor of dopamine and norepinephrine reuptake					
Bupropion☆ • Aplenzin, Forfivo XL, Wellbutrin SR, Wellbutrin XL • IR: 200–450 mg/day in 2–4 divided doses • SR: 150–400 mg in 2 divided doses • ER/XL: 150–450 mg daily • ER 12 hour tabs, ER/XL 24 hour tabs, IR tabs	• Hypersensitivity • Bulimia or anorexia • Abrupt discontinuation of alcohol, benzodiazepines, barbiturates, or AEDs • Seizure disorders • Use of MAOI within 2 wk • Concurrent use of linezolid or methylene blue	• Taste disturbance • Agitation • ↑ seizure activity • Hypertension • Psychotic symptoms • Anaphylaxis • Headache • Tachycardia • Weight loss	• Reduction or resolution of symptoms • Withdrawal symptoms from abrupt discontinuation • Worsening of depression, suicidality, or unusual behavior at initiation of therapy or when changing dose • Seizure activity	• CYP2B6 substrate • CYP2D6 inhibitor • CYP2B6 inhibitors may ↑ effects/toxicity • CYP2B6 inducers may ↓ effects • May ↑ effects/toxicity of CYP2D6 substrates • ↑ risk of hypertensive crises with MAOIs • May ↓ digoxin levels	Also used for smoking cessation (Zyban)
Mechanism of action – tetracyclic antidepressants: ↑ available synaptic concentrations of norepinephrine and/or serotonin					
Maprotiline • Only available as generic • 25–225 mg/day in 2–3 divided doses • Tabs	• Hypersensitivity • Seizure disorder • Use of MAOI within 2 wk • Acute recovery period post-MI	• ↑ seizure activity • Somnolence • Constipation • Nausea • Xerostomia	• Reduction or resolution of symptoms • Withdrawal symptoms from abrupt discontinuation • Worsening of depression, suicidality, or unusual behavior at initiation of therapy or when changing dose • Seizure activity	• CYP2D6 substrate • CYP2D6 inhibitors may ↑ effects/toxicity	None
Mirtazapine☆ • Remeron, Remeron SolTab • 15–45 mg at bedtime • ODTs, tabs	• Hypersensitivity • Use of MAOI within 2 wk	• ↑ appetite • Hyperlipidemia • Weight gain • Constipation • Somnolence • ↑ LFTs • Agranulocytosis • Serotonin syndrome	• Reduction or resolution of symptoms • Worsening of depression, suicidality, or unusual behavior at initiation of therapy or when changing dose • CBC • Weight • Lipid profile • Renal function • LFTs	• CYP1A2, CYP2D6, and CYP3A4 substrate • CYP1A2, CYP2D6, or CYP3A4 inhibitors may ↑ effects/toxicity • CYP1A2 or CYP3A4 inducers may ↓ effects	• Dosed at bedtime due to somnolence • Off-label use for appetite stimulation

ANXIETY

Summary of Treatment Recommendations

- Goals of therapy include improvement in overall functionality and quality of life through reduction of symptom frequency and intensity. Complete remission of illness is the long-term treatment goal.

- Treatment options are detailed in the medication charts and no consensus exists as to the preferred initial therapy or order of options thereafter. Not all medications are equivalent in the treatment of all anxiety disorders.

- Many clinicians prefer antidepressants (SSRIs, venlafaxine, duloxetine) as initial therapy due to their favorable side-effect profile as compared to other therapies. Benzodiazepines are commonly used, especially in acute situations. Although efficacious, these agents lend themselves to issues related to abuse/dependence, ↑ fall risk in the elderly, and potential for negative cognitive effects in general. Buspirone is a unique treatment option that is effective but requires 4 to 6 weeks to reach efficacy; thus, it is not useful in acute situations.

- Benzodiazepine selection should take into account varying pharmacokinetic profiles of agents. In elderly patients and those with hepatic impairment, preference is given to those agents that are shorter acting (less accumulation) and those metabolized by glucoronidation (e.g., lorazepam, oxazepam) versus oxidation (e.g., alprazolam, diazepam). Agents with a rapid onset and those with shorter half-lives have a greater potential for abuse.

Anxiolytics

Generic • Brand • Dose/Dosage Forms	Contraindications	Primary Side Effects	Key Monitoring Parameters	Pertinent Drug Interactions	Med Pearls
Mechanism of action – benzodiazepines: bind to GABA receptors, causing an influx of chloride which results in hyperpolarization and a less excitable state					
Alprazolam ☆ • Xanax, Xanax XR • IR: 0.75–4 mg/day in 2–3 divided doses • ER: 0.5–6 mg daily • ER tabs, ODTs, solution, tabs	• Hypersensitivity • Narrow-angle glaucoma • Concurrent use with ketoconazole or itraconazole (alprazolam) • Significant hepatic impairment (clonazepam) • Myasthenia gravis, severe respiratory impairment, severe hepatic impairment, or sleep apnea (diazepam)	• Somnolence • Ataxia • Dizziness • Changes in appetite • ↓ libido • Confusion • Constipation • Blurred vision • Dependence	• BP • Excessive sedation • Signs of withdrawal • LFTs (for chronic therapy)	• CYP3A4 substrates • CYP3A4 inhibitors may ↑ effects/ toxicity • CYP3A4 inducers may ↓ effects • Other CNS depressants, including alcohol, may ↑ CNS depressant effects • Use with opioids may lead to sedation, respiratory depression, coma, or death	• Schedule IV controlled substance • Adjust dose in severe hepatic impairment • Avoid use in pregnancy • Smoking ↓ concentration by up to 50% • Rapid onset, short-acting
Chlordiazepoxide • Librium • 5–25 mg 3–4 × /day • Caps					• Schedule IV controlled substance • Avoid in elderly • Avoid use in pregnancy • Slower-onset, long-acting
Clonazepam ☆ • Klonopin • 0.25–2 mg BID • ODTs, tabs					• Schedule IV controlled substance • Avoid use in pregnancy • Intermediate-onset, long-acting
Clorazepate • Tranxene T-Tab • 3.75–15 mg 2–4 × /day • Tabs					• Schedule IV controlled substance • Avoid in elderly • Avoid use in pregnancy • Rapid-onset, long-acting
Diazepam ☆ • Diastat, Valium • 2–10 mg PO 2–4 × /day • 2–10 mg IV/IM every 3–4 hr PRN • Injection, rectal gel, solution, tabs					• Schedule IV controlled substance • Avoid use in pregnancy • Rapid-onset, long-acting
Lorazepam ☆ • Ativan • 0.5–2 mg 2–3 × /day (max = 10 mg/day) • Injection, solution, tabs				• Hepatic conjugation • Not affected by CYP3A4 • Use with opioids may lead to sedation, respiratory depression, coma, or death	• Schedule IV controlled substance • Avoid use in pregnancy • Medium-onset, short-acting
Oxazepam • Only availably generically • 10–30 mg 3–4 × /day • Caps					• Schedule IV controlled substance • Avoid use in pregnancy • Medium-onset, short-acting

Anxiolytics *(cont'd)*

Generic • Brand • Dose/Dosage Forms	Contraindications	Primary Side Effects	Key Monitoring Parameters	Pertinent Drug Interactions	Med Pearls
Mechanism of action – SSRIs: selectively inhibit the reuptake of serotonin by presynaptic neuronal membranes with little to no effect on norepinephrine or dopamine reuptake					
Citalopram ☆ • Celexa • Details in antidepressants table	[See Antidepressants table]		Unlabeled use for panic disorder, GAD, posttraumatic stress disorder (PTSD), and OCD		
Escitalopram ☆ • Lexapro • Details in antidepressants table			Indicated for GAD		
Fluoxetine ☆ • Prozac, Sarafem • Details in antidepressants table			Indicated for OCD, panic disorder		
Paroxetine ☆ • Paxil, Paxil CR • Details in antidepressants table			Indicated for panic disorder, PTSD, GAD, OCD, social anxiety disorder (SAD)		
Sertraline ☆ • Zoloft • Details in antidepressants table			Indicated for OCD, panic disorder, SAD, PTSD		
Fluvoxamine • Luvox • Details in antidepressants table			Indicated for OCD		
Mechanism of action – nonselective β-adrenergic blocker which competitively blocks response to β_1- and β_2-adrenergic stimulation in the heart muscle, vascular smooth muscle, and bronchial muscles					
Propranolol ☆ (nonselective) • Inderal, Inderal LA, InnoPran XL • 10–80 mg 1 hr prior to anxiogenic event	• Hypersensitivity • Severe bradycardia • Heart block • Acute decompensated heart failure • Severe chronic obstructive pulmonary disease (COPD) or asthma	• Dizziness • Fatigue • Bradycardia • Gastrointesinal upset • Hypotension	• HR • BP	Use with other negative chronotropes (e.g., digoxin, verapamil, diltiazem, clonidine, or ivabradine) may ↑ risk of bradycardia	Unlabeled use for situational anxiety or acute panic attack

Anxiolytics *(cont'd)*

Generic • Brand • Dose/Dosage Forms	Contraindications	Primary Side Effects	Key Monitoring Parameters	Pertinent Drug Interactions	Med Pearls
Mechanism of action – exact mechanism is unknown; high affinity for 5-HT$_{1A}$ and 5-HT$_2$ receptors, mild affinity for dopamine (D$_2$) receptors					
Buspirone ☆ • Only available as generic • 7.5–30 mg BID • Tabs	• Hypersensitivity • Concurrent use with MAOI	• Headache • Dizziness • Nausea • Hostility • Confusion • Drowsiness • Restlessness	• Mental status • Symptoms of anxiety • Pseudo-parkinsonism	• CYP3A4 substrate • CYP3A4 inhibitors may ↑ effects/ toxicity • CYP3A4 inducers may ↓ effects	• Avoid use in severe renal or hepatic impairment • Takes 4–6 wk to reach efficacy
Mechanism of action – SNRIs: inhibit reuptake of neuronal serotonin and norepinephrine; may have weak inhibitory effect on reuptake of dopamine					
Venlafaxine XR ☆ • Effexor XR • Details in antidepressants table	[See Antidepressants table]		Indicated for GAD, panic disorder, SAD; unlabeled use for PTSD and OCD		
Duloxetine • Cymbalta • Details in antidepressants table			Indicated for GAD		
Mechanism of action – competes with histamine for H$_1$-receptor sites on effector cells in GI, blood vessels, and respiratory tract					
Hydroxyzine ☆ • Vistaril • 50–100 mg PO 4 ×/day • 50–100 mg IM every 4–6 hr PRN • Caps, injection, solution, tabs	• Hypersensitivity • Early pregnancy	• Dizziness • Drowsiness • Fatigue • Xerostomia • Blurry vision • Urinary retention	• BP • Mental status	Other CNS depressants, including alcohol, may ↑ CNS depressant effects	• Indicated for anxiety, pruritus, N/V, and as a perioperative adjunct • Use with caution in benign prostatic hyperplasia, respiratory disease, or glaucoma • Avoid in elderly • Adjust dose in renal impairment

BIPOLAR DISORDER

Guidelines Summary

- First-line treatment options for patient with acute manic episodes include lithium, divalproex, risperidone ER, paliperidone ER, olanzapine, quetiapine, aripiprazole, ziprasidone, and asenapine. Antipsychotic medications are detailed in medication charts later in the Schizophrenia section of this chapter.

- First-line treatment options for acute depressive episodes include lithium, lamotrigine or quetiapine monotherapy, olanzapine in combination with an SSRI, and lithium or divalproex plus SSRI/bupropion.

- First-line options for maintenance therapy include lithium, lamotrigine, valproate, olanzapine, quetiapine, aripiprazole, risperidone long-acting injection, and adjunctive ziprasidone.

Mood Stabilizers

Generic • Brand • Dose/Dosage Forms	Contraindications	Primary Side Effects	Key Monitoring Parameters	Med Pearls
Mechanism of action – lithium: altered sodium transport leads to a shift toward intraneuronal metabolism of catecholamines; the specific mechanism in mania is not fully understood				
Lithium ☆ • Lithobid • IR: 300–1,800 mg/day in 3–4 divided doses • ER: 450–900 mg BID • Caps, ER tabs, solution, tabs	• Severe renal or cardiovascular disease • Dehydration	• V/D • Drowsiness • Muscle weakness • Lack of coordination • Ataxia • Blurred vision • Tinnitus • Hypothyroidism	• Serum drug concentration 0.6–1.2 mEq/L • Renal function • Thyroid function tests • Serum Na+ concentrations	• Angiotensin-converting enzyme inhibitors, angiotensin II receptor blockers, diuretics, and nonsteroidal anti-inflammtory drugs may ↑ levels and risk of toxicity • Sodium depletion ↑ risk of toxicity
Mechanism of action – valproic acid: not fully understood; thought to ↑ GABA concentrations in the brain				
Valproic acid (divalproex sodium) ☆ • Depakote, Depakote ER, Depakene, Depacon • 10–60 mg/kg/day • Caps, delayed-release caps/tabs, ER tabs, injection, solution, sprinkle caps	[Specific drug details outlined in Epilepsy section of Neurological Disorders chapter]			
Mechanism of action – carbamazepine: inhibits voltage-gated sodium channels, thereby depressing electrical transmission in the nucleus ventralis anterior of the thalamus				
Carbamazepine ☆ • Equetro • 200–1,600 mg/day in 2 divided doses • ER caps	[Specific drug details outlined in Epilepsy section of Neurological Disorders chapter]			
Mechanism of action – lamotrigine: affects sodium channels stabilizing neuronal membranes; the exact mechanism in bipolar disorder is unknown				
Lamotrigine ☆ • Lamictal • 25–700 mg/day in 1–2 divided doses • Chewable tabs, ODTs, tabs	[Specific drug details outlined in Epilepsy section of Neurological Disorders chapter]			

SCHIZOPHRENIA

Guidelines Summary

For many years, atypical antipsychotics were considered the obvious first-line choice because of significantly reduced incidence of extrapyramidal side effects (EPS). Considerable controversy has surfaced, because of the ability of these medications to ↑ the risk of metabolic syndrome. Choice of either a typical or atypical antipsychotic is appropriate as first-line therapy. It should be considered, however, that atypical agents may have better efficacy in treating negative symptoms associated with schizophrenia.

- Goals of therapy include: Reduce or eliminate symptoms, minimize side effects of pharmacological treatment, and prevent relapse.
- Atypical and typical antipsychotics have similar efficacy profiles. Decision on first-line therapy is based on consideration of side-effect profiles, adherence issues, history of response, and cost.
- EPS are more likely to occur with typical antipsychotics but may be seen with atypical antipsychotics depending on the agent and dose. EPS include acute dystonic reactions, akathisia, parkinsonism, and tardive dyskinesia (TD).
- TD may occur at any time after taking an antipsychotic but generally occurs months to years after initiation. Symptoms include involuntary movements of the mouth, tongue, face, extremities, and trunk. TD may be irreversible; therefore, monitoring of abnormal involuntary movements in patients on antipsychotics is recommended. If TD occurs, the patient may be treated with with clonazepam or valbenazine.
- Neuroleptic malignant syndrome (NMS) is a rare side effect associated with antipsychotic use that presents in less than 1% of patients but may be life-threatening if left untreated. NMS is characterized by rigidity, hyperthermia, and autonomic instability; however, elevation of serum creatinine may also been seen. The onset of NMS is generally within a week of starting treatment with an antipsychotic but may also occur with an ↑ in dose of the antipsychotic. If NMS occurs, antipsychotics should be discontinued and supportive care can be implemented to target hydration as well as cardiovascular and renal symptoms.
- All antipsychotics carry a black box warning for use in patients with dementia-related psychosis due to an ↑ risk of death.

Antipsychotics

Generic • Brand • Dose/Dosage Forms	Contraindications	Primary Side Effects	Key Monitoring Parameters	Pertinent Drug Interactions	Med Pearls
Typical Antipsychotics					
Mechanism of action – phenothiazines: block postsynaptic mesolimbic dopaminergic receptors in the brain					
Chlorpromazine • Only available as generic • 30–800 mg/day PO in 2–4 divided doses • 25–100 mg IM every 4–6 hr PRN • Injection, tabs	• Hypersensitivity • Severe CNS depression • Coma	• Orthostatic hypotension • Falls • Drowsiness • Xerostomia • Constipation • Nausea • Urinary retention • Blurred vision • Photosensitivity • EPS • NMS • QT interval prolongation • Neutropenia	• BP • HR • Mental status • Lipid profile • Fasting blood glucose • Severity of EPS • Complete blood count (CBC) • LFTs • Involuntary movement • S/S of NMS • ECG	• CYP2D6 substrate (all but trifluoperazine and prochlorperazine) • CYP2D6 inhibitors may ↑ effects/toxicity • CYP1A2 substrate (tripfluoperazine only) • CYP1A2 inhibitors may ↑ effects/toxicity • CYP1A2 inducers may ↓ effects • CYP2D6 inhibitor (thio-ridazine only) • May ↑ effects/toxicity of CYP2D6 substrates • All may ↑ risk of torsades de pointes (TdP) with other drugs that prolong QT interval	May produce false-positive phenylketonuria and pregnancy test results
Fluphenazine • Only available as generic • 2.5–10 mg/day PO in 3–4 divided doses • 1.25–2.5 mg IM every 6–8 hr PRN • Decanoate (long-acting): 12.5–100 mg IM/subcut every 2–4 wk • Injection, injection (long-acting), solution, tabs	• Hypersensitivity • Severe CNS depression • Coma • Subcortical brain damage • Blood dyscrasias • Hepatic impairment				
Perphenazine • Only available as generic • 4–16 mg 2–4 ×/day • Tabs					
Trifluoperazine • Only available as generic • 2–20 mg BID • Tabs					May produce false-positive phenylketonuria test results
Prochlorperazine ☆ • Compro • 15–150 mg/day PO in 3–4 divided doses • 10–20 mg IM every 4–6 hr PRN • Injection, rectal suppository, tabs					May produce false-positive phenylketonuria and pregnancy test results

Antipsychotics   *(cont'd)*

Generic • Brand • Dose/Dosage Forms	Contraindications	Primary Side Effects	Key Monitoring Parameters	Pertinent Drug Interactions	Med Pearls
Thioridazine • Only available as generic • 300–800 mg/day in 2–4 divided doses • Tabs	[Same as above]	[Same as above]	[Same as above]	[Same as above]	May produce false-positive methadone and phencyclidine results
Mechanism of action — not well established; thought to block postsynaptic mesolimbic dopaminergic D_2 receptors in the brain					
Haloperidol ☆ • Haldol, Haldol Deconoate • 0.5–5 mg PO 2–3 ×/day • 2–5 mg IM every 4–8 hr PRN • Decanoate (long-acting): 10–15 × the daily PO dose (max = 200 mg) IM every 4 wk • Injection, injection (long-acting), solution, tabs	• Hypersensitivity • Parkinson's disease • Severe CNS depression • Coma	• Xerostomia • Drowsiness • Constipation • Nausea • Urinary retention • Blurred vision • Orthostatic hypotension • Falls • EPS • Priapism • QT interval prolongation • NMS • Neutropenia	• BP • HR • CBC • Mental status • ECG • EPS • Involuntary movement • S/S of NMS • LFTs	• CYP2D6 and CYP3A4 substrate • CYP2D6 or CYP3A4 inhibitors may ↑ effects/toxicity • CYP3A4 inducers may ↓ effects • May ↑ risk of TdP with other drugs that prolong QT interval	• IM decanoate form uses sesame oil • Immediate-release injection may also be given IV in ICU setting for treatment of delirium
Mechanism of action — a potent, centrally acting dopamine-receptor antagonist					
Pimozide • Orap • 1–2 mg/day in divided doses (max = 0.2 mg/kg/day or 10 mg/day, whichever is less) • Tabs	• Severe CNS depression • Coma • History of arrhythmias • Congenital long QT syndrome • Concurrent use with other QT interval prolonging medications • Hypokalemia or hypomagnesemia • Concurrent use with 3A4 inhibitors • Concurrent use with citalopram, escitalopram, or sertraline	• Somnolence • Drowsiness • Rash • Xerostomia • Constipation • Diarrhea • ↑ appetite • Taste disturbance • Impotence • Weakness • Visual disturbances • Speech disorder • Hypotension • QT interval prolongation • EPS • NMS • Neutropenia	• BP • HR • CBC • Mental status • ECG • EPS • Involuntary movement • S/S of NMS • LFTs	• CYP1A2, CYP2D6, and CYP3A4 substrate • CYP1A2, CYP2D6 or CYP3A4 inhibitors may ↑ effects/toxicity • CYP1A2 or CYP3A4 inducers may ↓ effects • May ↑ risk of TdP with other drugs that prolong QT interval	Only indicated for Tourette's disorder

Antipsychotics   *(cont'd)*

Generic • Brand • Dose/Dosage Forms	Contraindications	Primary Side Effects	Key Monitoring Parameters	Pertinent Drug Interactions	Med Pearls
Mechanism of action – blocks postsynaptic mesolimbic D_1 and D_2 receptors in the brain, and also possesses serotonin 5-HT_2 blocking activity					
Loxapine • Adasuve • 20–250 mg/day PO in 2–4 divided doses • 10 mg via inhalation daily • Caps, inhalation	*PO:* • Hypersensitivity • Severe CNS depression • Coma *Inhalation:* • Hypersensitivity • Asthma, COPD, or other bronchospastic disease • Acute wheezing	• Hypotension • Falls • N/V • Constipation • Xerostomia • Weakness • Sexual dysfunction • Dizziness • EPS • NMS • Seizures	• BP • HR • Mental status • EPS • S/S of NMS • CBC • Involuntary movement • S/S of bronchospasm (with inhalation)	No significant CYP450 interactions	May produce false-positive phenylketonuria test results
Mechanism of action – exerts effect on the ascending reticular activating system					
Molindone • Only available as generic • 30–100 mg/day in 3–4 divided doses • Tabs	• Hypersensitivity • Severe CNS depression • Coma	• Drowsiness • Xerostomia • Constipation • Hypotension • Tachycardia • EPS • NMS	• BP • HR • Mental status • EPS • Involuntary movement • S/S of NMS • CBC	No significant CYP450 interactions	None
Mechanism of action – blocks postsynaptic dopamine receptors, resulting in inhibition of dopamine-mediated effects; also has alpha-adrenergic blocking activity					
Thiothixene • Only available as generic • 6–60 mg/day in 2–3 divided doses • Caps	• Hypersensitivity • Severe CNS depression • Coma • Blood dyscrasias	• Hypotension • Dizziness • N/V • Constipation • Sexual dysfunction • Tachycardia • Insomnia • EPS • NMS	• BP • HR • CBC • Mental status • EPS • Involuntary movement • S/S of NMS	• CYP1A2 substrate • CYP1A2 inhibitors may ↑ effects/toxicity • CYP1A2 inducers may ↓ effects	May cause false-positive pregnancy test results

Antipsychotics *(cont'd)*

Generic • Brand • Dose/Dosage Forms	Contraindications	Primary Side Effects	Key Monitoring Parameters	Pertinent Drug Interactions	Med Pearls
Atypical Antipsychotics					
Mechanism of action – mixed and varied (per agent) D_2/5-HT$_2$ antagonist activity					
Aripiprazole☆ Abilify (PO): • 10–30 mg PO daily • ODTs, solution, tabs Abilify Maintena (ER IM injection): • 300–400 mg IM monthly (doses must be ≥26 days apart) Aristada (ER IM injection): • 441–882 mg IM every 4–6 wk Aristada Initio: • 675 mg IM × 1 dose	• Hypersensitivity • Severe hepatic impairment (asenapine)	• Weight gain • Constipation • N/V/D • Akathisia • Hyperglycemia • Hyperlipidemia • Anxiety • Sedation • QT interval prolongation • Orthostatic hypotension • Falls • Tachycardia • Neutropenia • Impulse control disorders • EPS (rare) • NMS	• Fasting plasma glucose • Fasting lipid panel • CBC • BP • HR • ECG • Weight/body mass index • Waist circumference • Mental status • EPS • S/S of NMS	Aripiprazole and brexpiprazole: • CYP2D6 and CYP3A4 substrates • ↓ dose with CYP2D6 or CYP3A4 inhibitors; may ↑ effects/toxicity • Avoid use with CYP3A4 inducers; may ↓ effects Olanzapine, asenapine, and clozapine: • CYP1A2 substrates • CYP1A2 inhibitors may ↑ effects/toxicity • CYP1A2 inducers may ↓ effects Quetiapine, lurasidone, and cariprazine: • CYP3A4 substrates • CYP3A4 inhibitors may ↑ effects/toxicity • CYP3A4 inducers may ↓ effects Iloperidone and risperidone: • CYP2D6 substrates • CYP2D6 inhibitors may ↑ effects/toxicity • All may ↑ risk of TdP with other drugs that prolong QT interval	• Partial D_2 agonist • Among the lowest risk of metabolic syndrome • Also indicated to treat acute manic and mixed episodes associated with bipolar I disorder, MDD (as adjunctive therapy), irritabilty with autistic disorder, and Tourette's disorder • Overlap oral antipsychotic for 21 days upon initiation of Aristada and 14 days upon initiation of Abilify Maintena • Aristada Initio injection is given in conjunction with an oral 30 mg dose and is not intended for repeat dosing
Olanzapine☆ Zyprexa (PO, immediate-release IM injection), Zyprexa Zydis (ODT): • 5–20 mg PO daily • 10–30 mg/dose IM • IM (immediate release), ODTs, tabs Zyprexa Relprevv (ER IM injection): • 150–405 mg IM (max = 300 mg every 2 wk or 405 mg every 4 wk)		• Weight gain • Constipation • N/V/D • Akathisia • Hyperglycemia • Hyperlipidemia • Anxiety • Sedation • QT interval prolongation • Orthostatic hypotension • Falls • Tachycardia • Neutropenia • Hyperprolac-tinemia (rare) • EPS (rare) • NMS			• Higher degree of weight gain than some other atypicals • Oral formulations also indicated to treat acute and chronic manic and mixed epi-sodes associated with bipolar I disorder • Immediate-release IM injection indicated to treat acute agita-tion associated with schizophrenia and bipolar I mania • Zyprexa Relprevv is associated with postinjection delirium/sedation

Antipsychotics *(cont'd)*

Generic • Brand • Dose/Dosage Forms	Contraindications	Primary Side Effects	Key Monitoring Parameters	Pertinent Drug Interactions	Med Pearls
Paliperidone☆ Invega (ER tabs): • 3–12 mg PO daily Invega Sustenna (monthly ER IM injection): • 39–234 mg IM monthly Invega Trinza (every 3 mo ER IM injection): • 273–819 mg IM every 3 mo	[Same as above]	[Same as above]	[Same as above]	[Same as above]	• Major active metabolite of risperidone • Invega Trinza should only be used in patients who have been stabilized with Invega Sustenna for ≥4 mo • Also indicated for schizoaffective disorder
Quetiapine☆ • Seroquel, Seroquel XR • IR: 50–750 mg/day in 2–3 divided doses • ER: 300–800 mg daily • ER tabs, tabs					• ER tabs usually dosed at bedtime due to somnolence • Also indicated for manic and depressive episodes associated with bipolar I disorder
Iloperidone • Fanapt • 1–12 mg BID • Tabs					• Lower risk of weight gain than many atypicals • Low risk of somnolence • May improve cognitive function
Asenapine • Saphris • 5–10 mg BID • SL tabs					• Very low incidence of EPS • Also indicated to treat acute manic and mixed episodes associated with bipolar I disorder

Antipsychotics   *(cont'd)*

Generic • Brand • Dose/Dosage Forms	Contraindications	Primary Side Effects	Key Monitoring Parameters	Pertinent Drug Interactions	Med Pearls
Risperidone ☆ Risperdal, Risperdal M-Tab: • 2–16 mg/day PO in 1–2 divided doses • ODTs, solution, tabs Risperdal Consta (ER IM injection) • 12.5–50 mg IM every 2 wk	[Same as above]	[Same as above]	[Same as above]	[Same as above]	• Sedation often leads to bedtime dosing • Oral formulations also indicated to treat acute manic and mixed episodes associated with bipolar I disorder and irritabilty with autistic disorder • ER IM injection also indicated for maintenance treatment of bipolar I disorder • Oral antipsychotic should be overlapped for 3 weeks upon initiation of Risperdal Consta
Ziprasidone ☆ • Geodon • 20–100 mg PO BID • 10 mg IM every 2 hr or 20 mg IM every 4 hr • Caps, injection	• Hypersensitivity • Decompensated heart failure • Recent MI • History of QT interval prolongation • Concurrent use of QT interval prolonging medications				• Must be administered with at least 500 calories • Lower risk of metabolic syndrome when compared to other atypicals • Oral formulation also indicated to treat acute manic and mixed episodes associated with bipolar I disorder and for maintenance treatment of bipolar I disorder • IM injection indicated to treat acute agitation associated with schizophrenia
Lurasidone • Latuda • 40–160 mg daily • Tabs	• Hypersensitivity • Concurrent use with strong 3A4 inhibitors or inducers				• Must be administered with at least 350 calories • Also indicated for treatment of depressive episodes associated with bipolar I disorder
Brexpiprazole • Rexulti • 1–4 mg daily • Tabs	Hypersensitivity				• Partial D_2 agonist • Also indicated as adjunctive therapy for major depressive disorder

Antipsychotics   *(cont'd)*

Generic • Brand • Dose/Dosage Forms	Contraindications	Primary Side Effects	Key Monitoring Parameters	Pertinent Drug Interactions	Med Pearls
Cariprazine • Vraylar • 1.5–6 mg daily • Caps	[Same as above]	[Same as above]	[Same as above]	[Same as above]	• Partial D$_2$ agonist • Also indicated to treat acute manic and mixed episodes associated with bipolar I disorder
Clozapine ☆ • Clozaril, FazaClo, Versacloz • 12.5–900 mg/day in 1–3 divided doses • ODTs, suspension, tabs	• Hypersensitivity • Seizures • Myocarditis, cardiomyopathy, mitral valve incompetence • Severe neutropenia • Orthostatic hypotension, bradycardia, syncope	• Orthostatic hypotension • Tachycardia • QT interval prolongation • Hyperglycemia • Hyperlipidemia • Weight gain • Agranulocytosis • NMS • Seizures • Myocarditis	• Absolute neutrophil count weekly for 6 mo, then every 2 wk for 6 mo, then every 4 wk • Fasting plasma glucose • Fasting lipid panel • BP • HR • ECG • Weight/body mass index • Mental status • S/S of NMS		• Prescribers, patients, and pharmacies must enroll in the Clozapine REMs program • Used less frequently than other atypicals due to requirement for frequent monitoring • Effective in treatment of refractory cases and in patients at high risk for suicide

Tardive Dyskinesia Treatment

Generic • Brand • Dose/Dosage Forms	Contraindications	Primary Side Effects	Key Monitoring Parameters	Pertinent Drug Interactions	Med Pearl
Mechanism of action – exact mechanism is unknown; thought to reversibly inhibit VMAT2					
Valbenazine • Ingrezza • 40–80 mg daily • Caps	Hypersensitivity	• Drowsiness • Fatigue • Sedation • Falls • Equilibrium disturbance • Abnormal gait • Akathisia • Vomiting	• AIMS scale • DISCUS scale • ECG	• CYP3A4 substrate • Avoid use with strong CYP3A4 inducers	Indicated for the treatment of TD

SLEEP DISORDERS

Insomnia

Guidelines Summary

- Goals of therapy: Improve quality and quantity of sleep and improve daytime sleep-related impairment.

- All patients should be educated about good sleep hygiene. Nonpharmacological measures are the preferred initial treatment.

- Pharmacological therapy should be combined with behavioral therapy to achieve the best results. Medication selection is based upon the following patient-specific elements: (1) symptom pattern, (2) patient preference, (3) availability, (4) cost, (5) prior response, (6) comorbid conditions, (7) contraindications, (8) concurrent medications, (9) side effect profile, and (10) treatment goals.

- Pharmacological classes for insomnia include benzodiazepines, benzodiazepine receptor agonists (BzRA), melatonin receptor agonists, and sedating antidepressants.

- Short-intermediate acting BzRAs, benzodiazepines, or melatonin receptor agonists are first-line therapy options for most patients. BzRAs and benzodiazepines ideally should be limited to short-term use (7–10 days); however, there is limited evidence to support use extended to 6–12 months.

- Inadequate response after an initial trial of the above agents can be followed with a trial on a second agent from within these therapeutic class options.

- Third-line options include sedating antidepressants or off-label combination therapy or self-care therapies such as antihistamines.

Treatment Algorithm

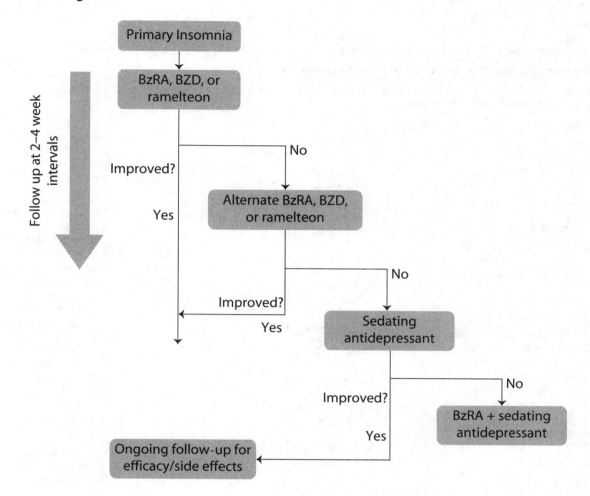

Medications for Insomnia

Generic • Brand • Dose/Dosage Forms	Contraindications	Primary Side Effects	Key Monitoring	Pertinent Drug Interactions	Med Pearl
Benzodiazepine receptor agonists (schedule IV controlled substances)					
Mechanism of action – enhances GABA through stimulation of the benzodiazepine 1 receptor, which results in hyperpolarization and a ↓ in neuronal excitabilty with sedative and hypnotic effects					
Eszopiclone ☆ • Lunesta • 1–3 mg at bedtime • Tabs	Hypersensitivity	• Headache • Xerostomia • Dizziness • Nausea • Somnolence • Sleep-related activities: hazardous activities such as sleep-driving and cooking have been reported (rare), incidence ↑ with alcohol use or using above max doses • Behavior changes such as ↓ inhibition, aggression, agitation, hallucinations, and depersonalization (rare)	• Improvement in sleep quality/ quantity • Presence of side effects	• CYP3A4 substrate • CYP3A4 inhibitors may ↑ effects/ toxicity • CYP3A4 inducers may ↓ effects • Other CNS depressants, including alcohol, may ↑ CNS depressant effects	• High-fat/heavy meal will delay absorption; administer on an empty stomach • Associated with taste disturbance
Zolpidem ☆ • Ambien, Ambien CR, Zolpimist • IR or oral spray: 5–10 mg PO at bedtime (max = 5 mg for females) • CR: 6.25–12.5 mg PO at bedtime (max = 6.25 mg for females) • ER tabs, oral spray, tabs • Edluar, Intermezzo (SL tabs) • Edluar: 5–10 mg/night SL (max = 5 mg for females) • Intermezzo: 1.75–3.5 mg/ night SL (max = 1.75 mg for females)					• Take IR tabs, ER tabs, oral spray, and SL tabs (Edluar only) immediately before bedtime • SL tabs (Intermezzo only) helpful for nighttime awakenings; take in bed if patient wakes in the middle of the night (only if ≥4 hr remain before desired wake-up time) and there is difficulty in returning to sleep • Heavy/high-fat meal will delay absorption; administer on an empty stomach
Zaleplon • Sonata • 5–20 mg at bedtime • Caps					• Heavy/high-fat meal will delay absorption; administer on an empty stomach • Headache incidence = 30–40%

Medications for Insomnia *(cont'd)*

Generic • Brand • Dose/Dosage Forms	Contraindications	Primary Side Effects	Key Monitoring	Pertinent Drug Interactions	Med Pearl
Benzodiazepines (schedule IV controlled substances)					
Mechanism of action – bind to GABA A receptors to enhance inhibitory effect of GABA on neuronal excitability					
Estazolam • Only available as generic • 1–2 mg PO at bedtime • Tabs	• Pregnancy • Narrow-angle glaucoma • Concurrent use with itraconazole or ketoconazole	• Somnolence • Dizziness • Hypokinesia • Hangover effect • Abnormal coordination • Confusion • Xerostomia • Constipation	• Improvement in sleep quality/ quantity • Presence of side effects	• CYP3A4 substrate • CYP3A4 inhibitors may ↑ effects/ toxicity • CYP3A4 inducers may ↓ effects • Other CNS depressants, including alcohol, may ↑ CNS depressant effects	• Time to peak 0.5–6 hr; $T_{1/2}$ 10–24 hr • Administer on an empty stomach
Temazepam ☆ • Restoril • 7.5–30 mg PO at bedtime • Caps	• Pregnancy • Narrow-angle glaucoma				Time to peak 1.2–1.6 hr; $T_{1/2}$ 3.5–18 hr
Triazolam • Halcion • 0.125–0.5 mg PO at bedtime • Tabs	• Pregnancy • Narrow-angle glaucoma • Concurrent use with itraconazole, ketoconazole, nefazodone, or protease inhibitors				• Time to peak 1–2 hr; $T_{1/2}$ 1.5–5.5 hr • Administer on an empty stomach
Flurazepam • Only available as generic • 15–30 mg PO at bedtime (max = 15 mg for females) • Caps	• Pregnancy • Narrow-angle glaucoma				Time to peak 3–6 hr; $T_{1/2}$ 2.5 hr (active metabolite ~70 hr)

Medications for Insomnia   *(cont'd)*

Generic • Brand • Dose/Dosage Forms	Contraindications	Primary Side Effects	Key Monitoring	Pertinent Drug Interactions	Med Pearl
Melatonin Receptor Agonists					
Mechanism of action – MT1 and MT2 receptor agonist					
Ramelteon • Rozerem • 8 mg within 30 min of bedtime • Tabs	• Angioedema with prior use • Concurrent use with fluvoxamine	• Anaphylaxis/ angioedema • Dizziness • Fatigue • Depression • Sleep-related activities: hazardous activities such as sleep-driving and cooking have been reported (rare), incidence ↑ with alcohol use • Behavior changes such as agitation, hallucinations, and mania	• Improvement in sleep quality/ quantity • Presence of side effects	• CYP1A2 substrate • CYP1A2 inhibitors may ↑ effects/ toxicity • CYP1A2 inducers may ↓ effects • Other CNS depressants, including alcohol, may ↑ CNS depressant effects	• Not a scheduled/ controlled substance • Heavy/high-fat meal will delay absorption; administer on an empty stomach
Tasimelteon • Hetlioz • 20 mg at bedtime • Caps	None	• Drowsiness • Headache • Abnormal dreams • ↑ LFTs	• Improvement in sleep quality/ quantity • Presence of side effects • LFTs	• CYP1A2 and CYP3A4 substrate • CYP1A2 and CYP3A4 inhibitors may ↑ effects/ toxicity • CYP1A2 and CYP3A4 inducers may ↓ effects • Other CNS depressants, including alcohol, may ↑ CNS depressant effects	• Indicated for non-24-hour sleep-wake disorder • Should be taken at the same time each night • Not a scheduled/ controlled substance • May take weeks to months to see effect • Administer on an empty stomach

Medications for Insomnia *(cont'd)*

Generic • Brand • Dose/Dosage Forms	Contraindications	Primary Side Effects	Key Monitoring	Pertinent Drug Interactions	Med Pearl
Orexin Receptor Antagonist					
Mechanism of action – antagonizes OX1R and OX2R which blocks the binding of wake-promoting compounds orexin A and orexin B					
Suvorexant • Belsomra • 10–20 mg at bedtime • Tabs	Narcolepsy	• Drowsiness • Headache • Dizziness • Sleep-related activities: hazardous activities such as sleep-driving and cooking have been reported (rare), incidence ↑ with alcohol or other CNS depressant use or using above max doses • Depression • Abnormal dreams	• Improvement in sleep quality/quantity • Presence of side effects	• CYP3A4 substrate • CYP3A4 inhibitors may ↑ effects/toxicity • CYP3A4 inducers may ↓ effects • Other CNS depressants, including alcohol, may ↑ CNS depressant effects	• Schedule IV controlled substance • Should be taken with ≥7 hr remaining before planned time of awakening • Heavy/high-fat meal will delay absorption; administer on an empty stomach

Restless Leg Syndrome

Guidelines Summary

- First-line options for the treatment of RLS include ropinirole and pramipexole.
- Other treatment options include carbidopa/levodopa, opioids, gabapentin enacarbil, gabapentin, and pregabalin.

Drug Treatment

Please see the medication chart in the Parkinson's Disease section of the Neurological Disorders chapter for more specific information on ropinirole, pramipexole, and carbidopa/levodopa. Please see the medication chart in the Epilepsy section of the Neurological Disorders chapter for more specific information on gabapentin and pregabalin.

Narcolepsy

Guidelines Summary

- First-line treatment options for excessive daytime sedation include modafinil, sodium oxybate, stimulants (amphetamine, methamphetamine, dextroamphetamine, methylphenidate), and selegiline. For information on the stimulants, please see the Attention-Deficit Hyperactivity Disorder (ADHD) section in this chapter. For information on selegiline, please see the Parkinson's Disease section in the Neurological Disorders chapter.

- TCAs and fluoxetine may be used for the treatment of cataplexy. Please see the Depression section of this chapter for more information regarding these medications.

- Nonpharmacologic treatment includes scheduled naps.

Medications for Narcolepsy

Generic • Brand • Dose/Dosage Forms	Contraindications	Primary Side Effects	Key Monitoring	Pertinent Drug Interactions	Med Pearl
Mechanism of action – binds to the dopamine receptor, inhibiting dopamine reuptake					
Modafinil • Provigil • 200 mg daily • Tabs	Hypersensitivity	• Rash (Stevens-Johnson syndrome possible) • Angioedema • Headache • Nervousness • Anxiety • Dizziness • Insomnia • Hypertension • N/D	• Level of alertness • BP • Exacerbation of agitation, anxiety, depression	• CYP3A4 substrate and inducer • CYP2C19 inhibitor • CYP3A4 inhibitors may ↑ effects/ toxicity • CYP3A4 inducers may ↓ effects • May ↑ effects/ toxicity of CYP2C19 substrates • May ↓ effects of 3A4 substrates • May ↓ effects of hormonal contraceptives during and for 1 mo after discontinuing treatment	• Schedule IV controlled substance • If used for narcolepsy or obstructive sleep apnea/ hypopnea, administer dose in the morning • If used for shift work sleep disorder, administer dose 1 hr before work
Armodafinil • Nuvigil • 150–250 mg daily • Tabs					• R-enantiomer of modafinil • Schedule IV controlled substance • If used for narcolepsy or obstructive sleep apnea, administer dose in the morning • If used for shift work sleep disorder, administer dose 1 hr before work
Mechanism of action – derivative of GABA that serves as an inhibitory transmitter					
Sodium oxybate • Xyrem • Initial: 2.25 g at bedtime after patient in bed, then 2.25 g 2.5–4 hr later; titrate dose to usual effective dose of 6–9 g per night • Solution	Concurrent use with alcohol or sedative hypnotic agents	• Dizziness • N/V • Somnolence • Enuresis • Tremor • Confusion • Anxiety • Sleepwalking • Depression	• Drug abuse • Depression or suicidality • Mental status	• CNS depressants, including alcohol, may ↑ CNS depressant effects • Divalproex sodium may ↑ effects/ toxicity; ↓ sodium oxybate dose by 20%	• Schedule III controlled substance • 1.1 g Na+ in 6 g nightly dose • Administer on an empty stomach • Also effective for the treatment of cataplexy • REMS program

ATTENTION-DEFICIT/HYPERACTIVITY DISORDER (ADHD)

Guidelines Summary

- First-line pharmacologic therapy for ADHD includes stimulant medications. Approved options included methylphenidate, dexmethylphenidate, dextroamphetamine, dextroamphetamine + amphetamine, and lisdexamfetamine.

- Nonstimulant options approved for ADHD are generally reserved for one of the following: concerns related to abuse/diversion, strong family/patient preference for nonstimulant medications, or as adjunctive therapy to stimulants. Options include atomoxetine, guanfacine, and clonidine. Of these options, atomoxetine monotherapy is preferred to guanfacine and clonidine, which are generally reserved for adjunctive therapy.

- When selecting a stimulant, patient-specific factors such as ability to swallow tablets/capsules, affordability, number of daily doses required, and presence of a tic disorder are considerations.

- Interpatient variability in efficacy is recognized and alternate stimulant agents are recommended as second- and third-line options after appropriate titration to maximal effective/tolerated dose of initial stimulant selected.

Medications for Attention-Deficit/Hyperactivity Disorder

Generic • Brand • Dose & Max	Contraindications	Primary Side Effects	Key Monitoring	Pertinent Drug Interactions	Med Pearl
Stimulants					
Mechanism of action – block reuptake of norepinepherine and dopamine					
Methylphenidate IR☆ • Ritalin, Methylin • 10–60 mg/day in 2–3 divided doses • Chewable tabs, solution, tabs Methylphenidate ER • Aptensio XR: 10–60 mg daily • Concerta: 18–72 mg every morning • Metadate CD: 10–60 mg daily • Quillichew ER: 10–60 mg every morning • Quillivant XR: 10–60 mg every morning • Ritalin LA: 10–60 mg daily • Ritalin SR: 10–60 mg/day in 2–3 divided doses • ER caps, ER chewable tabs, ER suspension, ER tabs Methylphenidate transdermal patch • Daytrana • Initial: 10-mg patch daily; titrate to effect	• Anxiety • Tension • Agitation • Glaucoma • Motor tics • Recent MAOI, linezolid, or methylene blue use (within 14 days) • Family history or diagnosis of Tourette's syndrome • Advanced arteriosclerosis • Moderate to severe HTN • Symptomatic cardiac disease	General • Anorexia • Nausea • Weight loss • Insomnia • Dizziness • Lightheadedness • Irritability • ↑ sweating • Blurred vision • Priapism • Growth suppression • Peripheral vasculopathy (Raynaud's) • Dependence Cardiovascular • ↑ BP • Tachycardia Psychiatric • May exacerbate anxiety, mania, aggression, hostility, or depression • Use with caution in patients with pre-existing psychiatric conditions	• Resolution of symptoms • BP • HR • Height/weight • ECG at baseline and if chest pain or syncope • Signs of misuse/abuse	• MAOIs require 14-day washout period prior to stimulant initiation • ↑ risk of serotonin syndrome with MAOIs, SSRIs, SNRIs, triptans, tricyclic anti-depressants (TCAs), fentanyl, lithium, dextromethorphan, meperidine, buspirone, linezolid, methylene blue, St. John's wort	• Schedule II controlled substance • Black box: Potential for dependency • Generally taken every morning to avoid insomnia • Remove patch after 9 hr of wear; alternate application site (hips) • Withdrawal potential; titrate slowly and taper upon discontinuation • Also indicated for narcolepsy
Dexmethylphenidate IR • Focalin, Focalin XR • IR: 2.5–10 mg BID • ER: 5–40 mg every morning • ER caps, tabs					• Schedule II controlled substance • Black box: Potential for dependency • ER generally taken q A.M. to avoid insomnia • For IR, 1st dose given q A.M., 2nd dose given at least 4 hr later • Withdrawal potential; titrate slowly and taper upon discontinuation • D-enantiomer of methylphenidate

Medications for Attention-Deficit/Hyperactivity Disorder   *(cont'd)*

Generic • Brand • Dose & Max	Contraindications	Primary Side Effects	Key Monitoring	Pertinent Drug Interactions	Med Pearl
Mechanism of action – promote the release of catecholamines					
Dextroamphetamine and amphetamine ☆ • IR only available generically, Adderall XR • IR: 5–40 mg/day in 1–3 divided doses • ER: 5–30 mg every morning • ER caps, tabs	• Anxiety • Tension • Agitation • Glaucoma • Motor tics • Recent MAOI, linezolid, or methylene blue use (within 14 days) • Family history or diagnosis of Tourette's syndrome • Advanced arteriosclerosis • Moderate to severe HTN • Symptomatic cardiac disease	General • Anorexia • Nausea • Weight loss • Insomnia • Dizziness • Lightheadedness • Irritability • ↑ sweating • Blurred vision • Priapism • Growth suppression • Peripheral vasculopathy (Raynaud's) • Dependence Cardiovascular • ↑ BP • Tachycardia Psychiatric • May exacerbate anxiety, mania, aggression, hostility, or depression • Use with caution in patients with pre-existing psychiatric conditions	• Resolution of symptoms • BP • HR • Height/weight • ECG at baseline and if chest pain or syncope • Signs of misuse/abuse	• MAOIs require 14-day washout period prior to stimulant initiation • ↑ risk of serotonin syndrome with MAOIs, SSRIs, SNRIs, triptans, tricyclic antidepressants (TCAs), fentanyl, lithium, dextromethorphan, meperidine, buspirone, linezolid, methylene blue, St. John's wort	• Schedule II controlled substance • Black box: Potential for dependency • ER generally taken q A.M. to avoid insomnia • Withdrawal potential; titrate slowly and taper upon discontinuation • IR also indicated for narcolepsy
Dextroamphetamine • IR only available generically, Dexedrine Spansules (ER) • IR: 2.5–40 mg/day in 1–2 divided doses • ER: 5–40 mg/day in 1–2 divided doses • ER caps, solution, tabs					• Schedule II controlled substance • Black box: Potential for dependency • ER generally taken q A.M. to avoid insomnia • For IR, 1st dose given q A.M., 2nd dose given 4–6 hr later • Withdrawal potential; titrate slowly and taper upon discontinuation • Also indicated for narcolepsy

Medications for Attention-Deficit/Hyperactivity Disorder (cont'd)

Generic • Brand • Dose & Max	Contraindications	Primary Side Effects	Key Monitoring	Pertinent Drug Interactions	Med Pearl
Lisdexamfetamine☆ • Vyvanse • 30–70 mg every morning • Caps, chewable tabs	[Same as above]	[Same as above]	[Same as above]	[Same as above]	• Schedule II controlled substance • Black box: Potential for dependency • Prodrug of dextroamphetamine; rapid effect muted if injected or snorted (designed to decrease abuse potential) • Contents can be mixed with water—drink immediately • Withdrawal potential; titrate slowly and taper upon discontinuation • Also indicated for binge eating disorder
Amphetamine • Adzensys XR-ODT, Dynavel XR, Evekeo • 2.5–20 mg/day • ER suspension, ER-ODT tabs, tabs					May use doses up to 30 mg/day for obesity or 60 mg/day for narcolepsy

Nonstimulants

Mechanism of action – selectively inhibits norepinephrine reuptake

Generic • Brand • Dose & Max	Contraindications	Primary Side Effects	Key Monitoring	Pertinent Drug Interactions	Med Pearl
Atomoxetine☆ • Strattera • 40–100 mg/day in 1–2 divided doses • Caps	• Narrow-angle glaucoma • Pheochromocytoma • Recent MAOI use (within 14 days) • Cardiovascular conditions that may worsen with ↑ BP or HR	• Headache • Insomnia • Nausea • Anorexia • Somnolence • Xerostomia • Menstrual changes • Orthostasis • Urinary hesitancy/retention • Growth suppression • Can exacerbate pre-existing psychiatric illness, including hallucinations/mania • Priapism • Suicidal ideation • Liver injury (rare)	• Resolution of symptoms • S/S liver injury (fatigue, abdominal pain, yellowed skin, darkened urine) • LFTs • BP • HR • Height/weight • ECG at baseline and if chest pain or syncope • Signs of misuse/abuse	• CYP2D6 substrate • CYP2D6 inhibitors may ↑ effects/toxicity; ↓ dose in patients who are CYP2D6 poor metabolizers if taking strong CYP2D6 inhibitor (paroxetine, fluoxetine, quinidine) • MAOIs require 14-day washout period prior to stimulant initiation	• Risk of suicidal ideation in children • Capsules cannot be opened

Medications for Attention-Deficit/Hyperactivity Disorder *(cont'd)*

Generic • Brand • Dose & Max	Contraindications	Primary Side Effects	Key Monitoring	Pertinent Drug Interactions	Med Pearl
Mechanism of action – selective alpha$_{2A}$ receptor agonist that reduces sympathetic outflow					
Guanfacine ☆ • Intuniv • 1–7 mg daily • ER tabs	Hypersensitivity	• Dizziness • Fatigue • Somnolence • Nausea • Xerostomia • Constipation • Bradycardia • Atrioventricular block • Headache • Hypotension • Syncope	• Resolution of symptoms • BP • HR • ECG	• CYP3A4 substrate • ↓ daily dose by 50% if used with strong or moderate CYP3A4 inhibitors; double daily dose if used with strong or moderate CYP3A4 inducers • Additive CNS depressant effects with other CNS depressants • Additive BP lowering with other antihypertensives	• High-fat meals ↑ medication absorption; administer on an empty stomach • Can be used as monotherapy or as adjunctive to stimulant therapy • Also used for hypertension (formulations not interchangeable) • Do not crush • Do not stop abruptly due to risk of rebound HTN
Mechanism of action – alpha$_2$ receptor agonist that results in reduced sympathetic outflow					
Clonidine • Kapvay • 0.1–0.4 mg at bedtime • ER tabs	Hypersensitivity	• Headache • Irritability • Nightmares • Insomnia • Constipation • Xerostomia • Somnolence • Bradycardia • Atrioventricular block • Hypotension • Rebound hypertension (if abruptly discontinued)	• Resolution of symptoms • BP • HR • ECG	• Additive CNS depressant effects with other CNS depressants • Additive BP lowering with other antihypertensives	• Do not crush • Do not stop abruptly due to risk of rebound HTN

Pain Management

11

This chapter covers the following drug classes:

- **Nonopioid oral and nonsteroidal anti-inflammatory drugs (NSAIDs)**
- **Opioid analgesics**
- **Analgesic adjuncts**
- **Skeletal muscle relaxants**

The text also provides an overview of basic treatment and management of pain.

PAIN MANAGEMENT

Guidelines Summary

- Drug therapy is the mainstay of management for acute pain. The drugs discussed in this review are classified into three categories: Nonopioid analgesics, including acetaminophen and nonsteroidal anti-inflammatory drugs (NSAIDs), opioid pain management, and co-analgesics. The drug classes can be used in monotherapy and combination for pain.

- As the pain ↑, so does the dose of medications, the migration to stronger medications, and the use of combinations of medications with different mechanisms of actions.

- Acetaminophen and NSAIDs are useful for acute and chronic pain arising from a variety of causes, including surgery, trauma, arthritis, and cancer.

- NSAIDs are indicated for pain involving inflammation because acetaminophen lacks clinically effective anti-inflammatory properties.

- Major differences between NSAIDs and opioid analgesics
  - NSAIDs are both analgesic and anti-inflammatory in nature and have some antipyretic effect.
  - NSAIDs have a dose ceiling of effect in relationship with adverse effects.
  - NSAIDs do not produce physical or psychological dependence.

- Initiation of opioid analgesics should be based on a pain-directed history and physical that includes repeated pain assessment.
  - Opioid analgesics should be added to nonopioids to manage acute pain and cancer-related pain that does not respond to nonopioids alone.
  - There is enormous variability in doses of opioids required to provide pain relief, even among opioid-naïve patients.
  - It is important to give each analgesic an adequate trial. As a result, a clinician may ↑ the opioid dose to establish analgesia or until unacceptable side effects appear before changing to another opioid.
  - It is recommended to administer analgesics on a regular schedule if pain is present most of the day. This approach allows the patient to stay ahead of the pain.
    - » For chronic pain, consider having a scheduled long-acting agent on board and a short-acting agent for times of breakthrough pain.
- Summary of Centers for Disease Control (CDC) guidelines for prescribing opioids for chronic pain
  - Nonopioids and nonpharmacologic treatment options are preferred for the treatment of chronic pain.
  - Goals of treatment, risks, expected benefits, and patient and clinician responsibilities should be discussed before opioids are started.
  - When starting treatment, start with immediate-release (IR) opioids at the lowest effective dose.
  - Use caution with doses >50 morphine milligram equivalents (MME)/day. Doses >90 MME/day should be avoided if possible or justified for chronic use.
  - For acute pain, provide only the quantity of opioids needed for the expected duration. A quantity for ≤3 days is often sufficient and patients will rarely need >7 days of opioids.
  - After starting opioids, reassess risks and benefits within 1–4 weeks. For chronic therapy, reassess risks and benefits every 3 months. Discontinue therapy if the risks outweigh the benefits.
- Patient-controlled analgesia (PCA) using an intravenous (IV) opioid for acute pain is a commonly used technique for pain control.
  - PCA is used with a computerized-controlled infusion pump.
  - PCA is most often used for the IV administration of opioids for acute pain and allows patients considerable control over the treatment of pain.
  - PCA is not recommended in situations in which oral opioids could readily manage pain or in patients with altered cognition.

- Skeletal muscle relaxants (SMRs) are classified as either antispastic agents (baclofen, dantrolene, tizanidine), which are used to treat cerebral palsy or multiple sclerosis, or as antispasmodic agents (carisoprodol, chlorzoxazone, cyclobenzaprine, metaxolone, methocarbamol, orphenadrine), which are used for the treatment of musculoskeletal conditions such as lower back pain.

  - SMRs should not be used as first-line agents in the treatment of musculoskeletal pain. SMRs should be used only for the short-term treatment of acute low back pain if the patient is unable to tolerate or is unresponsive to NSAIDs or acetaminophen.

Nonopioid Oral and Nonsteroidal Anti-Inflammatory Drugs (NSAIDs)

Generic • Brand • Dose/Dosage Forms	Contraindications	Primary Side Effects	Key Monitoring Parameters	Pertinent Drug Interactions	Med Pearls
Mechanism of action – ↓ pain through weak inhibition of prostaglandin synthesis					
Acetaminophen (APAP) • Tylenol, Ofirmev • Oral: 325–1,000 mg every 4–6 hr (max = 4,000 mg/day) • IV <50 kg: 12.5 mg/kg q 4 hr or 15 mg/kg q 6 hr (max = 3,750 mg/day) • IV >50 kg: 650 mg q 4 hr or 1,000 mg q 6 hr (max = 4,000 mg/day) • Tabs, chewable tabs, caps, caplets, IV, oral liquid, rectal suppository	• Hypersensitivity • Severe hepatic impairment	• Hepatotoxicity • Nausea (IV form)	Pain relief	Alcohol may ↑ risk of hepatotoxicity	• Oral products are OTC • Antipyretic properties
Salicylates					
Mechanism of action – irreversible inhibition of COX-1 & COX-2 enzymes, which decreases prostaglandin synthesis; inhibition of thromboxane A_2					
Aspirin • Ascription, Ecotrin, Bufferin • 325–1,000 mg q 4–6 hr (max = 4,000 mg/day) • Tabs, chewable tabs, caplets, ER caps, rectal suppository	• Allergy to aspirin or NSAIDs • Active bleeding • Age <19 years	• GI upset (dyspepsia, GI ulceration) • Bleeding	• Pain relief • GI symptoms • S/S bleeding	May ↑ risk of bleeding with anticoagulants, other antiplatelets, and NSAIDs	• OTC • Administer with food
Nonacetylated salicylates					
Mechanism of action – inhibits COX-1 & COX-2 enzymes, which decreases prostaglandin synthesis					
Diflunisal • Only available as generic • 500–1,000 mg daily in 2 divided doses (max = 1,500 mg/day) • Tabs	• Hypersensitivity • Allergy to aspirin or NSAIDs • Use in the setting of a CABG	• GI upset (dyspepsia, GI ulceration) • Bleeding • Rash • Edema • ↓ renal function	• Pain relief • GI symptoms • Renal function	May ↑ risk of bleeding with anticoagulants, antiplatelets, and NSAIDs	• Administer with food • May check salicylate levels with chronic use or high doses (range = 10–30 mg/dL)
Salsalate • Only available as generic • 500–3,000 mg/day in 2–3 divided doses (max = 3,000 mg/day) • Tabs					Administer with food

Nonopioid Oral and Nonsteroidal Anti-Inflammatory Drugs (NSAIDs)   *(cont'd)*

Generic • Brand • Dose/Dosage Forms	Contraindications	Primary Side Effects	Key Monitoring Parameters	Pertinent Drug Interactions	Med Pearls
NSAIDs					
Mechanism of action – reversible inhibition of COX-1 & COX-2 enzymes resulting in decreased prostaglandin synthesis					
Propionic Acids					
Ibuprofen • Motrin, Advil, Caldolor • PO: 200–3,200 mg/day in 3–4 divided doses (max = 3,200 mg/day) • IV: 400–800 mg q 6 hr (max = 3,200 mg/day) • Tabs, chewable tabs, caps, IV, oral suspension	• Hypersensitivity • Allergy to aspirin or NSAIDs • Use in the setting of a CABG	• GI upset (dyspepsia, GI ulceration) • Rash • Edema • ↑ BP • ↓ renal function	• Pain relief • GI symptoms • Renal function • BP	• May ↑ risk of bleeding with anticoagulants, antiplatelets, and NSAIDs • May ↑ risk of lithium toxicity	• Administer with food • Available OTC (200 mg) and Rx (400–800 mg) • Available in pediatric preparations (oral suspension, chewable tabs) • Ibuprofen lysine injection (Neo-Profen) indicated for closure of patent ductus arteriosus in premature infants
Fenoprofen • Nalfon • 200–3,200 mg/day in 3–4 divided doses (max = 3,200 mg/day) • Tabs, caps					Administer with food
Flurbiprofen • Only available as generic • 50–300 mg/day in 2–4 divided doses (max = 300 mg/day) • Tabs					
Naproxen • Naprosyn • IR: 250–1,500 • ER: 750–1,500 mg/daily (max dose for chronic use = 1,000 mg/day) • OTC: 200 mg q 8–12 hr (max = 400 mg/12 hr or 600 mg/24 hr) • Tabs, caps, oral suspension, DR tabs, ER tabs					• Administer with food • Preferred NSAID in patients with CVD

Nonopioid Oral and Nonsteroidal Anti-Inflammatory Drugs (NSAIDs) *(cont'd)*

Generic • Brand • Dose/Dosage Forms	Contraindications	Primary Side Effects	Key Monitoring Parameters	Pertinent Drug Interactions	Med Pearls
Naproxen sodium • Aleve • OTC: 220 mg q 8–12 hr (max = 440 mg/8–12 hr or 600 mg/24 hr) • Rx: 275–550 mg BID • Tabs	[Same as above]	[Same as above]	[Same as above]	[Same as above]	• Administer with food • Available Rx and OTC • Preferred NSAID in patients with CVD
Oxaprozin • Daypro • 600–1,200 mg/daily (max <50 kg = 1,200 mg/day; >50 kg 1,800 mg/day or 26 mg/kg/day) • Tabs					Administer with food
Acetic Acids					
Diclofenac • Cambia, Zipsor, Zorvolex • Max = 100 mg/day for all indications • IR tab: 25–100 mg in 2–4 divided doses • ER tab: 100 mg daily • Caps: 18–35 mg TID • IV: 37.5 mg q 6 hr PRN • Caps, tabs, ER tabs, oral powder, IV, cream, gel, patch	• Hypersensitivity • Allergy to aspirin or NSAIDs • Use in the setting of a CABG	• GI upset (dyspepsia, GI ulceration) • Rash • Edema • ↑ BP • ↓ renal function	• Pain relief • GI symptoms • Renal function • BP	• May ↑ risk of bleeding with anticoagulants, antiplatelets, and NSAIDs • May ↑ risk of lithium toxicity	• Administer with food • Cambia packet should be mixed with 1–2 oz of water
Etodolac • Only available as generic • 200–1,000 mg/day in 1–4 divided doses (max = 1,000 mg/day) • Tabs, ER tabs, caps					Administer with food
Indomethacin • Indocin, Tivorbex • IR: 20–200 mg day in 2 divided doses (max = 200 mg/day) • ER: 75–150 mg in 1–2 divided doses (max = 150 mg/day) • Caps, ER caps, IV, rectal suppository, oral suspension		• GI upset (dyspepsia, GI ulceration) • Rash • Edema • ↑ BP • ↓ renal function • Headache • Dizziness			• Administer with food • Most commonly used to treat gout • Fat-soluble, crosses blood-brain barrier

Nonopioid Oral and Nonsteroidal Anti-Inflammatory Drugs (NSAIDs)   *(cont'd)*

Generic • Brand • Dose/Dosage Forms	Contraindications	Primary Side Effects	Key Monitoring Parameters	Pertinent Drug Interactions	Med Pearls
Nabumetone • Only available as generic • 500–2,000 mg in 1–2 divided doses • Tabs	[Same as above]	[Same as above]	[Same as above]	[Same as above]	Administer with food
Ketorolac • Only available as generic • IR: 10 mg q 4–6 hr PRN (max = 40 mg/day) • IV/IM: 30 mg q 6 hr PRN (max = 120 mg/day) • NS: >50 kg: 1 spray (15.75 mg) in each nostril q 6–8 hr (max = 4 doses/126 mg/day) • NS: <50 kg: 1 spray (15.75 mg) in 1 nostril q 6–8 hr (max = 4 doses/63 mg/day) • IV, IM, tabs, nasal spray, eye drop	• Hypersensitivity • Active PUD • GI or cerebrovascular bleeding • Severe renal impairment • Allergy to aspirin or NSAIDs • Prophylactic analgesia before surgery • Labor and delivery • Use in the setting of a CABG	• GI upset (dyspepsia, GI ulceration) • Rash • Edema • ↑ BP • ↓ renal function		• May ↑ risk of bleeding with anticoagulants, antiplatelets, and NSAIDs • May ↑ risk of lithium toxicity • Use with probenecid • Use with pentoxifylline	• Administer with food • Maximum length of treatment for any formulation or combination of formulations <5 days

Oxicams

Generic • Brand • Dose/Dosage Forms	Contraindications	Primary Side Effects	Key Monitoring Parameters	Pertinent Drug Interactions	Med Pearls
Meloxicam • Mobic, Vivlodex • Mobic: 7.5–15 mg daily • Vivlodex: 5–15 mg daily • Caps, tabs, oral suspension	• Hypersensitivity • Allergy to aspirin or NSAIDs • Use in the setting of a CABG	• GI upset (dyspepsia, GI ulceration) • Rash • Edema • ↑ BP • ↓ renal function	• Pain relief • GI symptoms • Renal function • BP	• May ↑ risk of bleeding with anticoagulants, antiplatelets, and NSAIDs • May ↑ risk of lithium toxicity	• Administer with food • More COX-2 selective than other NSAIDs • Fewer GI symptoms
Piroxicam • Feldene • 10–20 mg daily • Caps					

Fenamates

Generic • Brand • Dose/Dosage Forms	Contraindications	Primary Side Effects	Key Monitoring Parameters	Pertinent Drug Interactions	Med Pearls
Meclofenamate • Only available as generic • 50–400 mg/day in 4–6 divided doses (max = 400 mg/day) • Caps	• Hypersensitivity • Allergy to aspirin or NSAIDs • Use in the setting of a CABG	• GI upset (dyspepsia, GI ulceration) • Rash • Edema • ↑ BP • ↓ renal function	• Pain relief • GI symptoms • Renal function • BP	• May ↑ risk of bleeding with anticoagulants, antiplatelets, and NSAIDs • May ↑ risk of lithium toxicity	Administer with food

Selective COX-2 Inhibitor

Mechanism of action – inhibits COX-2 enzyme resulting in decreased prostaglandin synthesis

Generic • Brand • Dose/Dosage Forms	Contraindications	Primary Side Effects	Key Monitoring Parameters	Pertinent Drug Interactions	Med Pearls
Celecoxib • Celebrex • 100–400 mg/day in 1–2 divided doses • Caps	• Hypersensitivity • Allergy to aspirin or NSAIDs • Use in the setting of a CABG • Sulfa allergy	• GI upset (dyspepsia, GI ulceration) • Rash • Edema • ↑ BP • ↓ renal function	• Pain relief • GI symptoms • Renal function • BP	• May ↑ risk of bleeding with anticoagulants, antiplatelets, and NSAIDs • May ↑ risk of lithium toxicity	Lower incidence of GI toxicity compared with nonselective NSAIDs

Opioid Analgesics

Generic • Brand • Initial Dose/Dosage Form	Contraindications	Primary Side Effects	Key Monitoring Parameters	Pertinent Drug Interactions	Med Pearls
Mechanism of action – stimulate opioid receptors (mu, kappa, delta) in the CNS					
Phenanthrenes					
Morphine • MS Contin, Arymo ER, Duramorph, Kadian, Morpha-Bond ER • IR: 5–30 mg q 4 hr PRN • IM: 5–20 mg q 4 hr PRN • IV: 2.5–15 mg q 4 hr PRN • Rectal: 10–20 mg q 4 hr PRN • Tabs, ER tabs, ER caps, IV, IM oral solution, caps	• Hypersensitivity • Respiratory depression • Acute or severe bronchial asthma • GI obstruction • Paralytic ileus	• Constipation • N/V • CNS depression • Sedation • Confusion • Respiratory depression • Hypotension • Bradycardia	• Pain relief • Constipation • Mental status • Signs of abuse/misuse • State prescription monitoring plan (PDMP) data • RR • BP • HR	• Other CNS depressants, including alcohol and benzodiazepines, may ↑ CNS depressant effects • MAOIs may ↑ adverse effects; avoid use if MAOIs have been used within past 14 days • ↑ risk of serotonin syndrome with MAOIs, SSRIs, SNRIs, TCAs, triptans, lithium, dextromethorphan, buspirone, linezolid, methylene blue, St. John's wort, tramadol, and tapentadol	• Schedule II controlled substance • High abuse potential • Start with IR product • May take with food to reduce nausea • Often need a stimulant laxative for constipation • Arymo ER and MorphaBond ER are FDA-labeled abuse-deterrent formulations
Morphine sulfate/naltrexone • Embeda • 20 mg/0.8 mg daily • ER caps					• Schedule II controlled substance • FDA-labeled abuse-deterrent formulation

Opioid Analgesics   *(cont'd)*

Generic • Brand • Initial Dose/Dosage Form	Contraindications	Primary Side Effects	Key Monitoring Parameters	Pertinent Drug Interactions	Med Pearls
Oxycodone • OxyContin, Oxaydo, Xtampza ER • IR: 5–15 mg q 4–6 hr • ER: 50% of total daily oral oxycodone dose administered q 12 hr • Caps, ER caps, oral solution, tabs, ER tabs	[Same as above]	[Same as above]	[Same as above]	• Oxycodone is a CYP3A4 substrate • CYP3A4 inhibitors may ↑ effects/toxicity • CYP3A4 inducers may ↓ effects • Other CNS depressants, including alcohol and benzodiazepines, may ↑ CNS depressant effects • MAOIs may ↑ adverse effects; avoid use if MAOIs have been used within past 14 days • ↑ risk of serotonin syndrome with MAOIs, SSRIs, SNRIs, TCAs, triptans, lithium, dextromethorphan, buspirone, linezolid, methylene blue, St. John's wort, tramadol, and tapentadol	• Schedule II controlled substance • High abuse potential • Start with IR product • May take with food to reduce nausea • Often need a stimulant laxative for constipation • OxyContin and Xtampza ER are FDA-labeled abuse-deterrent formulations • ER tabs are NOT bioequivalent to ER caps • ER caps should be administered with food and may be administered via a nasogastric or gastric tube
Oxycodone/acetaminophen • Endocet, Percocet, Xartemis XR • IR: 2.5 mg–10 mg/325 mg q 4–6 hr PRN • ER: 15 mg/650 mg q 12 hr • Dose is limited by APAP component (max APAP = 4 g/day) • Tabs, oral solution, ER tabs					
Oxycodone/naltrexone • Troxyca ER • 10 mg/1.2 mg–80 mg/9.6 mg q 12 hr • ER tabs					• Schedule II controlled substance • FDA-labeled abuse-deterrent formulation
Oxycodone/naloxone • Targiniq ER • 10 mg/5 mg–40 mg/20 mg q 12 hr					• Schedule II controlled substance • FDA-labeled abuse-deterrent formulation

Opioid Analgesics (cont'd)

Generic • Brand • Initial Dose/Dosage Form	Contraindications	Primary Side Effects	Key Monitoring Parameters	Pertinent Drug Interactions	Med Pearls
Hydrocodone • Hysingla ER, Vantrela ER, Zohydro ER • Hysingla ER: 20 mg daily • Vantrela ER & Zohydro ER: 10 mg q 12 hr (max = 180 mg/day) • ER caps, ER tabs	[Same as above]	[Same as above]	[Same as above]	• Hydrocodone is a CYP3A4 substrate • CYP3A4 inhibitors may ↑ effects/toxicity • CYP3A4 inducers may ↓ effects • Other CNS depressants, including alcohol and benzodiazepines, may ↑ CNS depressant effects • MAOIs may ↑ adverse effects; avoid use if MAOIs have been used within past 14 days • ↑ risk of serotonin syndrome with MAOIs, SSRIs, SNRIs, TCAs, triptans, lithium, dextromethorphan, buspirone, linezolid, methylene blue, St. John's wort, tramadol, and tapentadol	• Schedule II controlled substance • High abuse potential • Start with IR product • May take with food to reduce nausea • Often need a stimulant laxative for constipation • Hysingla ER is an FDA-labeled abuse-deterrent formulation
Hydrocodone/ acetaminophen • Lorcet, Norco, Vicodin, Xodol • 2.5 mg–10 mg/ 325 mg PO q 4–6 hr • Dose is limited by APAP component (max APAP = 4 g/ day) • Tabs, oral solution					
Hydromorphone • Dilaudid, Exalgo • IR: 2–4 mg q 4–6 hr PRN • XR: 8–64 mg q 24 hr • IV: 0.5–2 mg q 4 hr • IM: 1–2 mg q 4–6 hr • Supp: 3 mg q 6–8 hr • Tabs, ER tabs, oral liquid, IV, IM, rectal suppository				• Other CNS depressants, including alcohol and benzodiazepines, may ↑ CNS depressant effects • MAOIs may ↑ adverse effects; avoid use if MAOIs have been used within past 14 days • ↑ risk of serotonin syndrome with MAOIs, SSRIs, SNRIs, TCAs, triptans, lithium, dextromethorphan, buspirone, linezolid, methylene blue, St. John's wort, tramadol, and tapentadol	• Schedule II controlled substance • High abuse potential • Start with IR product • May take with food to reduce nausea • Often need a stimulant laxative for constipation

Opioid Analgesics *(cont'd)*

Generic • Brand • Initial Dose/Dosage Form	Contraindications	Primary Side Effects	Key Monitoring Parameters	Pertinent Drug Interactions	Med Pearls
Codeine • Only available as generic • IR: 15–60 mg q 4 hr PRN (max = 360 mg/day) • Tabs	[Same as above]	[Same as above]	[Same as above]	• Codeine is a CYP2D6 substrate • CYP2D6 inhibitors may ↓ effects • Other CNS depressants, including alcohol and benzodiazepines, may ↑ CNS depressant effects • MAOIs may ↑ adverse effects; avoid use if MAOIs have been used within past 14 days • ↑ risk of serotonin syndrome with MAOIs, SSRIs, SNRIs, TCAs, triptans, lithium, dextromethorphan, buspirone, linezolid, methylene blue, St. John's wort, tramadol, and tapentadol	• Schedule II controlled substance • Must be metabolized by CYP2D6 to morphine for analgesic effect • Good antitussive properties
Codeine/acetaminophen • Tylenol with codeine #3, Tylenol with codeine #4 • 15–60 mg/300 mg–600 mg q 4 hr PRN (max = 360 mg/day of codeine and 4,000 mg/day of acetaminophen) • Oral solution, tabs					
Oxymorphone • Opana • 5–10 mg q 4–6 hr • Tabs, IV, IM				• Other CNS depressants, including alcohol and benzodiazepines, may ↑ CNS depressant effects • MAOIs may ↑ adverse effects; avoid use if MAOIs have been used within past 14 days • ↑ risk of serotonin syndrome with MAOIs, SSRIs, SNRIs, TCAs, triptans, lithium, dextromethorphan, buspirone, linezolid, methylene blue, St. John's wort, tramadol, and tapentadol	• Schedule II controlled substance • High abuse potential • May take with food to reduce nausea • Often need a stimulant laxative for constipation • ER product removed from the market due to abuse concerns

Opioid Analgesics   *(cont'd)*

Generic • Brand • Initial Dose/Dosage Form	Contraindications	Primary Side Effects	Key Monitoring Parameters	Pertinent Drug Interactions	Med Pearls
Phenylpiperidines					
Meperidine • Demerol • IM: 50–150 mg q 3–4 hr (max = 600 mg/day) • IV, IM, tabs	• Hypersensitivity • Respiratory depression • Acute or severe bronchial asthma • GI obstruction • Paralytic ileus	• Constipation • N/V • CNS depression • Sedation • Confusion • Respiratory depression • Hypotension • Bradycardia	• Pain relief • Constipation • Mental status • Signs of abuse/misuse • State prescription monitoring plan (PDMP) data • RR • BP • HR	• Other CNS depressants, including alcohol and benzodiazepines, may ↑ CNS depressant effects • MAOIs may ↑ adverse effects; avoid use if MAOIs have been used within past 14 days • ↑ risk of serotonin syndrome with MAOIs, SSRIs, SNRIs, TCAs, triptans, lithium, dextromethorphan, buspirone, linezolid, methylene blue, St. John's wort, tramadol, and tapentadol	• NOT recommended for use as an analgesic • Limit use to <48 hours • Schedule II controlled substance • Maybe used for shivering or rigors • Renal accumulation of active metabolite normeperidine may cause seizures
Fentanyl • Duragesic • TD patch: 12–25 mcg applied q 72 hr • IV: 25–50 mcg/hr • Actiq transmucosal lozenge: 200 mcg over 15 minutes q 4 hr (max = 2 doses/breakthrough pain episode) • Lazanda nasal spray: 100 mcg q 2 hr PRN • Fentora buccal tablet: 100 mcg q 4 hr PRN • Abstral SL tablet: 100 mcg q 4 hr PRN • Onsolis buccal film: 200 mcg q 2 hr PRN (max = 4 applications/day) • Subsys SL spray: 100 mcg q 4 hr PRN (max = 2 doses/breakthrough pain episode)	• Hypersensitivity • Respiratory depression • Acute or severe bronchial asthma • GI obstruction • Paralytic ileus Opioid-intolerant patients			• CYP3A4 substrate • CYP3A4 inhibitors may ↑ effects/toxicity • CYP3A4 inducers may ↓ effects • Other CNS depressants, including alcohol and benzodiazepines, may ↑ CNS depressant effects • MAOIs may ↑ adverse effects; avoid use if MAOIs have been used within past 14 days • ↑ risk of serotonin syndrome with MAOIs, SSRIs, SNRIs, TCAs, triptans, lithium, dextromethorphan, buspirone, linezolid, methylene blue, St. John's wort, tramadol, and tapentadol	• Schedule II controlled substance • High abuse potential • Transdermal patch used for chronic pain, NOT for acute pain • Patch formulation indicated for opioid-tolerant patients • Patch takes 12–24 hours to begin working; to discard fold in half and flush • Abstral, Actiq, Fentora, Lazanda, Onsolis, and Subsys are transmucosal immediate-release fentanyl (TIRF) products for breakthrough pain and are a part of the TIRF REMS program for use • TIRF products are NOT interchangeable

Opioid Analgesics *(cont'd)*

Generic • Brand • Initial Dose/Dosage Form	Contraindications	Primary Side Effects	Key Monitoring Parameters	Pertinent Drug Interactions	Med Pearls
Diphenylheptane					
Methadone • Dolophine, Methadose • IR: 2.5–10 mg q 8–12 hr • IV, IM, oral solution, tabs	• Hypersensitivity • Respiratory depression • Acute or severe bronchial asthma • GI obstruction • Paralytic ileus	• Constipation • N/V • CNS depression • Sedation • Confusion • Respiratory depression • Hypotension • Bradycardia • QTc prolongation	• Pain relief • Constipation • Mental status • Signs of abuse/ misuse • State prescription monitoring plan (PDMP) data • RR • BP • HR • ECG	• CYP3A4 substrate • CYP3A4 inhibitors may ↑ effects/toxicity • CYP3A4 inducers may ↓ effects • Other CNS depressants, including alcohol and benzodiazepines, may ↑ CNS depressant effects • MAOIs may ↑ adverse effects; avoid use if MAOIs have been used within past 14 days • ↑ risk of serotonin syndrome with MAOIs, SSRIs, SNRIs, TCAs, triptans, lithium, dextromethorphan, buspirone, linezolid, methylene blue, St. John's wort • May ↑ risk of torsade de pointes with other QTc-prolonging drugs	• Schedule II controlled substance • Long half-life and may be difficult to titrate • Used for chronic pain • May be used for heroin and opioid abuse

Opioid Analgesics   *(cont'd)*

Generic • Brand • Initial Dose/Dosage Form	Contraindications	Primary Side Effects	Key Monitoring Parameters	Pertinent Drug Interactions	Med Pearls
Central Analgesics					
Tramadol • Ultram, ConZip • IR: 50–100 mg q 4–6 hr PRN (max = 400 mg/day) • ER: 100 mg q 24 hr (max = 300 mg/day)	• Hypersensitivity • Respiratory depression • Acute or severe bronchial asthma • GI obstruction • Paralytic ileus	• Constipation • N/V • CNS depression • Sedation • Confusion • Respiratory depression • Hypotension • Bradycardia • Serotonin syndrome • Seizures	• Pain relief • Constipation • Mental status • Signs of abuse/misuse • State prescription monitoring plan (PDMP) data • RR • BP • HR • S/S serotonin syndrome	• Other CNS depressants, including alcohol and benzodiazepines, may ↑ CNS depressant effects • MAOIs may ↑ adverse effects; avoid use if MAOIs have been used within past 14 days • ↑ risk of serotonin syndrome with MAOIs, SSRIs, SNRIs, TCAs, triptans, lithium, dextromethorphan, buspirone, linezolid, methylene blue, St. John's wort	• Schedule IV controlled substance • Adjust dose in renal impairment
Tramadol/acetaminophen • Ultracet • 37.5 mg/325 mg 2 tabs q 4–6 hr (max = 8 tabs/day) • Tabs					• Schedule IV controlled substance • Adjust dose in renal impairment • Treatment duration should not exceed 5 days
Tapentadol • Nucynta, Nucynta ER • IR: 50–100 mg q 4–6 hr • ER: 50 mg q 12 hr • Tabs, ER tabs		• Constipation • N/V • CNS depression • Sedation • Confusion • Respiratory depression • Hypotension • Bradycardia • Serotonin syndrome			• Schedule II controlled substance • Avoid use in severe renal impairment

Opioid Analgesics   *(cont'd)*

Generic • Brand • Initial Dose/Dosage Form	Contraindications	Primary Side Effects	Key Monitoring Parameters	Pertinent Drug Interactions	Med Pearls
Partial Opioid Agonists					
Buprenorphine • Belbuca, Buprenex, Butrans, Probuphine Implant, Sublocade • IM/IV: 0.3 mg q 6–8 hr • Transdermal patch: 5 mcg/hr applied weekly • Buccal film, transdermal patch, SQ implant, IV, IM, SL tab	• Hypersensitivity • Respiratory depression • Acute or severe bronchial asthma • GI obstruction • Paralytic ileus	• Constipation • Dizziness • Confusion • N/V • HTN • Hypotension • Respiratory depression • Fatigue • Hepatotoxicity • Pruritus (implant) • Erythema (implant)	• Pain relief • Constipation • Mental status • Signs of abuse/ misuse • State prescription monitoring plan (PDMP) data • RR • BP • LFTs	• CYP3A4 substrate • CYP3A4 inhibitors may ↑ effects/toxicity • CYP3A4 inducers may ↓ effects • Other CNS depressants, including alcohol and benzodiazepines, may ↑ CNS depressant effects • MAOIs may ↑ adverse effects; avoid use if MAOIs have been used within past 14 days • ↑ risk of serotonin syndrome with MAOIs, SSRIs, SNRIs, TCAs, triptans, lithium, dextromethorphan, buspirone, linezolid, methylene blue, St. John's wort, tramadol, and tapentadol	• Schedule III controlled substance • Can be used for pain management or opioid withdrawal/ dependence
Buprenorphine/ naloxone • Bunavail, Suboxone, Zubsolv • Bunavail buccal film: 2.1–12.6 mg/0.3–2.1 mg daily • Suboxone sublingual film target dose: 16 mg/4 mg daily • Zubsolv sublingual tablet target dose 11.4 mg/2.9 mg daily		• Pain • Withdrawal syndrome • Diaphoresis • Headache • Constipation • Dizziness • Confusion • N/V	• Pain • Constipation • Mental status • Signs of abuse/ misuse • State prescription monitoring plan (PDMP) data • S/S withdrawal		• Schedule III controlled substance • Indicated for the treatment of opioid dependence • Not recommended for heroin or opioid dependency induction treatment

Analgesic Adjuncts

Generic • Brand • Dose/Dosage Forms	Contraindications	Primary Side Effects	Key Monitoring Parameters	Pertinent Drug Interactions	Med Pearls
Mechanism of action – ↑ synaptic concentration of norepinephrine, desensitization of adenyl cyclase, and downregulation of serotonin receptors					
Desipramine • Norpramin • Initial: 10–25 mg/day (max = 300 mg/day) • Tabs / Amitriptyline ☆ • Only available generically • Initial: 25–50 mg/day (max = 150 mg) • Tabs	• Hypersensitivity • Use of MAOI within 2 wk • Concurrent use of linezolid or methylene blue • Acute recovery period post-myocardial infarction (MI)	• Anticholinergic symptoms • Weight gain • Bloating • Blurred vision • Xerostomia • Constipation • Dizziness • Somnolence • Headache • Fatigue • Serotonin syndrome	• Pain relief • Withdrawal symptoms from abrupt discontinuation • Suicidality • BP • ECG (in patients with cardiac disease or hyperthyroidism) • S/S of serotonin syndrome	• CYP2D6 substrate • CYP2D6 inhibitors may ↑ effects/toxicity • ↑ risk of serotonin syndrome with MAOIs, SSRIs, SNRIs, triptans, fentanyl, lithium, dextromethorphan, meperidine, buspirone, linezolid, methylene blue, St. John's wort, and tramadol	• Dangerous in overdose situations • Avoid in patients with high suicidality • Avoid dispensing large quantities • Neuropathic pain is an unlabeled indication • Taper off when medication is discontinued
Mechanism of action – structurally related to GABA, modulates the release of excitatory neurotransmitters through voltage-gated calcium channels					
Gabapentin ☆ • Neurontin • Initial 300 mg TID (max = 3,600 mg/day) • Caps, solution, tabs • Gralise • 300 mg daily on Day 1, then 600 mg daily on Day 2, then 900 mg daily on Days 3–6, then 1,200 mg daily on Days 7–10, then 1,500 mg daily on Days 11–14, then 1,800 mg daily • ER tabs • Horizant • 600 mg in AM × 3 days, then 600 mg every 12 hr • ER tabs	Hypersensitivity	• Dizziness • Fatigue • Somnolence • Ataxia • Weight gain • Angioedema • Behavioral disturbances (aggression, agitation, anger, anxiety, depression, hostility, nervousness) • Difficulty concentrating • Restlessness	• Pain relief • Suicidality	Other CNS depressants, including alcohol, may ↑ CNS depressant effects	• Adjust dose in renal impairment • Chronic neuropathic pain is not a labeled indication for IR product • Neurontin, Gralise, and Horizant indicated to treat post-herpetic neuralgia • Gralise and Horizant are NOT interchangeable with other gabapentin products

Analgesic Adjuncts *(cont'd)*

Generic • Brand • Dose/Dosage Forms	Contraindications	Primary Side Effects	Key Monitoring Parameters	Pertinent Drug Interactions	Med Pearls
Mechanism of action – modulates influx of calcium by binding to the alpha2-delta subunit on voltage-gated calcium channels					
Pregabalin ☆ • Lyrica, Lyrica CR • IR: 150 mg/day in 2–3 divided doses (max = 300–600 mg/day based on indication) • ER: 165–330 mg/ daily (max = 330 mg/day) • Caps, solution, ER caps	Hypersensitivity	• Angioedema • Somnolence • Dizziness • Peripheral edema	• Pain relief • Suicidality	[Same as above]	• Schedule V controlled substance • Adjust dose in renal impairment • Indicated for neuropathic pain associated with diabetes or spinal cord injury, fibromyalgia, and postherpetic neuralgia
Mechanism of action – SNRIs: inhibit the reuptake of serotonin and norepinephrine to allow higher available synaptic concentrations					
Duloxetine ☆ • Cymbalta • 30–60 mg/day in 1–2 divided doses (max = 60 mg/day) • ER caps	• Hypersensitivity • Use of MAOI within 2 wk • Concurrent use of linezolid or methylene blue • Hepatic impairment • Severe renal impairment (CrCl <30 mL/min)	• Hepatotoxicity • Orthostatic hypotension • Rash (Stevens-Johnson syndrome possible) • Palpitations • Diaphoresis • Constipation • ↓ appetite • N/D • Xerostomia • Asthenia • Dizziness • Insomnia or somnolence • Vertigo • Blurred vision • Polyuria • ↓ libido • Serotonin syndrome	• Pain relief • LFTs • BP • Withdrawal symptoms from abrupt discontinuation • Abnormal bleeding • Suicidality • S/S of serotonin syndrome	• CYP1A2 and CYP2D6 substrate • CYP1A2 or CYP2D6 inhibitors may ↑ effects/toxicity; avoid concomitant use with strong CYP1A2 inhibitors • CYP1A2 inducers may ↓ effects • ↑ risk of serotonin syndrome with MAOIs, SSRIs, triptans, TCAs, fentanyl, amphetamines, lithium, dextromethorphan, meperidine, buspirone, linezolid, methylene blue, St. John's wort, and tramadol • ↑ risk of bleeding when used with aspirin, NSAIDs, or anticoagulants	Indicated to treat diabetic neuropathy, fibromyalgia, and chronic musculoskeletal pain
Mechanism of action – induces the release of substance P, the principal chemomediator of pain impulses from the periphery					
Capsaicin • Salonpas, Zostrix-HP • Cream, gel, lotion: 0.025–0.1% applied 3–4 × daily • Patch: apply to affected area 3–4 × /day	Do not apply to wounds or damaged skin	Localized stinging	Pain relief	None	• OTC • Must be used regularly for ≥2 wk for maximal efficacy

Skeletal Muscle Relaxants

Generic • Brand • Dose & Max mg (frequency)	Contraindications	Primary Side Effects	Key Monitoring Parameters	Pertinent Drug Interactions	Med Pearls
Mechanism of action – inhibits reflexes at the level of the spinal cord by hyperpolarization of afferent fibers					
Baclofen • Gablofen, Lioresal • 5–20 mg PO TID–QID (max = 80 mg/day) • IT administration via infusion/implanted pump: 300–800 mcg/day	• Hypersensitivity • IV, IM, subcut, or epidural administration (for IT use)	• Hypotonia • Drowsiness • Confusion • Headache • N/V • Hypotension • Seizures • Dizziness	• Pain relief • Mental status	Other CNS depressants, including alcohol, may ↑ CNS depressant effects	Antispastic agent
Mechanism of action – depresses polysynaptic neuronal transmission in the spinal cord and reticular formation					
Carisoprodol • Soma • 250–350 mg 4 × /day • Tabs	• Hypersensitivity • Acute intermittent porphyria	• Drowsiness • Dizziness • Headache	• Pain relief • Mental status • Signs of abuse/ misuse/addiction	• CYP2C19 substrate • CYP2C19 inhibitors may ↑ effects/toxicity • CYP2C19 inducers may ↓ effects • Other CNS depressants, including alcohol, may ↑ CNS depressant effects	• Schedule IV controlled substance • Antispasmodic agent • Metabolized to meprobamate • Maximum recommended duration of treatment is 2–3 weeks
Mechanism of action – inhibits polysynaptic reflexes					
Chlorzoxazone • Only available generically • 250–750 mg 3–4 × /day • Tabs	Hypersensitivity	• Dizziness • Drowsiness • N/V/D • Urine discoloration • Hepatotoxicity	• Pain relief • LFTs	Other CNS depressants, including alcohol, may ↑ CNS depressant effects	Antispasmodic agent

Skeletal Muscle Relaxants *(cont'd)*

Generic • Brand • Dose & Max mg (frequency)	Contraindications	Primary Side Effects	Key Monitoring Parameters	Pertinent Drug Interactions	Med Pearls
Mechanism of action – reduces tonic somatic motor activity by altering alpha and gamma motor neurons					
Cyclobenzaprine • Amrix • IR: 5–10 mg TID • ER: 15–30 mg daily • ER caps, tabs	• Hypersensitivity • Use of MAOI within 2 wk • Hyperthyroidism • Heart failure • Arrhythmias • Atrioventricular block or conduction disturbance • Acute recovery of MI	• Drowsiness • Dizziness • Xerostomia • Fatigue • Constipation • Confusion • Weakness • Blurred vision • Irritability • Serotonin syndrome	• Pain relief • Mental status • S/S of serotonin syndrome	• CYP1A2 substrate • CYP1A2 inhibitors may ↑ effects/toxicity • CYP1A2 inducers may ↓ effects • Other CNS depressants, including alcohol, may ↑ CNS depressant effects • ↑ risk of serotonin syndrome with MAOIs, SSRIs, SNRIs, triptans, TCAs, fentanyl, lithium, dextromethorphan, meperidine, buspirone, linezolid, methylene blue, St. John's wort, and tramadol	• Antispasmodic agent • ER formulation should not be used in older adults (>65 yr) or patients with hepatic impairment
Mechanism of action – inhibits the release of calcium from sarcoplasmic reticulum					
Dantrolene • Dantrium • 25 mg daily × 7 days, then 25 mg TID × 7 days, then 50 mg TID × 7 days, then 100 mg TID (max = 400 mg/day) • Caps	• Hypersensitivity • Active liver disease • If spasticity is used to maintain upright posture/balance or function	• Hepatotoxicity • Drowsiness • Dizziness • Headache • Weakness • Diarrhea	• Pain relief • LFTs	• CYP3A4 substrate • CYP3A4 inhibitors may ↑ effects/toxicity • CYP3A4 inducers may ↓ effects • Concurrent use with estrogen may ↑ risk of hepatotoxicity • Other CNS depressants, including alcohol, may ↑ CNS depressant effects	• Antispastic agent • Females and patients >35 yr at ↑ risk for hepatotoxicity • IV formulation can also be used to treat malignant hyperthermia
Mechanism of action – general depression of the CNS					
Metaxalone • Skelaxin • 800 mg 3–4 × /day • Tabs	• Hypersensitivity • Severe renal or hepatic impairment • Predisposition to drug-induced, hemolytic, or other anemias	• Dizziness • Drowsiness • Headache • N/V • Hemolytic anemia • Jaundice • Rash	• Pain relief • Complete blood count	Other CNS depressants, including alcohol, may ↑ CNS depressant effects	Antispasmodic agent

Skeletal Muscle Relaxants   *(cont'd)*

Generic • Brand • Dose & Max mg (frequency)	Contraindications	Primary Side Effects	Key Monitoring Parameters	Pertinent Drug Interactions	Med Pearls
Mechanism of action – general depression of the CNS					
Methocarbamol • Robaxin • 4–6 g/day PO in 3–6 divided doses • 1 g IV/IM every 8 hr for no more than 3 consecutive days • Injection, tabs	• Hypersensitivity • Renal impairment (IV use because of polyethylene glycol in vehicle)	• Confusion • Impaired coordination • Headache • Sedation	• Pain relief • Presence of side effects	Other CNS depressants, including alcohol, may ↑ CNS depressant effects	Antispasmodic agent
Mechanism of action – central atropine-like effects for indirect skeletal muscle relaxation					
Orphenadrine • Only available generically • 100 mg PO BID • 60 mg IV/IM every 12 hr • ER tabs, injection	• Hypersensitivity • Glaucoma • GI obstruction • Peptic ulcer disease • Benign prostatic hyperplasia • Bladder obstruction • Megaesophagus • Myasthenia gravis	• Tachycardia • Palpitation • Dizziness • Syncope • Anaphylaxis • Drowsiness • Confusion • Constipation • N/V • Xerostomia • Urinary retention • Tremor • Blurred vision	• Pain relief • HR	• Additive effects with other anticholinergic medications • Other CNS depressants, including alcohol, may ↑ CNS depressant effects	Antispasmodic agent
Mechanism of action – alpha-2 receptor agonist					
Tizanidine • Zanaflex • 2–12 mg TID • Caps, tabs	Concurrent use with strong CYP1A2 inhibitors	• Somnolence • Hypotension • Syncope • Hepatotoxicity • Hallucinations • Anaphylaxis • Xerostomia • Weakness • Dizziness	• Pain relief • LFTs • BP	• CYP1A2 substrate • CYP1A2 inhibitors may ↑ effects/toxicity • CYP1A2 inducers may ↓ effects • Oral contraceptives may ↑ effects/toxicity • Concurrent use with clonidine may ↑ risk of hypotension • Other CNS depressants, including alcohol, may ↑ CNS depressant effects	Antispastic agent

Bone and Joint Disorders 12

This chapter covers the following disease states:

- **Osteoarthritis**
- **Rheumatoid arthritis**
- **Osteoporosis**
- **Gout**

OSTEOARTHRITIS

Guidelines Summary

The goals of therapy are to ↓ pain and stiffness, maintain/improve joint mobility and limit functional impairment, and ↑ quality of life.

- OA of the hand
  - First-line options: Topical capsaicin, topical nonsteroidal anti-inflammatory drugs (NSAIDs), oral NSAIDs, tramadol
  - Topical NSAIDs preferred over oral NSAIDs in patients ≥75 years of age
- OA of the knee or hip
  - First-line option: Acetaminophen (scheduled, up to maximum of 4 g/day for acute use in younger patients; maximum of 3 g/day for chronic use or use in patients >65 years of age)
  - Second-line options: Topical or oral NSAIDs (topical preferred in patients ≥75 years of age) or intra-articular corticosteroid injections
  - Third-line options: Duloxetine, tramadol, or intra-articular hyaluronan injections

Treatment Algorithm

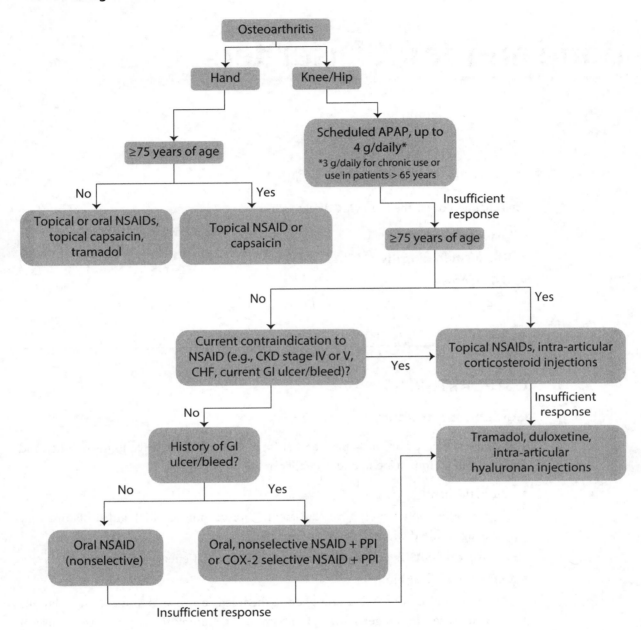

Drugs for Osteoarthritis

(See drug table in the Pain Management chapter for a review of acetaminophen and NSAIDs.)

Generic • Brand • Dose/Dosage Forms	Contraindications	Primary Side Effects	Key Monitoring Parameters	Pertinent Drug Interactions	Med Pearls
Adjunctive Therapies/Nutritional Supplements					
Glucosamine sulfate • Various • 500–1,500 mg/day in 1–2 divided doses daily	Unknown	• Itching • Gastrointestinal (GI) upset	• Pain relief • Presence of side effects	Unknown	• Nutritional supplement • Available OTC • Conflicting clinical trial data
Intra-Articular Injections					
Mechanism of action – serves as a lubricant for joint tissue					
Hyaluronate and derivates • Synvisc, Synvisc-One • Synvisc: Inject 16 mg (2 mL) once weekly for 3 wk (total of 3 injections) • Sinvisc-One: Inject 48 mg (6 mL) once per knee	Hypersensitivity	• Injection site reaction • Bruising • Erythema • Lumps • Pain • Swelling • Pruritus • Skin discoloration • Arthralgia • Infection	S/S of inflammation or infection	No known significant drug interactions	None

RHEUMATOID ARTHRITIS

Guidelines Summary

- Goals of therapy include achieving low disease activity or remission.

- A disease-modifying antirheumatic drug (DMARD) should be initiated within 3 months of diagnosis to retard disease progression.

- Leflunomide, sulfasalazine, hydroxychloroquine, and methotrexate are first-line DMARD options.

- In patients with moderate to severe disease activity, combination therapy may be considered initially.

- NSAIDs are useful for symptomatic relief during onset of DMARD and then can be used as needed otherwise. NSAIDs do not alter disease progression in RA.

- Corticosteroids are used as adjunctive therapy in patient with refractory symptoms.

- Biologic agents are used when initial monotherapy has been demonstrated to be ineffective or if moderate-to-high disease activity or poor prognostic features are present. Additional DMARDs may be tried prior to use of biologics.

- Biologic therapies ↑ the risk of serious infections and should not be initiated in a patient with an active infection or in combination with live vaccines.

Treatment Algorithm

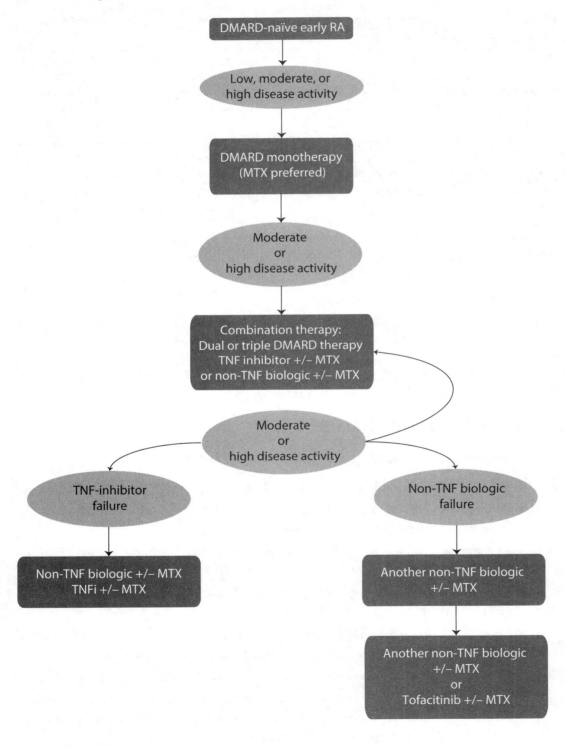

Medications for Rheumatoid Arthritis

Generic • Brand • Dose/Dosage Forms	Contraindications	Primary Side Effects	Key Monitoring Parameters	Pertinent Drug Interactions	Med Pearls
Mechanism of action – corticosteroids: exert anti-inflammatory and immunosuppressive effects by inhibiting prostaglandins and leukotrienes, which results in ↓ inflammation, ↓ pain, and a potential ↓ in joint destruction					
Prednisone☆ • Only available generically • 5–60 mg daily initially; individualized • Solution, tabs	• Systemic fungal infection • Hypersensitivity	• Hyperglycemia • ↑ blood pressure (BP) • ↓ bone mineral density (BMD) • Fluid retention • Impaired wound healing • Infection • Hyperglycemia • ↑ appetite • Irritability • Insomnia • Weight gain	• Blood sugar • BP • Electrolytes • BMD • Presence of edema/weight	May ↑ anticoagulant effect of warfarin	Side effects generally present with chronic and/or long-term use
DMARDs					
Mechanism of action – inhibit cytokine production, inhibit purine biosynthesis, thereby ↓ inflammation in affected joints					
Methotrexate☆ • Otrexup, Rasuvo, Rheumatrex, Trexall • 7.5 mg PO/subcut/IM weekly • Injection, tabs	• Hypersensitivity • Alcoholism • Liver disease • Immunodeficiency • Significant blood dyscrasias • Pregnancy • Lactation	• GI upset (nausea, diarrhea, abdominal pain) • Stomatitis • Thrombocytopenia • Leukopenia • Anemia • ↑ liver function tests (LFTs) • Interstitial lung disease • Rash (Stevens-Johnson syndrome possible) • Malaise • Fatigue • Fever/chills • Infection	• Pain relief • LFTs • Complete blood count (CBC) with differential • Renal function (sCr) • Folate concentrations • S/S of infection	• NSAIDs and salicylates ↑ risk of toxicity • Penicillins, sulfonamides, and tetracyclines may ↑ risk of toxicity	• May supplement with folic acid to ↓ side effects and prevent folate deficiency • Myelosuppression is biggest concern • Should be taken with food
Mechanism of action – not fully understood; thought to be related to immunosuppressant properties					
Hydroxychloroquine☆ • Plaquenil • 200–600 mg/day in 1–2 divided doses • Tabs	• Hypersensitivity • Retinal changes with agent in past • Children	• Macular damage • Corneal deposits • Retinopathy • Rash • Nausea • Diarrhea • Neutropenia • Thrombocytopenia • Anemia	• Ocular exams every 3 mo • CBC with differential	May ↑ serum digoxin concentrations	Hemolysis can occur in patients with glucose-6-phosphate dehydrogenase deficiency

Medications for Rheumatoid Arthritis *(cont'd)*

Generic • Brand • Dose/Dosage Forms	Contraindications	Primary Side Effects	Key Monitoring Parameters	Pertinent Drug Interactions	Med Pearls
Mechanism of action – inhibits pyrimidine synthesis, thereby ↓ lymphocyte proliferation and inflammation					
Leflunomide • Arava • 100 mg daily × 3 days, then 20 mg daily • Tabs	• Hypersensitivity • Severe hepatic impairment • Pregnancy	• Diarrhea • Hepatotoxicity • Alopecia • Rash (Stevens-Johnson syndrome possible) • Peripheral neuropathy • Interstitial lung disease • ↑ BP • Neutropenia • Thrombocytopenia • Anemia • Infection	• LFTs (monthly × 6 mo, then every 6–8 wk) • Renal function (sCr) • CBC with differential (monthly × 6 mo, then every 6–8 wk) • Pregnancy test (before therapy begins) • BP • S/S of infection	• CYP2C8 inhibitor • May ↑ effects/toxicity of CYP2C8 substrates • May ↓ effects of warfarin • May ↑ toxicity of rosuvastatin (max dose of rosuvastatin = 10 mg/day)	• Highly teratogenic • Appropriate contraception should be used • After stopping therapy, accelerated drug elimination procedure should be used to rapidly ↓ concentrations of active metabolite (comprised of cholestyramine or activated charcoal)
Mechanism of action – not fully understood; related to anti-inflammatory properties					
Sulfasalazine • Azulfidine, Azulfidine EN-tabs • 500–3,000 mg/day in 2 divided doses • ER tabs, tabs	• Hypersensitivity to any sulfa-containing drug or salicylates • Intestinal or urinary obstruction • Porphyria	• N/V/D • Rash (Stevens-Johnson syndrome possible) • Photosensitivity • Neutropenia • Anemia • Hepatotoxicity • Renal impairment • Alopecia • Stomatitis • Infection	• CBC with differential (every other wk × 3 mo, then every 2–3 mo × 3 mo, then every 3 mo) • LFTs (every other wk × 3 mo, then every 2–3 mo × 3 mo, then every 3 mo) • Renal function (sCr) (every other wk × 3 mo, then every 2–3 mo × 3 mo, then every 3 mo) • Folate concentrations	• May ↑ effects of warfarin • May ↓ serum digoxin concentrations	• May supplement with folic acid to ↓ side effects and prevent folate deficiency • Preferred option in pregnant patients

Medications for Rheumatoid Arthritis   *(cont'd)*

Generic • Brand • Dose/Dosage Forms	Contraindications	Primary Side Effects	Key Monitoring Parameters	Pertinent Drug Interactions	Med Pearls
Biologics					
Mechanism of action – binds to and inhibits the cytokine tumor necrosis factor (TNF), thereby inhibiting the subsequent inflammatory cascade					
Etanercept • Enbrel • 50 mg subcut weekly • Injection	Sepsis	• Injection site reactions • Anaphylaxis • Infection (especially latent tuberculosis [TB] reactivation, fungal infections, and hepatitis B virus [HBV] reactivation) • Lymphoma • Leukemia • Skin cancer • Heart failure (HF) exacerbation • Bone marrow suppression • Lupus-like syndrome • Demyelinating disorders	• PPD and HBV screening before initiating treatment • S/S of infection • S/S of heart failure • CBC with differential	Not to be given with live vaccines	• Store in refrigerator • Use within 14 days once at room temp • Discontinue if serious infection occurs • Use with caution in patients with HF • Can be self-administered • Can be used alone or in combination with methotrexate • Pneumococcal, influenza (IM), and HBV vaccines prior to initiating and/or after per CDC ACIP
Infliximab • Inflectra, Remicade • 3 mg/kg IV infusion at initiation, wk 2 and wk 6, then every 8 wk • Injection	• Hypersensitivity • Doses >5 mg/kg in moderate–severe HF	• Infusion reactions (hypotension, dyspnea, urticaria) • Delayed hypersensitivity reactions (fever, rash, myalgia, headache, sore throat, hand/facial edema, dysphagia, arthralgias) • Infection (especially latent TB reactivation, fungal infections, or HBV reactivation) • HF exacerbation • Bone marrow suppression • Lymphoma • Leukemia • Skin cancer • Hepatotoxicity	• PPD and HBV screening before initiating treatment • BP • LFTs • S/S of infection • S/S of HF • CBC with differential		• Delayed hypersensitivity reaction may occur as early as after 2nd dose • Premedicate with H_1 antagonist, H_2 antagonist, acetaminophen, and/or corticosteroid • Dose limited to ≤5 mg/kg in patients with HF • Discontinue if serious infection occurs • Indicated for use in combination with methotrexate • Pneumococcal, influenza (IM), and HBV vaccines prior to initiating and/or after per CDC ACIP

Medications for Rheumatoid Arthritis   *(cont'd)*

Generic • Brand • Dose/Dosage Forms	Contraindications	Primary Side Effects	Key Monitoring Parameters	Pertinent Drug Interactions	Med Pearls
Golimumab • Simponi, Simponi Aria • 50 mg subcut monthly or 2 mg/kg IV infusion at initiation and wk 4, then every 8 wk • Injection	None	• Injection site reactions • Anaphylaxis • Infection (especially latent TB reactivation, fungal infections, and HBV reactivation) • Lymphoma • Leukemia • Skin cancer • HF exacerbation • Bone marrow suppression • Lupus-like syndrome • Demyelinating disorders	• PPD and HBV screening before initiating treatment • S/S of infection • S/S of HF • CBC with differential	[Same as above]	• Use with caution in patients with HF • Discontinue if serious infection occurs • Subcut injection can be self-administered • Store subcut injection in refrigerator • Indicated for use in combination with methotrexate • Pneumococcal, influenza (IM), and HBV vaccines prior to initiating and/or after per CDC ACIP
Adalimumab • Humira • 40 mg subcut every other wk (if not taking methotrexate, may give weekly) • Injection					• Use with caution in patients with HF • Discontinue if serious infection occurs • Can be self-administered • Store in refrigerator • Use within 14 days once at room temp • Can be used alone or in combination with methotrexate or other non-biological DMARDs • Pneumococcal, influenza (IM), and HBV vaccines prior to initiating and/or after per CDC ACIP
Certolizumab pegol • Cimzia • 400 mg subcut at initiation, wk 2, and wk 4, then 200 mg subcut every other wk • Injection					• Use with caution in patients with HF • Discontinue if serious infection occurs • Can be self-administered • Store in refrigerator • Can be used alone or in combination with methotrexate or other non-biological DMARDs

Medications for Rheumatoid Arthritis *(cont'd)*

Generic • Brand • Dose/Dosage Forms	Contraindications	Primary Side Effects	Key Monitoring Parameters	Pertinent Drug Interactions	Med Pearls
Mechanism of action – binds to interleukin-1 (IL-1) receptors on target cells, thereby preventing release of chemotactic factors and adhesion molecules and subsequently ↓ inflammation and connective tissue damage					
Anakinra • Kineret • 100 mg subcut daily • Injection	Hypersensitivity	• Injection-site reactions (inflammation, ecchymosis) • Infection (including latent TB reactivation) • Neutropenia • Anaphylaxis	• PPD screening before initiating treatment • CBC with differential • S/S of infection	• Not to be given with TNF inhibitors • Not to be given with live vaccines	• Indicated for moderate–severe disease that has not responded to >1 DMARD • Can be self-administered • Store in refrigerator • Can be used alone or in combination with other non-biological DMARDs • Pneumococcal, influenza (IM), and HBV vaccines prior to initiating and/or after per CDC ACIP
Mechanism of action – IL-6 receptor antagonist					
Tocilizumab • Actemra • IV: 4 mg/kg IV infusion every 4 wk; may be ↑ to 8 mg/kg based on clinical response (max = 800 mg per infusion) • Subcut: <100 kg: 162 mg subcut every other wk (may be ↑ to every wk based on clinical response); ≥100 kg: 162 mg subcut weekly • Injection	• Hypersensitivity • Absolute neutrophil count <2,000/mm^3 • Platelets <150,000/mm^3 • ALT or AST >1.5× the upper limit of normal	• Infection (especially latent TB reactivation, fungal infections, and viral reactivation) • GI perforation • Neutropenia • Thrombocytopenia • ↑ LFTs • Dyslipidemia • Anaphylaxis • Demyelinating disorders	• PPD screening before initiating treatment • S/S of infection • CBC with differential • Lipid panel • LFTs	• Not to be given with TNF inhibitors • Not to be given with live vaccines	• Indicated for moderate–severe disease that has not responded to >1 DMARD • Discontinue if serious infection occurs • Subcut injection can be self-administered • Store subcut injection in refrigerator • Can be used alone or in combination with methotrexate or other non-biological DMARDs • Pneumococcal, influenza (IM), and HBV vaccines prior to initiating and/or after per CDC ACIP

Medications for Rheumatoid Arthritis *(cont'd)*

Generic • Brand • Dose/Dosage Forms	Contraindications	Primary Side Effects	Key Monitoring Parameters	Pertinent Drug Interactions	Med Pearls
Sarilumab • Kevzara • 150–200 mg subcut every 2 wk	• Absolute neutrophil count <2,000/mm³ • Platelets <150,000/mm³ • ALT or AST >1.5× the upper limit of normal	• ↑ LFTs • Pruritus at injection site • Infections (upper respiratory, pneumonia, urinary tract) • Hypertriglyceridemia	• PPD screening before initiating treatment • CBC with differential (prior to therapy, 4–8 wk after initiation, then every 3 mo) • LFTs (prior to therapy, 4–8 wk after initiation, then every 3 mo) • S/S of infection • Lipid panel • (4–8 wk after initiation)	Not to be given with live vaccines	• Indicated for moderate–severe disease that has not responded to ≥1 DMARD • Can be self-administered • Store in refrigerator • Use within 14 days once at room temp • Can be used alone or in combination with methotrexate or other non-biological DMARDs • Pneumococcal, influenza (IM), and HBV vaccines prior to initiating and/or after per CDC ACIP
Mechanism of action – selective costimulation modulator; inhibits T-cell activation					
Abatacept • Orencia • IV infusion administered at initiation, wk 2, and wk 4, then every 4 wk • IV weight-based dose: • <60 kg: 500 mg; • 60–100 kg: 750 mg; • >100 kg: 1,000 mg • Subcut: 125 mg subcut weekly (may be initiated with or without an IV loading dose)	None	• Anaphylaxis • Infection (especially latent TB reactivation, fungal infections, and HBV reactivation) • Chronic obstructive pulmonary disease (COPD) exacerbations • Headache • Nausea	• PPD and HBV screening before initiating treatment • S/S of infection	• Not to be given with TNF inhibitors • Not to be given with live vaccines	• Discontinue if serious infection occurs • Use with caution in patients with COPD • Subcut injection can be self-administered • Store subcut injection in refrigerator • Can be used alone or in combination with other non-biological DMARDs • Pneumococcal, influenza (IM), and HBV vaccines prior to initiating and/or after per CDC ACIP

Medications for Rheumatoid Arthritis   *(cont'd)*

Generic • Brand • Dose/Dosage Forms	Contraindications	Primary Side Effects	Key Monitoring Parameters	Pertinent Drug Interactions	Med Pearls
Mechanism of action – inhibits Janus kinase thereby reducing cytokine signaling					
Tofacitinib • Xeljanz, Xeljanz XR • IR: 5 mg BID • ER: 11 mg daily • ER tabs, tabs	None	• Infection (especially latent TB reactivation, fungal infections, and HBV reactivation) • Malignancy • GI perforation • Lymphocytopenia • Neutropenia • Anemia • ↑ LFTs • Dyslipidemia • Headache • Diarrhea • Increased risk of skin cancer	• PPD and HBV screening before initiating treatment • S/S of infection • Neutrophil/ platelet count (baseline, 1–2 mo, then Q 3 mo) • Lipid panel (4–8 wk after initiation; periodically) • LFTs • Lymphocyte count (baseline and Q 3 mo) • Hemoglobin (baseline, 1–2 mo, Q 3 mos) • Blood pressure • Heart rate • Skin examinations	• CYP3A4 substrate • CYP3A4 inhibitors may ↑ effects/ toxicity; dose when used with strong CYP3A4 inhibitors • CYP3A4 inducers may ↓ effects • Not to be given with TNF inhibitors • Not to be given with live vaccines	• Oral therapy offers advantage over many available biologics • Can be used alone or in combination with methotrexate or other non-biological DMARDs • Pneumococcal, influenza (IM), and HBV vaccines prior to initiating and/or after per CDC ACIP

OSTEOPOROSIS

Guidelines Summary

- Calcium and vitamin D are important prerequisites to pharmacological therapy. Dietary calcium is preferred to supplemental calcium. Without adequate calcium and vitamin D available, other therapies will be limited in their ability to improve bone architecture.

- In the absence of contraindications, alendronate, risedronate, zoledronic acid, and denosumab are the first-line therapy for the prevention and treatment of patients at increased risk of fractures.

- Teriparatide, denosumab, or zoledronic acid should be reserved for those patients unable to use oral therapy or for those with especially high fracture risk (i.e., previous osteoporotic fractures, multiple fracture risk factors, failed other therapies). Ibandronate has inferior efficacy data when compared to other bisphosphonates so should be reserved for those patients that cannot take a specific agent.

- Oral bisphosphonates are approved for prevention and treatment of osteoporosis (including glucocorticoid-induced osteoporosis) in men and women.

- Efficacy of bisphosphonates beyond 5 years is limited, with rare but serious side effects such as osteonecrosis of the jaw (ONJ) and atypical femur fractures. It is reasonable to reassess fracture risk and consider therapy discontinuation after 3–5 years.

- Raloxifene is recommended as an alternative choice for the treatment of osteoporosis in patients with contraindications to bisphosphonates or in patients who are unable to comply with the appropriate bisphosphonate administration instructions.

- Calcitonin is reserved for third-line therapy because of a lack of compelling evidence indicating fracture reductions and lack of long-term data. Calcitonin is approved for the treatment of acute pain secondary to vertebral fractures and is well tolerated; therefore, this medication may have a specific role in certain situations involving fractures of the spine.

- Estrogens and tissue-selective estrogen complex (conjugated estrogens/bazedoxifene) are approved for the prevention of osteoporosis in postmenopausal women but should only be considered in those patients unable to take nonestrogen medications. Patients should consider potential risks (cardiovascular, breast cancer, venous thromboembolism) before initiating therapy with these agents. If the decision is made to initiate estrogen-based therapy for osteoporosis prevention, the lowest effective dose should be used for the shortest duration.

Osteoporosis Treatment Summary

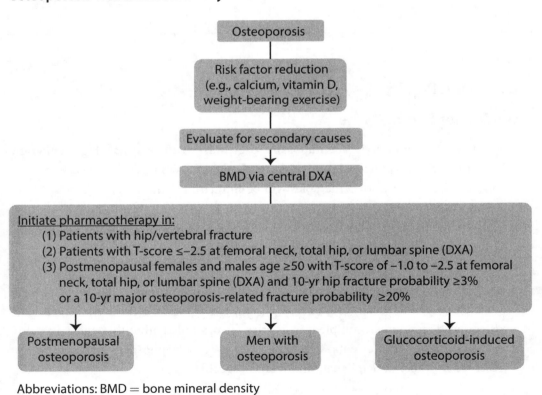

Osteoporosis

Risk factor reduction
(e.g., calcium, vitamin D,
weight-bearing exercise)

Evaluate for secondary causes

BMD via central DXA

Initiate pharmacotherapy in:
  (1) Patients with hip/vertebral fracture
  (2) Patients with T-score ≤−2.5 at femoral neck, total hip, or lumbar spine (DXA)
  (3) Postmenopausal females and males age ≥50 with T-score of −1.0 to −2.5 at femoral neck, total hip, or lumbar spine (DXA) and 10-yr hip fracture probability ≥3% or a 10-yr major osteoporosis-related fracture probability ≥20%

Postmenopausal osteoporosis

Men with osteoporosis

Glucocorticoid-induced osteoporosis

Abbreviations: BMD = bone mineral density

Management of Postmenopausal Osteoporosis

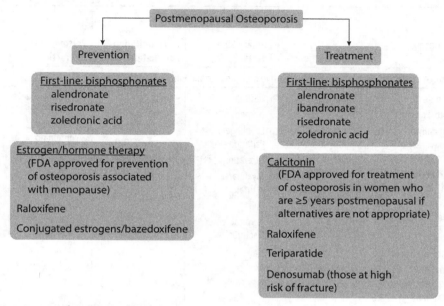

Postmenopausal Osteoporosis

Prevention

First-line: bisphosphonates
 alendronate
 risedronate
 zoledronic acid

Estrogen/hormone therapy
 (FDA approved for prevention
 of osteoporosis associated
 with menopause)

Raloxifene

Conjugated estrogens/bazedoxifene

Treatment

First-line: bisphosphonates
 alendronate
 ibandronate
 risedronate
 zoledronic acid

Calcitonin
 (FDA approved for treatment
 of osteoporosis in women who
 are ≥5 years postmenopausal if
 alternatives are not appropriate)

Raloxifene

Teriparatide

Denosumab (those at high
risk of fracture)

Management of Osteoporosis in Men

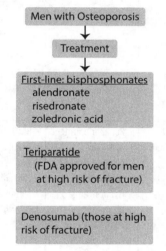

Men with Osteoporosis

Treatment

First-line: bisphosphonates
 alendronate
 risedronate
 zoledronic acid

Teriparatide
 (FDA approved for men
 at high risk of fracture)

Denosumab (those at high
risk of fracture)

Management of Glucocorticoid-Induced Osteoporosis

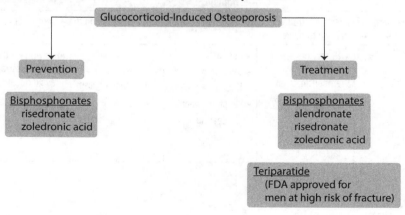

Glucocorticoid-Induced Osteoporosis

Prevention

Bisphosphonates
 risedronate
 zoledronic acid

Treatment

Bisphosphonates
 alendronate
 risedronate
 zoledronic acid

Teriparatide
 (FDA approved for
 men at high risk of fracture)

Medications for Osteoporosis

Generic • Brand • Dose/Dosage Forms	Contraindications	Primary Side Effects	Key Monitoring Parameters	Pertinent Drug Interactions	Med Pearls
Mechanism of action – bisphosphonates: adsorb to bone apatite and inhibit osteoclast activity					
Alendronate☆ • Binosto, Fosamax • 10 mg daily or 70 mg weekly (treatment) • 5 mg daily or 35 mg weekly (prevention) • Effervescent tabs, solution, tabs Risedronate☆ • Actonel, Atelvia • IR: 5 mg daily, 35 mg weekly, or 150 mg monthly • ER: 35 mg weekly • ER tabs, tabs Ibandronate☆ • Boniva • PO: 150 mg monthly • IV: 3 mg every • 3 mo • Injection, tabs	• Esophageal stricture • Hypersensitivity • Inability to sit upright or stand for ≥30 min • Creatinine clearance (CrCl) <35 mL/min • Hypocalcemia	• Nausea • Dyspepsia • Esophageal irritation • Ulceration • Myalgia/ arthralgia • ONJ • Atypical femur fractures	• BMD • Serum calcium concentrations • Serum 25(OH)D concentrations	• Absorption ↓ with antacids and products containing bi- or trivalent cations (e.g., iron, magnesium, aluminum, calcium, or zinc) (separate by ≥30 min) • NSAIDs may ↑ risk of GI symptoms	• Alendronate and risedronate IR tabs must be taken with 6–8 oz of water ≥30 minutes (60 min for ibandronate) prior to other medications/food • Alendronate oral solution should be followed by ≥2 oz of water; effervescent tabs should be dissolved in 4 oz of room-temperature water • Risedronate ER tabs must be taken with ≥4 oz of water immediately after breakfast • Patient should remain upright for ≥30 min (60 min for ibandronate) (for alendronate, must also remain upright until after first food of day)
Zoledronic acid • Reclast • 5 mg IV infusion yearly (every 2 yr for prevention) • Injection	• Hypersensitivity • CrCl <35 mL/min • Hypocalcemia	• Renal impairment • ONJ • Atypical femur fractures • Hypocalcemia • Myalgia/ arthralgia • Acute-phase reaction (fever, myalgia, flu-like symptoms)	• BMD • Renal function • Serum calcium concentrations • Serum 25(OH)D concentrations	• ↑ risk of hypocalcemia with loop diuretics • ↑ risk of nephrotoxicity with other nephrotoxic drugs (aminoglycosides, NSAIDs)	Acetaminophen may be given after drug is administered to minimize acute-phase reaction symptoms
Mechanism of action – selective estrogen receptor modulators: through selective binding to estrogen receptors, ↓ bone resorption and ↓ biochemical markers of bone turnover					
Raloxifene☆ • Evista • 60 mg daily • Tabs	• History of pulmonary embolism, deep vein thrombosis, or retinal vein thrombosis • Pregnancy/ lactation	• Hot flashes • Leg cramps • Thromboembolism • Peripheral edema • ↑ sweating	• BMD • S/S of thromboembolism	Absorption ↓ by bile acid sequestrants (avoid concurrent use)	Lipid effects include ↓ low-density lipoprotein cholesterol (LDL-C) with no effect on high-density lipoprotein cholesterol (HDL-C)/triglycerides

Medications for Osteoporosis *(cont'd)*

Generic • Brand • Dose/Dosage Forms	Contraindications	Primary Side Effects	Key Monitoring Parameters	Pertinent Drug Interactions	Med Pearls
Miscellaneous Agents					
Mechanism of action – inhibits bone resorption through inhibition of osteoclast activity, to a small degree, stimulates bone formation through stimulation of osteoblast activity					
Calcitonin • Miacalcin • 1 spray (200 units) in 1 nostril daily intranasally • 100 units IM or subcut daily • Injection, nasal spray	Hypersensitivity	• Anaphylaxis • Hypocalcemia • Nasal irritation and dryness • Rhinitis • Malignancy	BMD	None	• Refrigerate injection and unopened nasal spray bottle; once opened, keep nasal spray at room temp while in use • Discard unused nasal spray after 30 days
Mechanism of action – acts as a parathyroid hormone (PTH) agonist; thereby ↑ bone formation by the stimulation of osteoblast activity and ↑ renal reabsorption of calcium					
Teriparatide • Forteo • 20 mcg subcut daily • Injection	Hypersensitivity	• Orthostatic hypotension • Dizziness • Nausea • Hypercalcemia • Hyperuricemia • Hypercalciuria	• BMD • BP • Urinary calcium • Serum calcium concentrations • Serum 25(OH)D concentrations	May predispose to digoxin toxicity	• ↓ risk of vertebral and nonvertebral fractures • Should not use for >2 yr • Black box warning: osteosarcoma • Store in refrigerator
Abaloparatide • Tymlos • 80 mcg subcut daily • Injection	None			None	
Mechanism of action – monoclonal antibody, bone-modifying agent					
Denosumab • Prolia • 60 mg subcut every 6 mo • Injection	• Hypersensitivity • Hypocalcemia • Pregnancy	• Anaphylaxis • Hypocalcemia • ONJ • Atypical femur fractures • Skin infections • Rash • Myalgia/ arthralgia • Hyperlipidemia	• BMD • Serum calcium concentrations • Serum 25(OH)D concentrations • Serum phosphorus concentrations • Serum magnesium concentrations	None	Store in refrigerator

GOUT

Treatment of Acute Gouty Arthropathy

- Asymptomatic hyperuricemia does not require therapy.
- First-line treatment for acute gout
  - Corticosteroids: Preferred unless contraindicated due to low cost and tolerability when used short-term
  - NSAIDs: Also appropriate; any NSAID can be used (see the medication charts in the Pain Management chapter for more specific NSAID information)
  - Colchicine:
    » More expensive and less well tolerated but may be considered first line in patients without contraindications
    » Should be used at low dose (1.2 mg, then 0.6 mg 1 hour later); high-dose therapy (1.2 mg PO, then 0.6 mg/hour for 6 hours) does not improve efficacy and results in more frequent side effects
  - The use of oral (preferred) or parenteral corticosteroids is recommended for multijoint involvement, while an intra-articular corticosteroid can be used to target one specific symptomatic joint.
  - Urate-lowering therapy should not be used in most patients after a first acute gout attack or in patients with infrequent attacks.

Prophylaxis of Gout

- Patients with >2 gout flares/year or those with complicated gout (may be considered for urate-lowering therapy)
- Pharmacists should discuss benefits, harms, costs, and individual preferences with patients regarding use of urate-lowering therapy in patients with recurrent attacks.
- Urate-lowering with allopurinol or febuxostat should be combined with prophylactic therapy (low-dose NSAID or low-dose colchicine) for the first 8–12 weeks of therapy to avoid exacerbations.
- Routine monitoring of serum uric acid in patients on urate-lowering therapy is not recommended. Treatment should be guided by frequency of gout attacks.
- Pegloticase is indicated for refractory chronic gout in patients with insufficient response or contraindications to traditional therapy.

Drugs for Gout

Generic • Brand • Dose & Max	Contraindications	Primary Side Effects	Key Monitoring Parameters	Pertinent Drug Interactions	Med Pearls
Mechanism of action – colchicine: inhibits lactic acid production, decreases uric acid deposition, reduces phagocytosis, and decreases inflammation					
Colchicine • Colcrys, Mitigare • 1.2 mg, then 0.6 mg 1 hr later (max = 1.8 mg) • Caps, tabs	• Hypersensitivity • Serious GI, renal, hepatic, or cardiac disorders	• N/V/D • Rare: bone marrow suppression, aplastic anemia, thrombocytopenia	• Serum uric acid • GI symptoms • Periodic CBC	• CYP3A4 and P-glycoprotein substrate • CYP3A4 inhibitors may ↑ effects/ toxicity • CYP3A4 inducers may ↓ effects	• Patients may be provided with a prescription to be filled on a PRN basis and used during an exacerbation • Used for treatment and prophylaxis
Mechanism of action – xanthine oxidase inhibitor: by inhibition of xanthine oxidase, impairs the conversion of xanthine to uric acid, thereby ↓ the production of uric acid					
Allopurinol☆ • Zyloprim • 100–800 mg daily • Tabs	Hypersensitivity	• Rash (Stevens-Johnson syndrome possible) • Leukopenia • GI upset	• Serum uric acid concentrations • Renal function	May ↑ levels/ risk of toxicity of mercaptopurine and azathioprine (↓ dose of mercaptopurine and azathioprine to 25% of usual dose)	Adjust dose in renal impairment
Febuxostat • Uloric • 40–80 mg daily • Tabs	Concurrent use with azathioprine or mercaptopurine	• ↑ LFTs • Arthralgia	• LFTs (2 and 4 months after initiation and periodically thereafter) • Serum uric acid concentrations	• May ↑ levels/ risk of toxicity of mercaptopurine and azathioprine (contraindicated) • May ↑ levels/ risk of toxicity of theophylline	• No renal dose adjustment necessary • Not to be used during acute gout flares
Mechanism of action – uricosuric agents: ↑ the renal clearance of uric acid by inhibiting tubular reabsorption					
Probenecid • Only available generically • 250–1,000 mg BID • Tabs	• Hypersensitivity • CrCl <50 mL/min • History of renal calculi • Overproducers of uric acid • Peptic ulcer disease	• GI upset • Rash • Nephrolithiasis	• Serum uric acid concentrations • Renal function	• May ↑ levels/ risk of toxicity of methotrexate • May ↑ levels of penicillins	May precipitate acute gouty attacks; avoid use during acute gouty arthritis
Mechanism of action – catalyzes oxidation of uric acid to allantoin, thereby ↓ serum uric acid concentrations					
Pegloticase • Krystexxa • 8 mg IV infusion (over >2 hr) every 2 wk • Injection	• Glucose-6-phosphate-dehydrogenase deficiency • Risk of hemolysis • Methemoglobinemia	• Acute gout exacerbation • Infusion reactions • Anaphylaxis • HF exacerbation	• Serum uric acid concentrations • S/S of anaphylaxis/ infusion reactions 1 hr after infusion • S/S of HF exacerbation	None	• Indicated only for refractory cases • Patient should receive pre-treatment with antihistamine and corticosteroid • Gout flare prophylaxis with colchicine or NSAID 1 wk prior to administration is recommended

Drugs for Gout *(cont'd)*

Generic • Brand • Dose & Max	Contraindications	Primary Side Effects	Key Monitoring Parameters	Pertinent Drug Interactions	Med Pearls
Mechanism of action – inhibits the transporter proteins involved in renal uric acid reabsorption, uric acid transporter 1 (URAT1), and organic anion transporter 4 (OAT4), which ↓ serum uric acid concentrations and ↑ renal clearance of uric acid					
Lesinurad • Zurampic • 200 mg daily • Tabs	• CrCl <45 mL/min • Kidney transplant recipients • Tumor lysis syndrome	• Headache • ↑ serum creatinine • Acute renal failure • Nephrolithiasis • Gastroesophageal reflux disease	• Serum uric acid concentrations • Renal function	• CYP2C9 substrate • CYP2C9 inhibitors may ↑ effects/ toxicity • CYP2C9 inducers may ↓ effects • May ↓ effects of hormonal contraceptives	Must be used in combination with xanthine oxidase inhibitor
Lesinurad/ allopurinol • Duzallo • 200 mg/200 mg or 200 mg/300 mg daily tabs	• CrCl <45 mL/min • Kidney transplant recipients • Tumor lysis syndrome • Hypersensitivity to allopurinol	• Rash (Stevens-Johnson syndrome possible) • Leukopenia • GI upset • Headache • ↑ serum creatinine • Acute renal failure • Nephrolithiasis • Gastroesophageal reflux disease	• Serum uric acid concentrations • Renal function	May ↑ levels/ risk of toxicity of mercaptopurine and azathioprine (↓ dose of mercaptopurine and azathioprine to 25% of usual dose) • CYP2C9 substrate • CYP2C9 inhibitors may ↑ effects/ toxicity • CYP2C9 inducers may ↓ effects • May ↓ effects of hormonal contraceptives	Only indicated for patients on >300 mg allopurinol daily

Hematologic Disorders

14

This chapter covers the following diseases:

- **Iron deficiency anemia**
- **Anemia of chronic kidney disease and dialysis**
- **Megaloblastic anemias**
- **Sickle cell disease**

IRON DEFICIENCY ANEMIA

Guidelines Summary

In children, adolescents, and women of reproductive age, a trial of iron is a reasonable approach if the review of symptoms, history, and physical examination are negative; however, the Hgb should be checked at one month. If there is not a 1 g/dL ↑ in the Hgb level in that time, possibilities include malabsorption of oral iron, lack of compliance, continued bleeding, or presence of an unknown lesion.

- Dose of elemental iron needed to treat IDA is 120 mg/day for 3 months in adults and 3 mg/kg/day in children (max of 60 mg/day).

- An ↑ in the Hgb level of 1 g/dL after 1 month of treatment is an indicator of adequate response to iron therapy.

- Therapy should be continued for 3 months after correction of IDA to allow for replenishment of iron stores.

- Iron sulfate in a dose of 325 mg provides 65 mg of elemental iron, whereas 30 mg of iron gluconate provides 38 mg of elemental iron.

- GI absorption of elemental iron is enhanced in the presence of an acidic gastric environment, which can be accomplished through simultaneous intake of ascorbic acid (i.e., vitamin C).

- Patients should be counseled to take iron 2 hours before or 4 hours after antacids to minimize the potential for chelation and decreased absorption.

- Although iron absorption occurs more readily when taken on an empty stomach, this ↑ the likelihood of iron-induced stomach upset. The increased patient adherence that may result from taking the iron with food should be weighed against the inferior iron absorption that may occur.

- Laxatives, stool softeners, and adequate intake of liquids can alleviate the constipating effects of oral iron therapy.

- Indications for the use of intravenous (IV) iron include:
  - Intestinal malabsorption
  - Intolerance to oral iron, which often results in patient nonadherence

Medications for Iron Deficiency Anemia

Generic • Brand • Dose/Dosage Forms	Contraindications	Primary Side Effects	Key Monitoring	Pertinent Drug Interactions	Med Pearl
Mechanism of action – replaces iron found in Hgb, myoglobin; allows the transportation of oxygen via Hgb					
Ferrous sulfate, gluconate, fumarate • Sulfate: Fer-In-Sol, Fer-Iron, Slow-Fe • Gluconate: Ferate • Fumarate: Ferretts • Sulfate: 300 mg 2–4 × /day • Gluconate/fumarate: 60 mg 2–4 × /day • ER tabs, solution, tabs	• Hypersensitivity to iron salts • Hemochromatosis (GI tract absorbs excess iron) • Hemolytic anemia	• GI irritation • Epigastric pain • Nausea/ vomiting (N/V) • Dark stools • Stomach cramping • Constipation	• Serum iron • TIBC • Serum ferritin • Reticulocyte count • Hgb/Hct	• ↓ absorption of tetracyclines, fluoroquino- lones, levodopa, methyldopa, and penicillamine • Proton pump inhibitors (PPIs), H_2 blockers, and antacids can ↓ iron absorption	Administer with vita- min C or orange juice to ↑ absorption

Medications for Iron Deficiency Anemia *(cont'd)*

Generic • Brand • Dose/Dosage Forms	Contraindications	Primary Side Effects	Key Monitoring	Pertinent Drug Interactions	Med Pearl
Mechanism of action – iron complex taken up by reticuloendothelial system and then released for storage or for transport and incorporation into Hgb; eventually replenishes depleted iron stores in the bone marrow					
Iron dextran complex • Infed (IM or IV) • Dose (in mL) = 0.0442 (desired Hgb − observed Hgb) × lean body weight (LBW) + (0.26 × LBW) • Max dose = 100 mg/day	Hypersensitivity	• Anaphylaxis • Hypotension • Tightness in the chest • Wheezing • Flushing	• Anaphylactic reaction • Serum iron • TIBC • Serum ferritin • Transferrin saturation • Reticulocyte count • Hgb/Hct • Blood pressure • Heart rate	None	• Test dose is required • Anaphylaxis may still occur despite having an uneventful test dose • If flushing or hypotension occur, ↓ infusion rate
Sodium ferric gluconate • Ferrlecit • 125 mg via IV infusion (usually × 8 doses) • Injection		• Anaphylaxis • Tachycardia • Hypotension • Chest pain • Dizziness		May ↓ absorption of oral iron	• A safer form of parenteral iron compared to iron dextran • No test dose required
Ferumoxytol • Feraheme • 510 mg via IV infusion followed by 510 mg via IV infusion 3–8 days later • Injection	• Hypersensitivity • History of allergic reaction to any IV iron product	• Anaphylaxis • Diarrhea • Constipation • Hypotension • Dizziness			• Patients with multiple drug allergies at ↑ risk for anaphylactic reaction • May interfere with MRI readings for up to 3 mo after use • No test dose required
Iron sucrose • Venofer • Hemodialysis-dependent: 100 mg IV 1–3 ×/wk during dialysis until cumulative dose of 1,000 mg achieved (10 doses) • Peritoneal dialysis-dependent: 300 mg IV, then 300 mg IV 14 days later, then 400 mg IV 14 days later • No dialysis: 200 mg IV administered on 5 separate occasions during a 14-day time period • Injection	Hypersensitivity	• Anaphylaxis • Hypotension • Headache • Chest pain • Dizziness			• Can be administered as a slow IV injection (2–5 min) or as an IV infusion (time is dose dependent) • No test dose required
Ferric carboxymaltose • Injectafer • <50 kg: 15 mg/kg IV, then 15 mg/kg IV ≥7 days later (max = 1500 mg/treatment course) • ≥50 kg: 750 mg IV, then 750 mg IV ≥7 days later • Injection		• Anaphylaxis • Hypertension • Nausea • Flushing • Hypophosphatemia • Dizziness		Unknown	• Can be administered as a slow IV injection (100 mg/min) or as an IV infusion (over ≥15 min) • No test dose required

ANEMIA OF CHRONIC KIDNEY DISEASE AND DIALYSIS

Guidelines Summary

- Treatment guidelines are based on Hgb.
- ESAs should be used with caution in patients with malignancy if cure of malignancy is an option or if anemia can be managed via transfusion.
- The upper limit of Hgb should not exceed 11.5 g/dL in adults.
- In adults, ESAs should not be used to intentionally ↑ the Hgb >13 g/dL.
- In pediatric patients, the range of Hgb should be 11–12 g/dL.
- Iron therapy may be used if transferrin saturation is <30% and ferritin is <500 ng/mL.

Medications for Anemia of Chronic Kidney Disease and Dialysis

Generic • Brand • Dose/Dosage Forms	Contraindications	Primary Side Effects	Key Monitoring	Pertinent Drug Interactions	Med Pearl
Erythropoietin Stimulating Agents					
Mechanism of action – induce erythropoiesis by stimulating the division and differentiation of committed erythroid progenitor cells; induce the release of reticulocytes from the bone marrow into the bloodstream					
Epoetin alfa • Procrit, Epogen • Initial: 50–100 units/kg IV or subcut 3 × /wk • Injection Darbepoetin alfa • Aranesp • CKD patients on dialysis: 0.45 mcg/kg IV or subcut weekly or 0.75 mcg/kg IV or subcut every 2 wk • CKD patients not on dialysis: 0.45 mcg/kg IV or subcut every 4 wk • Injection	• Hypersensitivity • Uncontrolled hypertension • Pure red cell aplasia	• Hypertension • ↑ mortality, myocardial infarction, stroke, or thromboembolism (if target Hgb >11 g/dL) • Seizures • Peripheral edema • Headache • Nausea • Arthralgia	• Hgb • Ferritin • Transferrin saturation • Iron stores • Blood pressure	None	• IV route preferred for patients on hemodialysis • In patients with CKD on dialysis, initiate treatment if Hgb <10 g/dL • Do not ↑ dose more frequently than every 4 wk • If Hgb ↑ by >1 g/dL in a 2-wk period, ↓ dose by ≥25% • If Hgb has not ↑ by >1 g/dL in 4-wk period, ↑ dose by 25% • For CKD patients on dialysis, if Hgb >11 g/dL, ↓ or interrupt dose • For CKD patients NOT on dialysis, if Hgb >10 g/dL, ↓ or interrupt dose

Medications for Anemia of Chronic Kidney Disease and Dialysis *(cont'd)*

Generic • Brand • Dose/Dosage Forms	Contraindications	Primary Side Effects	Key Monitoring	Pertinent Drug Interactions	Med Pearl
Dialysate Iron Replacement					
Mechanism of action – binds to transferrin for incorporation into hemoglobin					
Ferric pyrophosphate citrate • Triferic • 1 ampule: 2.5 gal. bicarbonate concentrate; 2 micromolar concentration	Hypersensitivity	• Peripheral edema • Urinary tract infection • Pain • Headache • Fatigue • Fistula thrombosis • Fistula hemor-rhage	Predialysis iron status	None	Only used in dialysis patients

MEGALOBLASTIC ANEMIAS

Medications for Megaloblastic Anemias

Generic • Brand • Dose/Dosage Forms	Contraindications	Primary Side Effects	Key Monitoring	Pertinent Drug Interactions	Med Pearl
Mechanism of action – coenzyme for various metabolic functions, cell replication, and hematopoiesis					
Cyanocobalamin (vitamin B$_{12}$) • Nascobal • IM: Initial: 100–1,000 mcg daily for 1 wk, then 100–1,000 mcg every 1–3 months • PO: 500–2,000 mcg daily, maintenance 1,000 mcg daily • Intranasal: 500 mcg in 1 nostril weekly • Tab, ER tab, SL tab, injection, lozenge, SL liquid	Hypersensitivity	• Anxiety • Itching • Diarrhea	• Serum vitamin B$_{12}$ • Hgb/Hct • Reticulocyte count • Serum folate • Serum iron	Metformin and PPIs may ↓ vitamin B$_{12}$ absorption	Hydroxocobalamin is a longer-acting form of vitamin B$_{12}$
Mechanism of action – coenzyme in many metabolic systems, particularly for purine and pyrimidine synthesis					
Folic acid (folate) ☆ • Only available generically • 0.4–1 mg daily • Prevention of neural tube defects: 0.4–0.8 mg daily • Tabs, injection, caps	Hypersensitivity	• Allergic reaction • Bronchospasm • Flushing • Malaise • Pruritus • Rash	• Serum folate • Hgb/Hct • Reticulocyte count • Serum iron	• May ↓ phenytoin and phenobarbital levels • Phenytoin and sulfasalazine may ↓ folate absorption	Products containing >0.8 mg of folic acid are Rx only

SICKLE CELL DISEASE

Guidelines Summary

Medication related considerations for patients with SCD:

- Prevent pneumococcal disease with the use of immunizations. Penicillin may also be used as a prophylactic agent up to age 5.
- Progestin-only hormonal contraceptives, levonorgestrel and intrauterine devices can be used in patients with SCD without concern.
- Rapidly assess and treat pain using nonopioid and opioid analgesics.
- May consider the use of hydroxyurea if an adult patient experiences three or more moderate-to-severe pain crises in a 12-month period.

Antidotes

16

The following chapter addresses drugs that are used as antagonist drugs:

- **Antidotes**
- **Acute poisoning**
- **General antidotes**

GENERAL ANTIDOTES

Activated Charcoal

Activated charcoal absorbs a wide range of toxins and is often given to reduce absorption within the GI tract. A single dose is generally effective, particularly if it is given within 1 hour of ingestion. Delayed use, however, may be beneficial for modified-release preparations or for drugs that slow GI transit time, such as those with antimuscarinic properties. Charcoal is generally well tolerated, although vomiting is common, and there is a risk of aspiration if the airway is not adequately protected. Repeated doses may be useful in eliminating some substances even after systemic absorption has occurred.

Active removal of poisons from the stomach by induction of emesis or gastric lavage has been widely used, but there is little evidence to support its role. Emesis should not be induced if the poison is corrosive or petroleum-based, or if the poison is removable by treatment with activated charcoal.

Gastric Lavage

Gastric lavage may occasionally be indicated for ingestion of noncaustic poisons that are not absorbed by activated charcoal, but only if less than 1 hour has elapsed since ingestion. Gastric lavage should not be attempted if the airway is not adequately protected.

Whole-bowel irrigation using a nonabsorbable osmotic agent such as a macrogol has also been used, particularly for substances that pass beyond the stomach before being absorbed (e.g., iron preparations or enteric-coated or modified-release formulations); however, its role is not established.

Antidotes

Toxic/Overdose Substance	Generic Name for Antidote • Brand Name/Dosage Form • Dose	Contraindications	Primary Side Effects	Key Monitoring	Med Pearl
Mechanism of action – pure opioid antagonist that competes and displaces narcotics at opioid receptor sites					
Opioids	Naloxone • Narcan, Evzio • 0.4–2 mg IV/IM/subcut every 2–3 min PRN; after reversal, repeat dose every 20–60 min PRN • Evzio: 0.4 mg IM/subcut every 2 min until emergency medical assistance is available • Narcan Nasal Spray: 1 spray (4 mg) every 2–3 min in alternating nostrils until emergency medical assistance is available • Injection, nasal spray	Hypersensitivity	• Tachycardia • Anxiety • Diaphoresis • Agitation • ↑ blood pressure (BP)	• Respiratory rate (RR) • Heart rate (HR) • BP	• Adverse effects can occur secondarily to reversal (withdrawal) • IV route is preferred due to quick effect • Nasal spray onset is longest (~8–13 min)
Mechanism of action – acts as a competitive antagonist at opioid receptor sites					
Opioids	Naltrexone • Vivitrol • PO: 25 mg initially, then 50 mg daily on weekdays with 100 mg on Saturdays **OR** 100 mg every other day; **OR** 150 mg every 3 days • IM: 380 mg every 4 wk • Injection, tabs	• Hypersensitivity • Acute opioid withdrawal • Failure to pass naloxone challenge • Positive urine drug screen for opioids	• Hepatotoxicity • Syncope • Headache • Sedation • Nausea/ vomiting (N/V) • Depression • Suicidality • Injection site reactions • Muscle cramps	• Opioid withdrawal • Liver function tests (LFTs) • Mental status	• Do not give until patient is opioid-free for 7–10 days (to minimize risk of withdrawal) • Indicated for treatment of alcohol and opioid dependence • Highest affinity for mu receptors

Antidotes   *(cont'd)*

Toxic/Overdose Substance	Generic Name for Antidote • Brand Name/Dosage Form • Dose	Contraindications	Primary Side Effects	Key Monitoring	Med Pearl
Mechanism of action – competitively inhibits the activity at the benzodiazepine recognition site on the GABA/benzodiazepine complex					
Benzodiazepines	Flumazenil • Only available generically • 0.2 mg IV over 30 sec; if desired consciousness not achieved 30 sec after dose, repeat with 0.3 mg IV over 30 sec; if desired consciousness not achieved, can then repeat with 0.5 mg IV over 30 sec every minute • Injection	• Hypersensitivity • Receiving benzodiazepine for potentially life-threatening condition • Showing signs of serious cyclic antidepressant overdosage	• Palpitations • Blurred vision • Ataxia • Agitation • Dizziness • Seizures • ↑ sweating • Headache	• BP • HR • RR • Benzodiazepine reversal may result in seizures in some patients • May cause return of residual effects of benzodiazepines	• If patient has not responded 5 min after receiving a cumulative dose of 5 mg, the sedation is likely not due to benzodiazepines • Reversal may affect nonbenzodiazepines (eszopiclone, zaleplon, zolpidem)
Mechanism of action – competitively inhibits alcohol dehydrogenase, an enzyme that catalyzes the metabolism of ethanol, methanol, and ethylene glycol					
• Methanol • Ethylene glycol	Fomepizole • Antizol • 15 mg/kg IV, then 10 mg/kg IV every 12 hr × 4 doses, then 15 mg/kg IV every 12 hr until ethylene glycol levels <20 mg/L and patient asymptomatic (with normal pH) • Injection	Hypersensitivity	• Headache • Nausea • Metallic taste • Drowsiness • Dizziness	• Plasma/urinary ethylene glycol or methanol concentrations • Plasma/urinary osmolality • Renal function • LFTs • Electrolytes • Arterial blood gas • Anion/osmolar gaps • S/S of methanol or ethylene glycol toxicity	• Therapy should be initiated immediately upon suspicion of methanol or ethylene glycol ingestion • Can be used alone or with hemodialysis
Mechanism of action – inhibits destruction of acetylcholine by acetylcholinesterase which prolongs effects of acetylcholine					
Anticholinergic drugs	Physostigmine • Only available generically • 0.5–2 mg IM/IV to start; repeat every 10–30 min until response • Injection	• GI or genitourinary obstruction • Asthma • Gangrene • Severe cardiovascular disease • Concurrent use of depolarizing neuromuscular blocking agents	• Palpitation • Bradycardia • Restlessness • Seizure	• HR • RR • Electrocardiogram (ECG)	

Antidotes *(cont'd)*

Toxic/Overdose Substance	Generic Name for Antidote • Brand Name/Dosage Form • Dose	Contraindications	Primary Side Effects	Key Monitoring	Med Pearl
Mechanism of action – antigen-binding fragments (Fab) are specific for the treatment of digitalis intoxication					
Digoxin	Digoxin immune Fab • DigiFab • 40 mg will bind to 0.5 mg of digoxin • Injection	Hypersensitivity to sheep products	• Exacerbation of heart failure • Rapid ventricular response • Hypokalemia	• Serum potassium • BP • ECG • Renal function	Serum digoxin levels will greatly ↑ with digoxin immune Fab use and are not an accurate determination of body stores; do not monitor serum digoxin concentrations for several days to >1 wk
Mechanism of action – supplies a free thiol group which binds to and inactivates acrolein, the urotoxic metabolite of ifosfamide and cyclophosphamide					
• Cyclophospha-mide • Ifosfamide	Mesna • Mesnex • IV-only regimen: 20% of ifosfamide dose IV at time of ifosfamide dose, and then at 4 and 8 hr after ifosfamide dose • IV and PO regimen: 20% of ifosfamide dose IV at time of ifosfamide dose, then 40% of ifosfamide dose PO at 2 and 6 hr after ifosfamide dose • Injection, tabs	Hypersensitivity	• Anaphylaxis • Rash (including Stevens-Johnson syndrome) • N/V/D • Constipation • Leukopenia • Thrombocyto-penia • Anemia • Fatigue • Fever	• Urinalysis • Inputs/outputs	Only indicated for prevention of hemor-rhagic cystitis induced by ifosfamide; off-label use for prevention of hemor-rhagic cystitis induced by cyclophosphamide
Mechanism of action – cardioprotective by converting intracellularly to a ring-opened chelating agent that interferes with iron-mediated oxygen free radical generation					
Doxorubicin	Dexrazoxane • Zinecard, Totect • 10:1 ratio of dexrazoxane: doxorubicin IV administered before doxorubicin • Injection	Hypersensitivity	• Myelosuppres-sion (additive to chemo-therapy) • Phlebitis	• Complete blood count with differential • LFTs • Renal function • Echocardiogram	• Only used if patients have received cumulative doxorubicin dose of 300 mg/m^2 and are continu-ing with doxorubicin therapy • Can also be used to treat anthracycline-induced extravasation (Totect)

Antidotes *(cont'd)*

Toxic/Overdose Substance	Generic Name for Antidote • Brand Name/Dosage Form • Dose	Contraindications	Primary Side Effects	Key Monitoring	Med Pearl
Mechanism of action – free thiol metabolite is available to bind to and detoxify reactive metabolites of cisplatin					
Cisplatin	Amifostine • Ethyol • 910 mg/m² IV daily given 30 min prior to chemotherapy • Injection	Hypersensitivity	• Hypotension • N/V • Rash (including Stevens-Johnson syndrome) • Anaphylaxis • Hypocalcemia	• BP (every 5 min during the infusion) • Serum calcium	• Indicated to ↓ cumulative renal toxicity associated with repeated cisplatin administration (in ovarian cancer) • Antiemetic recommend prior to and in conjunction with amifostine • Hold antihypertensive medications for 24 hr before amifostine therapy
Mechanism of action – combines with strongly acidic heparin to form a stable complex (salt) neutralizing the anticoagulant activity of both drugs					
Heparin	Protamine • Only available generically • 1 mg of protamine IV neutralizes ~100 units of heparin (max dose = 50 mg) • Injection	Hypersensitivity	• Hypersensitivity • Hypotension • Flushing • Dyspnea • Thromboembolism	• Activated partial thromboplastin time (aPTT) • BP • S/S of bleeding • S/S of thromboembolic events	Will also partially reverse anticoagulant effects of low-molecular weight heparins
Mechanism of action – promotes liver synthesis of clotting factors (II, VII, IX, X) which counteracts the mechanism of warfarin					
Warfarin	Vitamin K (phytonadione) • Mephyton • Depends on international normalized ratio (INR) and bleeding risk factors (i.e., INR >10: hold warfarin and give 2.5–5 mg vitamin K PO) • Injection, tabs	Hypersensitivity	• Anaphylaxis (especially with IV administration) • Thromboembolism	• Prothrombin time (PT) • INR • S/S of bleeding • S/S of thromboembolic events	• IM route should be avoided due to hematoma formation • Subcut is the preferred parenteral route • IV recommended only when major bleeding present at any INR • Expect INR to ↓ within 24–48 hr
Mechanism of action – monoclonal antibody fragment that binds to dabigatran and its metabolites					
Dabigatran	Idarucizumab • Praxbind • 5 g administered as 2 separate doses of 2.5 g IV ≤15 min apart • Injection	None	• Headache • Thromboembolism • Hypersensitivity	• aPTT • S/S of bleeding • S/S of thromboembolic events	Will not reverse effects of apixaban, edoxaban, or rivaroxaban

Antidotes *(cont'd)*

Toxic/Overdose Substance	Generic Name for Antidote • Brand Name/Dosage Form • Dose	Contraindications	Primary Side Effects	Key Monitoring	Med Pearl
Mechanism of action – binds factor Xa inhibitors (rivaroxaban and apixaban)					
• Rivaroxaban • Apixaban	Andexanet alfa • Andexxa • Low dose: Rivaroxaban ≤10 mg or apixaban ≤5 mg or administration of rivaroxaban or apixaban >8 hours: IV bolus of 400 mg at a target rate of 30 mg/min followed by 4 mg/min for up to 120 minutes • High dose: Rivaroxaban >10 mg or apixaban >5 mg: IV bolus of 800 mg at a target rate of 30 mg/min followed by 8 mg/min for up to 120 minutes	None	• Infusion site reactions • DVT • MI • PE • UTI	• S/S arterial or venous thromboembolic events • S/S ischemic events • S/S cardiac arrest	• Used for reversal of anticoagulation for life-threatening or uncontrolled bleeding • Not indicated at this time for Xa inhibtors other than rivaroxaban and apixaban
Mechanism of action – reduced form of folic acid: supplies the necessary cofactor blocked by methotrexate					
Methotrexate	Leucovorin • Only available generically • 15 mg PO/IM/IV every 6 hr × 10 doses until levels normalize • Injection, tabs	Vitamin B12-deficient megaloblastic anemias	• Anaphylaxis • Rash	Plasma methotrexate concentrations	Continue leucovorin until plasma methotrexate level <0.05 mmol/L
Mechanism of action – absorbs toxic substances or irritants, thus inhibiting GI absorption					
Numerous toxic substances	Activated charcoal • Actidose • 25–100 g/dose	• Unprotected airway • Non-intact GI tract • GI perforation • Intestinal obstruction	• Hypernatremia • Hypokalemia	• Constipation • Diarrhea	Sorbitol accelerates bowel evacuation
Mechanism of action – exact mechanism of benefit in countering acetaminophen toxicity is unknown					
Acetaminophen	Acetylcysteine • Acetadote, Cetylev • PO: 140 mg/kg, then 70 mg/kg every 4 hr × 17 doses • IV: 150 mg/kg (max = 15 g) over 60 min, then 50 mg/kg (max = 5 g) over 4 hr, then 100 mg/kg (max = 10 g) over 16 hr • Effervecent tabs, injection	Hypersensitivity	• Anaphylaxis • N/V • Rash	• Serum acetaminophen concentrations • LFTs • Bilirubin • PT/INR • Hemoglobin/hematocrit • Renal function	• Therapy should continue until acetaminophen levels are undetectable and there is no evidence of hepatotoxicity • Treatment should begin within 8 hr of acute ingestion

Antidotes   *(cont'd)*

Toxic/Overdose Substance	Generic Name for Antidote • Brand Name/Dosage Form • Dose	Contraindications	Primary Side Effects	Key Monitoring	Med Pearl
Mechanism of action – blocks the action of acetylcholine at parasympathetic sites in the smooth muscle, secretory glands, and the central nervous system					
Cholinergics	Atropine • AtroPen • 2 mg IM; may repeat with 2 additional doses every 10 min	None	• Anaphylaxis • N/V • Fatigue • Insomnia • Weakness • Tachycardia	• ECG • Respiratory status • HR • BP	Dose until symptoms subside
Mechanism of action – stimulates adrenergic receptors resulting in relaxation of smooth muscle of the bronchial tree, cardiac stimulation and dilation of skeletal muscle vasculature					
Hypersensitivity reactions	Epinephrine • Adrenalin, EpiPen, EpiPen Jr. • 0.2–0.5 mg IM or subcut every 5–15 min until improvement • EpiPen Jr.: 0.15 mg IM/subcut every 5–15 min until improvement	None	• Angina • Arrhythmias • Anxiety • Flushing • Dyspnea	• RR • HR • BP	IM administration in the anterolateral aspect of the middle third of the thigh is preferred
Mechanism of action – stimulates adenylate cyclase to produce increased cyclic AMP, which promotes hepatic glycogenolysis and gluconeogenesis					
Hypoglycemia	Glucagon • GlucaGen • 1 mg IV, IM, or subcut; may repeat in 15 min as needed	• Hypersensitivity • Insulinoma • Pheochromocy-toma	• Hypersensi-tivity • Hypotension • Nausea	• BP • Blood glucose • ECG • HR • Mental status	IV dextrose should be given as soon as available

Reproductive Health and Urologic Disorders

17

This chapter covers the following topics:

- **Contraception**
- **Hormone replacement therapy**
- **Erectile dysfunction**
- **Benign prostatic hyperplasia**
- **Urinary incontinence**

CONTRACEPTION

Therapy Selection

Available Prescription Therapies

- Combination estrogen and progestin
  - Monophasic
  - Multiphasic
- Progestin only
- Implantable
- Emergency contraception
  - Start within 72 hours of unprotected intercourse
  - Approved over-the-counter (OTC) (regardless of age)
  - Plan B (OTC)
    - » 2 tablets 0.75 mg levonorgestrel (taken every 12 hr × 2 doses)
  - Plan B One Step (OTC)
    - » 1 tablet by mouth, levonorgestrel 1.5 mg
  - Ella (Rx only)
    - » Ulipristal acetate 30 mg by mouth within 120 hr of unprotected intercourse

Advantages and Disadvantages of Contraception

Product Type	Advantages	Disadvantages
Combination products	Long history of superior efficacy; multiple formulations allow opportunity to try multiple-dose combination of estrogen/progestin components in different dosage forms (transdermal patch, oral, multiphasic, continuous); ↓ length of menses; ↓ incidence of cramping; ↓ risk of ectopic pregnancy	Drug interactions present; need for backup contraception with missed pills
Progestin only	Can be used safely in patients who are breastfeeding, are >35 years of age, and/or have systemic lupus erythematosus or intolerable estrogen-related side effects	Slightly less effective; require even stricter compliance than combinations; higher incidence of breakthrough bleeding; need for backup contraception with missed pills
Implantable	Longer-term efficacy	Not readily reversible; requires insertion at medical office

Adverse Effects Associated with Hormonal Imbalance

Estrogen Excess	Estrogen Deficiency	Progestin Excess	Progestin Deficiency
• Breast tenderness • Cyclic weight gain • Edema • Bloating • Hypertension • Melasma • Migraine • Nausea	• Vasomotor symptoms (hot flashes) • Spotting • Breakthrough bleeding (early) • ↓ libido • Dyspareunia	• ↓ libido • Depression • Fatigue • Weight gain • Acne • Hypomenorrhea • Vaginal candidiasis	• Heavy menstruation • Weight loss • Delayed menses • Spotting • Breakthrough bleeding (late)

Pharmacologic Contraceptives

Generic • Brand • Dose & Max	Contraindications	Primary Side Effects	Key Monitoring Parameters	Pertinent Drug Interactions	Med Pearls
Hormonal Contraceptives					
Oral monophasic/high-dose estrogen					
Ethinyl estradiol and norgestrel ☆ • Ogestrel • 50 mcg E. estradiol/0.5 mg norgestrel Ethinyl estradiol and ethynodiol diacetate • Zovia 1/50 • 50 mcg E. estradiol/1 mg E. diacetate Mestranol and norethindrone ☆ • Necon 1/50, Norinyl 1/50 • 50 mcg mestranol/1 mg norethindrone	• Pregnancy • Breast cancer • History of deep vein thrombosis (DVT) or pulmonary embolism (PE) • Lactation (<6 wk postpartum) • Smoker >35 years old	• Breast tenderness • ↑ breast size • Nausea • Edema • Bloating • Cyclic weight gain • DVT/PE • Headaches during active pills • Thrombophlebitis (rare) *Estrogen-excess side effects most common*	• Presence of side effects • Pregnancy	↓ effect of oral contraceptive: • Antibiotics (ampicillin, sulfonamides, tetracycline) • Anticonvulsants (phenytoin, topiramate, barbiturates) • Protease inhibitors • Rifampin Need backup method of contraception during use and for ≥1 wk after; for chronic therapy with above medications use another form of contraception	Take 1 tablet daily at the same time of day for 21 days, followed by 7 days of inactive placebo pills

Pharmacologic Contraceptives *(cont'd)*

Generic • Brand • Dose & Max	Contraindications	Primary Side Effects	Key Monitoring Parameters	Pertinent Drug Interactions	Med Pearls
Oral monophasic/low-dose estrogen					
Ethinyl estradiol and levonorgestrel • Afirmelle, Aviane, Falmina, Lessina, Orsythia • 20 mcg E. estradiol/ 0.1 mg levonorgestrel • Altavera, Ayuna, Introvale, Kurvelo, Levora, Marlissa, Portia, Seasonale, Setlakin, Quasense • 30 mcg E. estradiol/0.15 mg levonorgestrel	• Pregnancy • Breast cancer • History of DVT or PE • Lactation (<6 wk postpartum) • Smoker >35 years old	• Nausea/vomiting (N/V) • Breakthrough bleeding • Spotting • Melasma • Headache • Weight change • Edema • DVT/PE • Side effects associated with hormonal imbalance (see preceding Adverse Effects table)	• Presence of side effects • Pregnancy	↓ effect of oral contraceptive: • Antibiotics (ampicillin, sulfonamides, tetracycline) • Anticonvulsants (phenytoin, topiramate, barbiturates) • Protease inhibitors • Rifampin Need backup method of contraception during use and for ≥1 wk after; for chronic therapy with above medications use another form of contraception	Seasonale is taken continuously for 84 days with 7 placebo pills; menses only every 3 mo
Ethinyl estradiol and drospirenone ☆ • Beyaz (has added folate), Loryna, Melamisa, Nikki, Safyral (has added folate), Syeda, Yaela, Yasmin, Yaz • 20–30 mcg E. estradiol/3 mg drospirenone			• Serum potassium • Pregnancy		• ↓ duration of menses • Drospirenone is a structural analog to spironolactone
Ethinyl estradiol and norgestrel ☆ • Cryselle, Elinest, Low-Ogestrel • 30 mcg E. estradiol/0.3 mg norgestrel			• Presence of side effects • Pregnancy		Take 1 tablet daily at the same time of day for 21 days, followed by 7 days of inactive placebo pills
Ethinyl estradiol and norethindrone acetate ☆ • Aurovela 1/20, Aurovela 24 Fe, Aurovela Fe 1/20, Blisovi 24 Fe, Gildess 1/20, Gildess 24 Fe, Gildess Fe 1/20, Junel 1/20, Junel Fe 1/20, Larin 1/20, Larin 24 Fe, Larin Fe 1/20, Lo Loestrin Fe, Loestrin 21 1/20, Loestrin 24 Fe, Loestrin Fe 1/20, Microgestin 1/20, Microgestin Fe 1/20 • 10–20 mcg E. estradiol/1 mg norethindrone acetate					
Ethinyl estradiol and norethindrone ☆ • Balziva, Briellyn, Femcon Fe, Gildagia, Nexesta Fe, Philith, Vyfemla, • 35 mcg E. estradiol/0.4 mg norethindrone • Brevicon ☆, Cyclafem 0.5/35, Cyonanz, Modicon, Nortrel 0.5/35, Wera • 35 mcg E. estradiol/0.5 mg norethindrone • Alyacen 1/35, Cyclafem 1/35, Dasetta 1/35, Necon 1/35 ☆, Norinyl 1/35, Nortrel 1/35, Nylia 1/35, Ortho-Novum 1/35, Pirmella 1/35 • 35 mcg E. estradiol/1 mg norethindrone					
Ethinyl estradiol and desogestrel • Bekyree, Kariva, Kimidess, Pimtrea, Viorele, Volnea • 10–20 mcg E. estradiol/0.15 mg desogestrel • Desogen, Emoquette, Enskyce, Isibloom, Kalliga • 30 mcg E. estradiol, 0.15 mg desogestrel					

Pharmacologic Contraceptives *(cont'd)*

Generic • Brand • Dose & Max	Contraindications	Primary Side Effects	Key Monitoring Parameters	Pertinent Drug Interactions	Med Pearls
Oral monophasic/low-dose estrogen *(cont'd)*					
Ethinyl estradiol and levonorgestrel • Ashlyna, Daysee, Seasonique, Simpesse • 30 mcg E. estradiol/0.15 mg levonorgestrel/10 mcg E. estradiol	[Same as above]	[Same as above]	[Same as above]	[Same as above]	[Same as above]
Ethinyl estradiol and norgestimate ☆ • Estarylla, Mili, Mono-Linyah, Ortho-Cyclen, Previfem, Sprintec • 35 mcg E. estradiol/0.25 mg norgestimate					
Oral biphasic					
Ethinyl estradiol and norethindrone ☆ • Necon 10/11 • 35 mcg E. estradiol, 0.5–1 mg norethindrone	• Pregnancy • Breast cancer • History of DVT or PE • Lactation (<6 wk postpartum) • Smoker >35 years old	• N/V • Breakthrough bleeding • Spotting • Melasma • Headache • Weight change • Edema • DVT/PE • Side effects associated with hormonal imbalance (see Table 2)	• Presence of side effects • Pregnancy	↓ effect of oral contraceptive: • Antibiotics (ampicillin, sulfonamides, tetracycline) • Anticonvulsants (phenytoin, topiramate, barbiturates) • Protease inhibitors • Rifampin Need backup method of contraception during use and for ≥1 wk after; for chronic therapy with above medications use another form of contraception	• Created to ↓ overall hormone exposure • High incidence of breakthrough bleeding

Pharmacologic Contraceptives *(cont'd)*

Generic • Brand • Dose & Max	Contraindications	Primary Side Effects	Key Monitoring Parameters	Pertinent Drug Interactions	Med Pearls
Oral triphasic					
Ethinyl estradiol and norethindrone ☆ • Alyacen 7/7/7, Aranelle, Cyclafem 7/7/7, Dasetta 7/7/7, Necon 7/7/7, Nortrel 7/7/7, Nylia 7/7/7, Ortho-Novum 7/7/7, Pirmella 7/7/7, Tri-Norinyl • 35 mcg E. estradiol/0.5–1 mg norethindrone Ethinyl estradiol and desogestrel • Cyclessa, Velivet • 25 mcg E. estradiol/0.1–0.15 mg desogestrel Ethinyl estradiol and norgestimate ☆ • Ortho Tri-Cyclen, Tri-Estarylla, Tri-Linyah, Tri-Mili, Tri-Previfem, Tri-Sprintec • 35 mcg E. estradiol/0.18–0.25 mg norgestimate • Ortho-TriCyclen Lo, Tri-Lo-Estarylla, Tri-Lo-Sprintec • 25 mcg E. estradiol/0.18–25 mg norgestimate Ethinyl estradiol and levonorgestrel • Elifemme, Enpresse, Levonest, Myzilra, Trivora • 30–40 mcg E. estradiol/0.075–0.125 mg levonorgestrel	• Pregnancy • Breast cancer • History of DVT or PE • Lactation (<6 wk postpartum) • Smoker >35 years old	• N/V • Breakthrough bleeding • Spotting • Melasma • Headache • Weight change • Edema • DVT/PE • Side effects associated with hormonal imbalance (see Table 2)	• Presence of side effects • Pregnancy	Same as biphasic	• Many triphasics approved for treatment of acne as well • More difficult to deal with missed pills • ↓ overall hormone exposure
Oral four-phasic					
Estradiol valerate and dienogest • Natazia • Days 1–2: 3 mg estradiol valerate • Days 3–7: 2 mg estradiol valerate + 2 mg dienogest • Days 8–24: 2 mg estradiol valerate + 3 mg dienogest • Days 25–26: 1 mg estradiol valerate • Days 27–28: inactive	• Pregnancy • Lactation • Breast cancer • History of DVT or PE • Hepatic disease • Abnormal uterine bleeding • Vascular disease • Hypercoagulopathy	• N/V • Breakthrough bleeding • Spotting • Melasma • Headache • Weight change • Edema • DVT/PE • Side effects associated with hormonal imbalance (see preceding Adverse Effects table)	• Presence of side effects • Pregnancy	Same as triphasic	• Only 4-phasic option available • ↑ efficacy for heavy menstrual bleeding

Pharmacologic Contraceptives *(cont'd)*

Generic • Brand • Dose & Max	Contraindications	Primary Side Effects	Key Monitoring Parameters	Pertinent Drug Interactions	Med Pearls
Transdermal					
Ethinyl estradiol and norelgestromin • Xulane • 35 mcg E. estradiol/0.15 mg norelgestromin	• Pregnancy • Breast cancer • History of DVT or PE • Lactation (<6 wk postpartum) • Smoker >35 years old	• N/V • Breakthrough bleeding • Spotting • Melasma • Headache • Weight change • Edema • DVT/PE • Side effects associated with hormonal imbalance (see preceding Adverse Effects table)	• Presence of side effects • Pregnancy	Same as oral contraceptives	• Safe with usual activities • Do not apply lotion to site of application • Improved compliance over oral • Apply weekly for 3 wk • Avoid if >90 kg
Other					
Ethinyl estradiol and etonogestrel ☆ • NuvaRing • 0.015 mg E. estradiol and 0.12 mg etonogestrel released daily • Inserted by patient intravaginally every 4 wk (active for 3 wk)	Negative pregnancy test needed for initiation	Same as oral contraceptives (systemic absorption occurs)	Same as oral contraceptives (systemic absorption occurs)	Same as oral contraceptives (systemic absorption occurs)	• May be removed before intercourse • Not to be used >4 mo after being dispensed
Oral progestin-only					
Norethindrone • Camila, Errin, Heather, Incassia, Jencycla, Micronor, Nor-QD • 0.35 mg daily	Negative pregnancy test prior to initiation	• ↓ libido depression • Fatigue • Weight gain • Acne • Hypomenorrhea	Presence of side effects	None	Can be used in breastfeeding women, those >35 yr who smoke, and those at risk of coronary heart disease
Norgestrel • Ovrette • 0.075 mg daily					
Parenteral progestin-only					
Medroxyprogesterone ☆ • Depo-Provera, Depo-Subq Provera 104 • 150 mg IM every 12 wk; or 104 mg subcut every 12 wk	• Must have negative pregnancy test to start therapy or to continue therapy if >14 wk since last injection • Breast cancer • Liver disease	• Weight gain • ↓ bone mineral density • Acne • Delayed return of fertility after discontinuation	Bone mineral density	None	• Supplement calcium and vitamin D due to potential bone loss • Do not use for >2 yr unless unable to use other forms of contraception

Pharmacologic Contraceptives   *(cont'd)*

Generic • Brand • Dose & Max	Contraindications	Primary Side Effects	Key Monitoring Parameters	Pertinent Drug Interactions	Med Pearls
Implantable/intrauterine					
Levonorgestrel ☆ • Mirena • 20 mcg released daily • Intrauterine • Kyleena • 17.5 mcg released daily • Intrauterine	• History or high risk of pelvic inflammatory disease (PID) or ectopic pregnancy • Breast cancer • Abnormal uterine bleeding • High risk for sexually transmitted infections (STIs) (multiple sexual partners) • Uterine or cervical cancer	• Spotting • Breakthrough bleeding • Amenorrhea • Mastalgia • Headache • Abdominal pain • PID	• Presence of side effects • Pregnancy	None	Remains in place for up to 5 yr
Levonorgestrel • Skyla • 6 mcg released daily • Intrauterine • Liletta • 15.6 mcg released daily • Intrauterine					Remains for 3 yr
Etonogestrel • Nexplanon • 68 mg subdermal implant in upper arm • Replace every 3 yr	History or high risk of PID or ectopic pregnancy	• Amenorrhea • Infrequent menses • Weight gain			Not studied in women >130% ideal body weight
Nonhormonal					
Copper–T380 • ParaGard • Intrauterine placement for up to 10 yrs	History or high risk of PID or ectopic pregnancy	• Heavy bleeding • Cramping	None	None	Can remain in place for up to 8–10 yr with efficacy

Doses Missed	Instructions for Patient
1	Take missed dose immediately and next dose at regular time
2 (during first 2 wk)	Take two doses daily for the next 2 days, then resume taking; use backup method for 7 days
2 (during third wk)	Sunday start: Take one dose daily until Sunday, dispose of current pack, then begin next pack without placebo pills. Backup method required for 7 days.
≥3	Other: Dispose of current pack and begin new pack. Backup method required for 7 days.

HORMONE REPLACEMENT THERAPY

Guidelines Summary

- All women should undergo careful evaluation prior to initiation of hormone replacement therapy (HRT), including comprehensive history and physical, mammography, and, potentially, bone densitometry.

- The benefit:risk ratio for HRT is highly individualized and based on a patient's symptoms, impact on quality of life, and degree of risk for adverse effects.

- The primary indications for HRT are vasomotor symptoms (VMS) of hot flashes and night sweats and genitourinary syndrome of menopause (GSM).

- Benefits are more likely to outweigh risks when therapy is initiated in symptomatic women who are either younger than 60 years or within 10 years of menopause onset.

- For women with early menopause, HRT is recommended until at least the median age of menopause (52 years).

- Local vaginal therapy is recommended over systemic therapy when vaginal symptoms are the only complaint.

- Prevention of osteoporosis with HRT should be considered only for women with a very strong risk of osteoporosis in whom other available therapies are not options.

- In women with an intact uterus who are receiving HRT, progestogen or combination conjugated equine estrogens with bazedoxefine is indicated to decrease the risk of endometrial hyperplasia and cancer that exists with unopposed estrogen use in these patients.

- Lowering doses of HRT or switching to transdermal formulation is appropriate as patients age or in those with hypertriglyceridemia at risk for pancreatitis.

- Due to an unclear evidence-based benefit:risk ratio, HRT is not recommended for any of the following indications: cardiovascular disease, stroke prevention, hyperlipidemia, or dementia prevention.

- The Women's Health Initiative (WHI) indicated increased risks of venous thromboembolism, stroke, coronary disease, and breast cancer in women who receive HRT for an extended period of time. The risk was greatest in patients on estrogen-progestogen combination therapy and lower in estrogen-only therapy.

- In women with a family history of breast cancer, evidence supports that HRT does not further increase the risk of breast cancer; family history should be one consideration when weighing the benefits and risks of therapy.

- Combination therapy should be limited to 3–5 years or less whenever possible. Longer-term use of estrogen only therapy may be considered.

- Nonhormonal options are available for the treatment of vasomotor symptoms in patients with contraindications to hormone therapy or preference to avoid hormone therapy. Evidence-based options include venlafaxine, paroxetine, fluoxetine, and gabapentin. (These agents are detailed in drug tables in the Neurological Disorders and Psychiatric Disorders chapters.) Brisdelle is a low-dose paroxetine product that is approved by the Food and Drug Administration solely for the treatment of vasomotor symptoms related to menopause.

Hormone Replacement Therapy

Generic • Brand • Dose/Dosage Form	Contraindications	Primary Side Effects	Key Monitoring Parameters	Med Pearls
Oral Preparations				
Estrogens				
Conjugated equine estrogens ☆ • Premarin • 0.3–2.5 mg daily	• Hypersensitivity • Abnormal bleeding • Breast cancer • History of DVT or PE • Pregnancy • Estrogen-dependent tumor • History of stroke or myocardial infarction (MI) • Hepatic impairment • Protein C, protein S, or antithrombin deficiency	• Nausea • Fluid retention • Bloating • Headaches • Mood changes • Breast tenderness • ↑ risk of DVT/PE, stroke, MI, and breast cancer • ↑ blood pressure (BP)	• Vaginal bleeding • S/S of DVT/PE • S/S of stroke • S/S of MI • BP • Pap smear • Breast exam • Mammogram	• Most studied • No generic equivalent • Should not be abruptly discontinued; taper
Micronized estradiol • Only available generically • 1–2 mg daily				• Long half-life • Most potent hepatic effects • Should not be abruptly discontinued; taper
Estropipate • Only available generically • 0.75–6 mg daily				
Esterified estrogens • Menest • 0.3–2.5 mg daily				Should not be abruptly discontinued; taper
Progestins				
Medroxyprogesterone ☆ • Provera • 2–10 mg daily	• Hypersensitivity • Abnormal bleeding • Breast cancer • History of DVT or PE • Pregnancy • Estrogen- or progesterone-dependent tumor • History of stroke or MI • Hepatic impairment	• ↓ libido • Cramping • Mood changes • Bloating • Nausea • Depression • Headache • ↑ risk of DVT/PE, stroke, MI, and breast cancer	• Vaginal bleeding • S/S of DVT/PE • S/S of stroke • S/S of MI • Pap smear • Breast exam • Mammogram	None
Micronized progestin • Prometrium • 200 mg daily				Primary use in patients with adverse effects associated with synthetic progestin

Hormone Replacement Therapy *(cont'd)*

Generic • Brand • Dose/Dosage Form	Contraindications	Primary Side Effects	Key Monitoring Parameters	Med Pearls
Selective Estrogen Receptor Modulator/Estrogen Agonist–Antagonist				
Ospemifene • Osphena • 60 mg daily	• Hypersensitivity • Abnormal bleeding • Breast cancer • History of DVT or PE • Pregnancy • Estrogen-dependent tumor • History of stroke or MI	• ↑ risk of DVT/PE, stroke, MI, and breast cancer • Vasomotor symptoms	• Vaginal bleeding • S/S of DVT/PE • S/S of stroke • S/S of MI • Pap smear • Breast exam • Mammogram	None
Combination Oral Preparations				
Conjugated equine estrogens and medroxyprogesterone ☆ • Prempro • 0.3–0.625 mg estrogen/ 1.5–2.5 mg progestin • Premphase • 0.625 mg/0 mg × 14 days then 0.625/5 mg × 14 days Estradiol and drospirenone • Angelique • 0.5–1 mg/0.25–0.5 mg daily Ethinyl estradiol and norethindrone acetate • FemHRT, Leribane, Fyavolv • 2.5–5 mcg/0.5–1 mg daily • Activella, Amabelz • 0.5–1 mg/0.1–0.5 mg daily	• Hypersensitivity • Abnormal bleeding • Breast cancer • History of DVT or PE • Pregnancy • Estrogen-dependent tumor • History of stroke or MI • Hepatic impairment • Protein C, protein S, or antithrombin deficiency	• Nausea • Fluid retention • Bloating • Headaches • Mood changes • Breast tenderness • ↑ risk of DVT/PE, stroke, MI, and breast cancer • ↑ BP	• Vaginal bleeding • S/S of DVT/PE • S/S of stroke • S/S of MI • BP • Pap smear • Breast exam • Mammogram	None
Transdermal and Topical Preparations				
17β Estradiol transdermal ☆ • Alora, Climara, Minivelle, Vivelle, Vivelle-Dot • 25–50 mcg/24 hours • Applied 1–2 × wk 17β Estradiol gel • Divigel, Elestrin, Estrogel • 0.25–1.25 g daily 17β Estradiol topical emulsion • Estrasorb • 2 packets (3.48 g) daily 17β Transdermal spray • Evamist • 1 spray (1.53 mg) daily; may ↑ to 2–3 sprays daily	• Hypersensitivity • Abnormal bleeding • Breast cancer • History of DVT or PE • Pregnancy • Estrogen-dependent tumor • History of stroke or MI • Hepatic impairment • Protein C, protein S, or antithrombin deficiency	• Skin irritation • Nausea • Fluid retention • Bloating • Headaches • Mood changes • Breast tenderness • ↑ risk of DVT/PE, MI, and breast cancer • ↑ BP	• Vaginal bleeding • S/S of DVT/PE • S/S of stroke • S/S of MI • BP • Pap smear • Breast exam • Mammogram	• Limited hepatic effects • Useful in patients with gastrointestinal disturbances • Side effects less common in general

Hormone Replacement Therapy   *(cont'd)*

Generic • Brand • Dose/Dosage Form	Contraindications	Primary Side Effects	Key Monitoring Parameters	Med Pearls
Vaginal Preparations				
Conjugated estrogen cream • Premarin • 0.5 g 1–2 × /wk to daily intravaginally (for 21 days, 7 days off)	• Hypersensitivity • Abnormal bleeding • Breast cancer • History of DVT or PE • Pregnancy • Estrogen-dependent tumor • History of stroke or MI • Hepatic impairment • Protein C, protein S, or antithrombin deficiency	Systemic side effects possible but rare	• Presence of adverse effects • Efficacy	• Used in cases of vaginal symptoms only • Effective for stress incontinence
Estradiol ring • Estring • 2 mg intravaginally; should remain in place for 90 days • Femring • 0.05–0.1 mg intravaginally; should remain in place for 90 days				Long-term use associated with endometrial hyperplasia
17β Estradiol cream • Estrace • 2–4 g intravaginally daily × 1–2 wk, then 1–2 g daily × 1–2 wk, then 1 g/day 1–3 × /wk				• Used in cases of vaginal symptoms only • Effective for stress incontinence
Estradiol tablet • Vagifem • 1 tab (10 mcg) intravaginally daily × 2 wk, then 1 tab (10 mcg) twice weekly				Used in cases of vaginal symptoms only

Drug Interactions

	Interacting Drug(s)	Result
Estrogen	3A4 inducers: barbiturates, carbamazepine, phenytoin rifampin, St. John's wort	↓ effect of estrogen
	Levothyroxine, warfarin	↓ effect of interacting drug
	3A4 inhibitors: azole antifungals, macrolide antibiotics, ritonavir, grapefruit juice	↑ effect of estrogen
	Corticosteroids	↑ effect of interacting drug
Progestin	3A4 inducers: barbiturates, carbamazepine, phenytoin rifampin, St. John's wort	↓ effect of progestin

ERECTILE DYSFUNCTION

Guidelines Summary

- Initial treatment for most patients will consist of therapy with a phosphodiesterase-5 (PDE-5) inhibitor because these agents are known to be efficacious and are minimally invasive.

- PDE-5 inhibitors are contraindicated in patients who are currently taking nitrates, due to a risk of significant, dangerous hypotension when these agents are used concomitantly.

- If a patient does not respond to therapy with a PDE-5 inhibitor, alternate therapy options should be considered, including a different PDE-5 inhibitor, alprostadil intraurethral suppositories, intracavernous injection, vacuum constriction devices, and penile prostheses.

- Lifestyle modification and treatment of underlying cause/secondary cause should also be encouraged (hypertension, diabetes, hyperlipidemia).

Erectile Dysfunction Treatment Summary

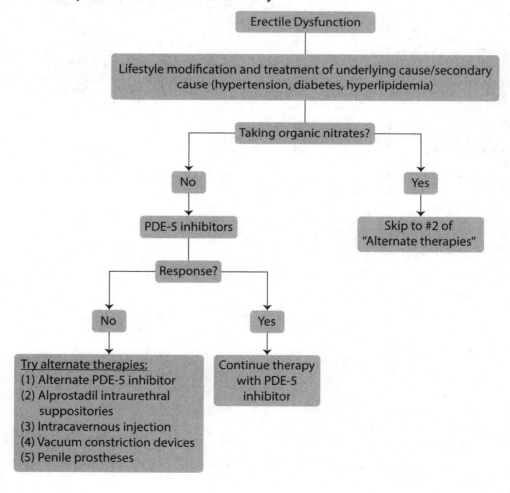

Medications for Erectile Dysfunction

Generic • Brand • Dose/Dosage Forms	Contraindications	Primary Side Effects	Key Monitoring Parameters	Pertinent Drug Interactions	Med Pearls
Oral					
Mechanism of action – PDE-5 inhibitors: enhance the activity of nitric oxide by inhibiting an enzyme (PDE-5) responsible for its degradation; enhanced nitric oxide allows relaxed smooth muscles and ↑ vasodilation and blood flow to the penis following stimulation					
Sildenafil☆ • Viagra • 25–100 mg PRN 0.5–4 hr prior to sexual activity (max = 1 dose daily) • Tabs Tadalafil☆ • Cialis • 5–20 mg PRN ≥30 min prior to sexual activity; or 2.5–5 mg daily • Tabs Vardenafil • Levitra, Staxyn • 5–20 mg (max = 10 mg for ODTs) PRN ~1 hr prior to sexual activity • ODTs, tabs Avanafil • Stendra • 50–200 mg PRN 15–30 min prior to sexual activity • Tabs	• Use with nitrates (continuous or intermittent) • Hypersensitivity • Concurrent use with riociguat	• Hypotension • Dizziness • Headache • Flushing • Dyspepsia • Priapism (not common) • Vision changes • Hearing changes	• Efficacy • Presence of side effects • BP	***Nitrates— Combination results in potentially fatal hypotension. Avoid concomitant use within 24 hours; 48 hours with tadalafil.*** • Concurrent use with alpha-blockers may ↑ risk of hypotension; avoid combination or use lowest dose of each agent used with close monitoring • 3A4 substrates • 3A4 inhibitors may ↑ effects/toxicity • 3A4 inducers may ↓ effects	Dose adjustments when used with strong 3A4 inhibitors: sildenafil (use initial dose of 25 mg); tadalafil (max dose = 10 mg every 72 hr; or 2.5 mg daily); vardenafil (max dose = 2.5–5 mg every 24–72 hr based on CYP3A4 inhibitor; do not use with ODTs); avanafil (avoid concurrent use)

Medications for Erectile Dysfunction *(cont'd)*

Generic • Brand • Dose/Dosage Forms	Contraindications	Primary Side Effects	Key Monitoring Parameters	Pertinent Drug Interactions	Med Pearls
Topical					
Testosterone transdermal patch • Androderm • 2.5–6-mg patch daily • Transdermal patch	• Hypersensitivity • Breast or prostate cancer	• ↑ liver function tests (LFTs) • ↑ risk of DVT/PE, stroke, and MI • Edema • Hyperlipidemia • Depression • Aggression	• LFTs • Serum testosterone concentrations • Prostate-specific antigen • Lipid panel	May ↑ effects/toxicity of warfarin	• Only useful in ED due to hypogonadism • Schedule III controlled substance • Risk of abuse
Testosterone gel ☆ • AndroGel, Fortesta, Testim, Vogelxo • AndroGel 1%: 50–100 mg daily • AndroGel 1.62%: 40.5–81 mg daily • Fortesta: 40–70 mg daily • Testim: 50–100 mg daily • Vogelxo: 50–100 mg daily					
Testosterone intranasal gel • Natesto • 1 pump per nostril (total = 11 mg) TID					
Testosterone buccal • Striant • 30 mg BID (apply to gum, above incisor)					
Testosterone solution • Axiron • 60–120 mg daily (apply to axilla)					

Medications for Erectile Dysfunction *(cont'd)*

Generic • Brand • Dose/Dosage Forms	Contraindications	Primary Side Effects	Key Monitoring Parameters	Pertinent Drug Interactions	Med Pearls
Intramuscular					
Testosterone • Depo-Testosterone (cypionate), Generic (enanthate), Aveed (undecanoate) • Cypionate or enanthate: 50–400 mg IM every 2–4 wk • Undecanoate: 750 mg IM, then 750 mg IM 4 wk later, then 750 mg IM every 10 wk	• Hypersensitivity • Breast or prostate cancer • Serious cardiac, renal or hepatic disease	• ↑ LFTs • ↑ risk of DVT/PE, stroke, and MI • Edema • Hyperlipidemia • Depression • Aggression	• LFTs • Serum testosterone concentrations • PSA • Lipid panel	May ↑ effects/toxicity of warfarin	• Only useful in ED due to hypogonadism • Schedule III controlled substance
Intraurethral					
Alprostadil • Muse • 125–250 mcg pellets 5–10 min before intercourse	• Hypersensitivity • Urethral stricture • Chronic urethritis	• Urethral pain • Burning • Priapism • Hypotension	• Presence of side effects • Efficacy • BP	None	Duration of effect is 30–60 min
Intracavernosal					
Alprostadil • Caverject, Edex • 1–40 mcg 5–20 min before intercourse injected intracavernosal	• Hypersensitivity • Sickle-cell trait • Multiple myeloma • Leukemia	• Pain at injection site • Erythema • Priapism • Hypotension	• Presence of side effects • Efficacy • BP periodically	None	Self-injection training should be done in physician's office

BENIGN PROSTATIC HYPERPLASIA

Guidelines Summary

- Watchful waiting (no pharmacologic therapy) is appropriate for patients with mild symptoms (AUA-SI scores <8).

- In general, pharmacologic therapy is considered for patients with moderate–severe symptoms (AUA-SI scores ≥8).

- Alpha-antagonists are the treatment of choice for patients with LUTS and are used as monotherapy or in combination with 5-alpha reductase inhibitors or anticholinergics.

  - Nonselective alpha-antagonists such as terazosin and doxazosin are equally effective as the alpha 1A selective antagonists, tamsulosin, alfuzosin, and silodosin.

  - Nonselective alpha-antagonists require slow dose titration and lower BP; therefore, these agents should be used with caution in patients at risk for hypotension.

  - First-dose syncope and dizziness are common side effects, especially with the nonselective alpha-antagonists. Dosing at bedtime can minimize this side effect, but patients should be educated to stand up slowly to avoid falls.

  - Intraoperative floppy iris syndrome (IFIS) is a potential side effect of the alpha-antagonists that can significantly complicate cataract surgery. Patients with planned cataract surgery should not initiate new alpha-antagonist therapy until cataract surgery is complete.

- 5-alpha reductase inhibitors are appropriate as monotherapy or in combination with alpha-antagonists in patients with enlarged prostate glands. Concomitant therapy with alpha-antagonists will allow symptoms to improve during the initial 6 months of therapy when the 5-alpha reductase inhibitor is reaching maximal efficacy.

  - Although earlier guidelines suggested use of 5-alpha reductase inhibitors in patients with prostate glands >50 mL (50 g), newer studies have demonstrated benefits in patients with prostate glands >30 mL (30 g).

- Anticholinergic agents such as tolterodine may be considered in patient with LUTS (primarily irritative) and without an elevated postvoid residual (<250 mL). Please see the Urinary Incontinence section of this chapter for specifics related to anticholinergic medications.

PDE-5 inhibitors are now clinically indicated for daily use for the treatment of LUTS/BPH (tadalafil is approved by the Food and Drug Administration for this indication) but are generally reserved for patients who have not responded to more conventional therapies. Because PDE-5 inhibitors exhibit a significant drug interaction with non-selective alpha-antagonists, special care should be taken to monitor for and avoid this combination.

BPH Treatment Summary

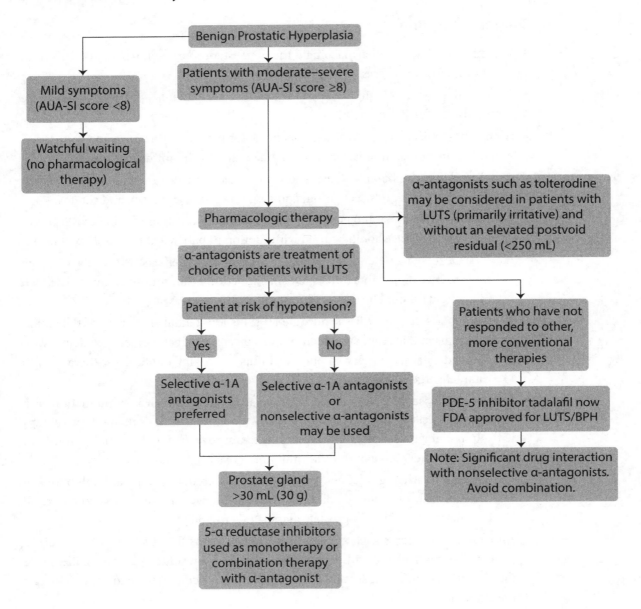

Medications for BPH

Generic • Brand • Dose/Dosage Forms	Contraindications	Primary Side Effects	Key Monitoring Parameters	Pertinent Drug Interactions	Med Pearls
Nonselective Alpha-1 Antagonists					
Doxazosin ☆ • Cardura, Cardura XL • IR: 1–8 mg at bedtime • ER: 4–8 mg in A.M. • ER tabs, tabs Terazosin ☆ • Only available generically • 1–10 mg at bedtime • Caps	Hypersensitivity	• Orthostatic hypotension • Dizziness • Reflex tachycardia • Peripheral edema • Headache • Drowsiness • Priapism (rare)	• BP • Heart rate • LUTS	↑ risk of hypotension with PDE-5 inhibitors (avoid concurrent use)	• Dosed at bedtime (except for doxazosin ER which is dosed in A.M.) to prevent dizziness/falls during the day • ↑ risk of IFIS in patients undergoing cataract surgery
Selective Alpha-1A Antagonists					
Tamsulosin ☆ • Flomax • 0.4–0.8 mg daily	Hypersensitivity	• Orthostatic hypotension • Dizziness • Headache • Priapism (rare)	• BP • LUTS	• CYP2D6 and CYP3A4 substrate • CYP2D6 and CYP3A4 inhibitors may ↑ effects/toxicity; avoid use with strong CYP3A4 inhibitors • CYP3A4 inducers may ↓ effects • ↑ risk of hypotension with PDE-5 inhibitors • Cimetidine may ↑ levels	• Take ~30 min after a meal • Expensive relative to nonselective agents • ↑ risk of IFIS in patients undergoing cataract surgery
Alfuzosin • Uroxatral • 10 mg daily • ER tabs	• Hypersensitivity • Moderate to severe hepatic impairment • Concurrent use with strong 3A4 inhibitors			• CYP3A4 substrate • CYP3A4 inhibitors may ↑ effects/toxicity; concurrent use with strong CYP3A4 inhibitors contraindicated	• Take with food • Do not crush or chew • Expensive relative to nonselective agents • ↑ risk of IFIS in patients undergoing cataract surgery
Silodosin • Rapaflo • 8 mg daily • Caps	• Hypersensitivity • Severe renal or hepatic impairment • Concurrent use with strong 3A4 inhibitors	• Orthostatic hypotension • Dizziness • Headache • Diarrhea • Retrograde ejaculation • Priapism (rare)		• CYP3A4 inducers may ↓ effects • ↑ risk of hypotension with PDE-5 inhibitors	• Adjust dose in renal impairment • Take with food • Expensive relative to nonselective agents • ↑ risk of IFIS in patients undergoing cataract surgery

Medications for BPH (cont'd)

Generic • Brand • Dose/Dosage Forms	Contraindications	Primary Side Effects	Key Monitoring Parameters	Pertinent Drug Interactions	Med Pearls
5-Alpha Reductase Inhibitors					
Finasteride ☆ • Proscar • 5 mg daily • Tabs	• Hypersensitivity • Pregnant women or women of reproductive potential	• ↓ libido • ED • Gynecomastia	• PSA • LUTS	None	• Cause significant ↓ in PSA; should establish new PSA baseline ≥6 mo after initiation of therapy • Dutasteride caps and crushed/broken finasteride tabs should not be handled by pregnant women or women of childbearing potential (potentially teratogenic for male infants) • Men taking dutasteride should not donate blood for ≥6 mo after discontinuing therapy • Onset of effect can be up to 6 mo
Dutasteride ☆ • Avodart • 0.5 mg daily • Caps				• CYP3A4 substrate • CYP3A4 inhibitors may ↑ effects/ toxicity • CYP3A4 inducers may ↓ effects	

Combination Products: See individual drug components for important points.		
Brand	**Components**	**Dosing**
Jalyn	Dutasteride + Tamsulosin	1 cap (0.5 mg dutasteride/0.4 mg tamsulosin) daily (~30 min after a meal)

URINARY INCONTINENCE

Summary of Treatment Recommendations

- General
  - Nonpharmacological therapy is important as either monotherapy or an adjunct to pharmacotherapy. Options such as pelvic floor muscle training (PFMT) exercises and scheduled voiding are common.
- Stress incontinence
  - First-line recommendation is nonpharmacological PFMT.
  - Options for treatment include topical estrogen, alpha agonists, and tricyclic antidepressants. Alpha agonists carry the risk of ↑ BP and heart rate, and should

be used with extreme caution in patients with pre-existing hypertension or heart conditions.

- Urge incontinence
  - Options for treatment include antimuscarinic medications, mirabegron, and imipramine.
- Overflow incontinence
  - Treatment options are varied based upon the determined etiology. Since many cases of overflow incontinence are secondary to BPH, see the BPH section of this chapter for recommendations.

Medications for Urinary Incontinence

Generic • Brand • Dose/Dosage Forms	Contraindications	Primary Side Effects	Key Monitoring Parameters	Pertinent Drug Interactions	Med Pearls
Topical vaginal estrogen preparations: used in the treatment of stress incontinence (first-line) and urge incontinence (third-line); refer to the Hormone Replacement Therapy section of this chapter for more detailed information					
Tricyclic antidepressants: imipramine and desipramine are most commonly used in incontinence; used primarily in urge incontinence and stress incontinence; refer to the Psychiatric Disorders chapter for more detailed information					
Anticholinergic/Antimuscarinic Agents					
Oxybutynin ☆ • Ditropan XL • IR: 5 mg 2–4 × /day • ER: 5–30 mg daily • ER tabs, tabs • Oxytrol • Apply 1 patch (3.9 mg/day) twice weekly • Transdermal patch • Gelnique • 10%: Apply contents of 1 sachet (100 mg/g) daily • Transdermal gel	• Hypersensitivity • Urinary retention • Gastric retention • Narrow-angle glaucoma	• Dry mouth • Dry eyes • Constipation • Urinary retention • Dizziness • Somnolence • Hallucinations • Agitation • Confusion • Blurred vision • ↑ intraocular pressure • Angioedema	• S/S of incontinence • Presence of side effects	Additive effects with other anticholinergic medications	• Side effects less common with ER tabs and transdermal formulations • Transdermal patch available over-the-counter
Tolterodine ☆ • Detrol, Detrol LA • IR: 1–2 mg BID • ER: 2–4 mg daily • ER caps, tabs				• CYP2D6 and CYP3A4 substrate • CYP2D6 and CYP3A4 inhibitors may ↑ effects/toxicity • CYP3A4 inducers may ↓ effects • Additive effects with other anticholinergic medications	• Side effects less common with ER tabs • Adjust dose in renal or hepatic impairment

Medications for Urinary Incontinence *(cont'd)*

Generic • Brand • Dose/Dosage Forms	Contraindications	Primary Side Effects	Key Monitoring Parameters	Pertinent Drug Interactions	Med Pearls
Anticholinergic/Antimuscarinic Agents (cont'd)					
Darifenacin ☆ • Enablex • 7.5–15 mg daily • ER tabs	[Same as above]	[Same as above]	[Same as above]	• CYP3A4 substrate • CYP3A4 inhibitors may ↑ effects/ toxicity • CYP3A4 inducers may ↓ effects • Additive effects with other anticholinergic medications	• Adjust dose in renal or hepatic impairment • Max dose = 7.5 mg daily with strong CYP3A4 inhibitors
Solifenacin ☆ • Vesicare • 5–10 mg daily • Tabs					• Adjust dose in hepatic impairment • Max dose = 5 mg daily with strong CYP3A4 inhibitors
Fesoterodine ☆ • Toviaz • 4–8 mg daily • ER tabs					• Adjust dose in renal impairment • Max dose = 4 mg daily with strong CYP3A4 inhibitors
Trospium ☆ • Only available generically • IR: 20 mg BID • ER: 60 mg daily • ER caps, tabs				• Metformin may ↓ levels • Additive effects with other anticholinergic medications	• Take 30 min before meals or on an empty stomach • Adjust dose in renal impairment and in patients ≥75 yr

Medications for Urinary Incontinence *(cont'd)*

Generic • Brand • Dose/Dosage Forms	Contraindications	Primary Side Effects	Key Monitoring Parameters	Pertinent Drug Interactions	Med Pearls
Mechanism of action – beta-3 adrenergic receptor agonist					
Mirabegron • Myrbetriq • 25–50 mg daily • ER tabs	Hypersensitivity	• Hypertension • Angioedema • Headache	• BP • S/S of incontinence	• CYP2D6 inhibitor • May ↑ effects/ toxicity of CYP2D6 substrates • May ↑ serum digoxin concentrations • May ↑ effects of warfarin • Additive effects with other anticholinergic medications	• Adjust dose in renal or hepatic impairment • Fewer anticholinergic side effects; may be a good option in elderly patients with anticholinergic side effects • Hypertension may limit use • Very expensive
Alpha Agonists					
Pseudoephedrine • Sudafed • 30–60 mg every 4–6 hr PRN (max = 240 mg/24 hrs) Phenylephrine • Many • 10–20 mg every 4 hr PRN	• Hypersensitivity • Concurrent use of monoamine oxidase inhibitors (MAOIs) • Uncontrolled hypertension	• ↑ BP • ↑ heart rate • ↑ blood sugar • Irritability • Insomnia	• BP • Heart rate • Fasting plasma glucose (if diabetes)	Concurrent use with MAOIs may ↑ risk of hypertensive crises	Use with caution in hypertension or pre-existing cardiac conditions

Preventive Medicine

This chapter covers the following preventive healthcare measures:

- **Immunizations**
- **Weight loss**
- **Smoking cessation**

IMMUNIZATIONS

Immunizations

Vaccine • Brand Name • Route of Administration	Contraindications	Adverse Effects	Target Population	Medication Pearls
Live vaccines				
Herpes zoster (shingles) • Zostavax • Subcut	• History of anaphylaxis to gelatin or neomycin • Immunosuppression or immunodeficiency	• Injection site reactions • Headache • Flu-like symptoms • Fever	All patients ≥60 years of age	None
Live attenuated influenza • FluMist Quadrivalent • Intranasal	• Anaphylaxis to previous influenza vaccination • Hypersensitivity to egg protein • Children 2–17 years of age taking aspirin	• Runny nose • Nasal congestion • Fever • Sore throat • Headache • ↓ appetite • Weakness	All patients 2–49 years of age yearly	
Measles, mumps, rubella (MMR) • M-M-R II • Subcut	• Hypersensitivity to any vaccine component • Febrile illness • Immunosuppression or immunodeficiency • Pregnancy	• Injection site reactions • Arthralgia • Myalgia • Rash	Children ≥12 months	

Immunizations *(cont'd)*

Vaccine • Brand Name • Route of Administration	Contraindications	Adverse Effects	Target Population	Medication Pearls
Live vaccines *(cont'd)*				
Rotavirus • Rotarix, RotaTeq • Oral	• Hypersensitivity • History of intussusception • Severe combined immunodeficiency disease	• Fever • Diarrhea • Vomiting • Otitis media • Nasopharyngitis	• Infants and children 6–24 weeks (Rotarix) • Infants and children 6–32 weeks (RotaTeq)	None
Varicella (chickenpox): • Varivax • Subcut	• Allergic reaction to vaccine, gelatin, or neomycin • Immunodeficiency or immunosuppression • Active, untreated tuberculosis • Pregnancy	• Injection site reactions • Rash • Fever • Malaise • Arthralgia	Children ≥12 months of age	
Inactivated vaccines				
Influenza • Afluria, Fluad, Fluarix Quadrivalent, Flucelvax, Flucelvax Quadrivalent, Flulaval Quadrivalent, Fluvirin, Fluzone High-Dose, Fluzone Intradermal Quadrivalent, Fluzone Quadrivalent • Intradermal (Fluzone Intradermal Quadrivalent) • IM (remainder)	• Allergy to previous influenza vaccination • Allergy to eggs (except for Flucelvax)	• Fever • Malaise • Myalgia • Injection site reactions	All patients ≥6 months of age	Yearly vaccination to account for antigenic drifts and ↓ antibody levels over time

Immunizations *(cont'd)*

Vehicle • Brand Name • Route of Administration	Contraindications	Adverse Effects	Target Population	Medication Pearls
Inactivated vaccines *(cont'd)*				
Diphtheria, tetanus, acelluar pertussis • DTaP: Daptacel, Infanrix • IM • Tdap: Adacel, Boostrix • IM • Td: Decavac, Tenivac • IM	**DTaP** • Serious allergic reaction to previous dose of diphtheria toxoid-, tetanus toxoid-, or pertussis-containing vaccine • Encephalopathy within 7 days of previous vaccination • Progressive neurologic disorders **Tdap** • Serious allergic reaction to diphtheria toxoid, tetanus toxoid and pertussis antigen-containing vaccine • Encephalopathy within 7 days of previous vaccination **Td** • Serious allergic reaction to tetanus toxoid or diphtheria toxoid containing vaccine	• Injection site reactions • Arthus reactions • Swelling • Fever	• DTaP: Children 6 week–6 years of age • Tdap: Single dose once >7 years of age or in third trimester of each pregnancy • Td: 1 dose every 10 years once ≥7 years of age	Tdap is needed only once per lifetime (except should be given during each pregnancy)
Human papillomavirus (HPV) • Cervarix (HPV2), Gardasil (HPV4), Gardasil 9 (HPV9) • IM	• Hypersensitivity • Allergy to yeast (Gardasil, Gardasil 9)	• Injection site reactions • Headache • Fever • Fatigue • Myalgia	• Cervarix: Females 9–25 years of age • Gardasil: Females and males 9–26 years of age • Gardasil 9: Females and males 9–26 years of age	• Cervarix protects against HPV types 16 and 18 • Gardasil protects against HPV types 6, 11, 16, and 18 • Gardasil 9 protects against HPV types 6, 11, 16, 18, 31, 33, 45, 52, and 58

Immunizations *(cont'd)*

Vaccine • Brand Name • Route of Administration	Contraindications	Adverse Effects	Target Population	Medication Pearls
Inactivated vaccines (cont'd)				
Streptococcus pneumoniae • Pneumovax 23 (PPSV23) • IM, subcut • Prevnar 13 (PCV13) • IM	• Severe allergic reaction to pneumococcal vaccine • Severe allergic reaction to any diphtheria toxoid-containing vaccine (PCV13)	• Injection site reactions • Fever • Myalgia	• PCV13: children 2–59 months of age; children 60–71 months of age with chronic heart disease, asthma, diabetes, asplenia, or immunosuppressive conditions; children ≥6 years of age, adolescents, and adults with asplenia or immunosuppressive conditions; and all patients ≥65 years of age • PPSV23: All patients ≥65 years of age; children, adolescents, and adults ≥2 years of age at ↑ risk for pneumococcal disease (asplena, sickle cell disease, heart failure, chronic obstructive pulmonary disease, asthma, diabetes, chronic liver disease, cigarette smokers, and immunosuppressed)	• PPSV23 not indicated for children <2 years of age • Second dose of PPSV23 recommended for patients ≥65 years of age with previous dose given ≥5 years ago
Meningococcal • MCV4: Menactra, Menveo • IM • MPSV4: Menomune • Subcut	• Hypersensitivity • Hypersensitivity to diphtheria toxoid (MCV4)	• Injection site reactions • Headache • Fever • Malaise	• MCV4: Adolescents 11–18 years of age with a booster dose after 5 years (if initial dose given before age 16); patients ≥2 months of age at ↑ risk of meningococcal disease (can be used up to age 55) • MPSV4: Unvaccinated adults >56 years of age who are at ↑ risk of meningococcal disease	MPSV4 should not be used in children <2 years of age

Immunizations *(cont'd)*

Vaccine • Brand Name • Route of Administration	Contraindications	Adverse Effects	Target Population	Medication Pearls
Inactivated vaccines (cont'd)				
Hepatitis A • Havrix, VAQTA • IM	• Hypersensitivity • Allergic reaction to vaccine or neomycin	• Injection site reactions • Fever	• All children ≥12 months of age • International travel other than Canada, Europe, Japan, New Zealand, or Australia • Men who have sex with men (MSM) • Illicit drug users • Laboratory workers • Patients with chronic liver disease or clotting disorders	None
Hepatitis B • Engerix-B, Recombivax HB • IM	• Hypersensitivity • Allergic reaction to previous hepatitis B vaccination or yeast	• Injection site reactions • Headache • Fatigue • Fever	• Infants at birth • All infants and children • Healthcare workers • International travel • Patients with multiple sexual partners • MSM • Injection drug users • Adults with diabetes mellitus • HIV • Chronic liver disease • End-stage renal disease	
Haemophilus influenzae type B • ActHIB, Hiberix, PedvaxHIB • IM	• Hypersensitivity • Hypersensitivity to tetanus toxoid (ActHIB and Hiberix)	Injection site reactions	All infants and children through age 59 months	
Polio • IPOL • IM, subcut	Hypersensitivity		All infants and children >2 months of age	
Recombinant zoster • Shingrix • IM	Hypersensitivity	• Injection site reactions • Fatigue • Headache • Myalgia • Fever	Adults >50 years of age	Recommended for patients who have already received Zostavax, but must be separated by ≥8 wk

WEIGHT LOSS

Guidelines Summary

Healthcare providers should evaluate a patient's BMI at each visit and create an individualized treatment plan. Weight loss plans need to include moderate caloric reduction, increased physical activity, and behavioral strategies that patients can use to sustain weight loss.

Medications for Weight Loss

Generic • Brand • Dose/Dosage Form	Contraindications	Primary Side Effects	Key Monitoring	Pertinent Drug Interactions	Med Pearls
Mechanism of action – inhibits gastric and pancreatic lipase to inhibit dietary fat					
Orlistat • Xenical, Alli (over-the-counter [OTC]) • Xenical: 120 mg TID with each meal • Alli: 60 mg TID with each meal • Caps	• Hypersensitivity • Chronic malabsorption syndrome • Pregnancy • Cholestasis	• Oily discharge/ spotting • Fecal urgency • Hepatotoxicity • Nephrolithiasis • Cholelithiasis • Flatulence	• Weight • BMI • Serum glucose • Thyroid function • Liver function tests (LFTs) • Renal function	• May ↓ absorption of cyclosporine, warfarin, anticonvulsants, amiodarone, levothyroxine, and antiepileptic drugs levels • ↓ absorption of fat-soluble vitamins (A, D, E, K)	• Available OTC • Should supplement with multivitamin
Mechanism of action – stimulates hypothalamus to release norepinephrine (phentermine); suppresses appetite and ↑ satiety through inhibition of neuronal sodium channels and ↑ GABA activity (topiramate)					
Phentermine with topiramate • Qsymia • 3.75 mg/23 mg daily × 14 days, then 7.5 mg/46 mg daily × 12 wk; if 3% of baseline body weight has not been lost, discontinue therapy or ↑ dose to 11.25 mg/69 mg daily × 14 days, then 15 mg/92 mg daily • Caps	• Hypersensitivity to phentermine or sympathomimetics • Pregnancy • Hyperthyroidism • Glaucoma • Use of monoamine oxidase inhibitor (MAOI) within 2 wk	• Tachycardia • Headache • Insomnia • Xerostomia • Constipation • Paresthesia • Difficulty concentrating • Confusion • Memory issues • Speech problems • Depression • Dizziness • Kidney stones • Angle closure glaucoma • Visual field defects • ↓ sweating • Hyperthermia • Metabolic acidosis • ↑ SCr • Hypokalemia	• Weight • BMI • Heart rate (HR) • Blood pressure (BP) • Serum bicarbonate • Serum potassium • Serum glucose • Renal function • Suicidality • Intraocular pressure	• ↑ risk of hypertensive crisis with MAOIs • Other central nervous system (CNS) depressants, including alcohol, may ↑ CNS depressant effects • Concurrent use with loop or thiazide diuretics may ↑ risk of hypokalemia • Phenytoin or carbamazepine may ↓ topiramate levels • Concurrent use with valproic acid may ↑ risk of hyperammonemia or hypothermia • Concurrent use with zonisamide or acetazolamide may ↑ risk of metabolic acidosis or nephrolithiasis	• Schedule IV controlled substance • Adjust dose in renal or hepatic impairment • Teratogenic • Give in A.M. to minimize risk of insomnia • If patient has not lost 5% of baseline body weight by wk 12 of phentermine 15 mg/topiramate 92 mg daily, discontinue therapy

Medications for Weight Loss   (cont'd)

Generic • **Brand** • **Dose/Dosage Form**	**Contraindications**	**Primary Side Effects**	**Key Monitoring**	**Pertinent Drug Interactions**	**Med Pearls**
Mechanism of action – stimulates hypothalamus to release norepinephrine					
Phentermine • Adipex-P • 15–37.5 mg/day in 1–2 divided doses • Caps, tabs	• Hypersensitivity to phentermine or sympathomimetics • History of cardiovascular disease (e.g., coronary artery disease, stroke, arrhythmias, heart failure, uncontrolled hypertension) • Pregnancy • Breast feeding • Hyperthyroidism • Glaucoma • Use of MAOI within 2 wk • Agitation • History of drug abuse	• Hypertension • Tachycardia • Primary pulmonary hypertension • Valvular heart disease • Euphoria • Dizziness • Insomnia • Psychosis • Tremor	• Weight • BMI • BP • HR • S/S of valvular heart disease	↑ risk of hypertensive crisis with MAOIs	• Schedule IV controlled substance • Give before breakfast or 1–2 hr after breakfast
Mechanism of action – activates 5-HT2c receptors which stimulates pro-opiomelanocortin neurons that stimulate alpha-melanocortin-4 receptors which lead to ↑ satiety and ↓ appetite					
Lorcaserin • Belviq, Belviq XR • IR: 10 mg BID • ER: 20 mg daily • ER tabs, tabs	• Hypersensitivity • Pregnancy	• Headache • Dizziness • Nausea • Xerostomia • Constipation • Hypoglycemia • Difficulty concentrating • Memory issues • Priapism • Bradycardia • Leukopenia • Hyperprolactinemia • Serotonin syndrome	• Weight • BMI • Complete blood count • Serum glucose • Prolactin levels • S/S of valvular heart disease	• CYP2D6 inhibitor • May ↑ effects/toxicity of CYP2D6 substrates • ↑ risk of serotonin syndrome with MAOIs, selective serotonin reuptake inhibitors, serotonin-norepinephrine reuptake inhibitors, triptans, tricyclic antidepressants, fentanyl, lithium, dextromethorphan, meperidine, buspirone, linezolid, methylene blue, St. John's wort, and tramadol • Thioridazine • Antipsychotics • Ergot derivatives • Bupropion • Metoprolol • Tamoxifen • Serotonin modulators	• Schedule IV controlled substance • If patient has not lost ≥5% of baseline body weight by wk 12, discontinue therapy

Medications for Weight Loss *(cont'd)*

Generic • Brand • Dose/Dosage Form	Contraindications	Primary Side Effects	Key Monitoring	Pertinent Drug Interactions	Med Pearls
Mechanism of action – not fully understood, weight loss thought to result from regulation of food intake via hypothalmus and mesolimbic influence.					
Naltrexone/ bupropion • Contrave • 8 mg/90 mg daily × 1 wk, then BID × 1 wk, then 16 mg/ 180 mg every A.M. and 8 mg/ 90 mg every P.M. × 1 wk, then 16 mg/180 mg BID • ER tabs	• Hypersensitivity to naltrexone or bupropion • Concurrent use of other products containing bupropion • Chronic opioid use • Uncontrolled hypertension • Seizure disorders • Bulimia • Anorexia nervosa • Abrupt discontinuation of alcohol, benzodiazepines, barbiturates, or antiepileptic drugs • Use of MAOI within 2 wk • Pregnancy	• Headache • Insomnia • Nausea/vomiting (N/V) • Constipation • Dizziness • Xerostomia • Seizures • Hypertension • Tachycardia • Anaphylaxis • Hepatotoxicity	• Weight • BMI • BP • HR • Renal function • LFTs • Suicidality	• CYP2B6 substrate • CYP2D6 inhibitor • CYP2B6 inhibitors may ↑ effects/toxicity • CYP2B6 inducers may ↓ effects • May ↑ effects/toxicity of CYP2D6 substrates • ↑ risk of hypertensive crisis with MAOIs	• Do not administer with a high-fat meal • Adjust dose in renal or hepatic impairment
Mechanism of action – GLP-1 analog which ↑ glucose-dependent insulin secretion, ↓ inappropriate glucagon secretion, slows gastric emptying, and ↓ food intake					
Liraglutide • Saxenda • 0.6 mg subcut daily × 1 wk, then ↑ by 0.6 mg daily at weekly intervals to target of 3 mg subcut daily • Injection	• Hypersensitivity • History of medullary thyroid carcinoma • Multiple endocrine neoplasia syndrome type 2 • Pregnancy	• Tachycardia • Headache • Hypoglycemia • N/V/D • Constipation • Fatigue • Dyspepsia • Dizziness • ↓ appetite • Anaphylaxis • Cholelithiasis • Pancreatitis • Thyroid tumors	• Weight • BMI • HR • Serum glucose • Renal function • S/S of pancreatitis • S/S hypoglycemia • Thyroid tumors	• May delay absorption of other drugs due to ↑ gastric emptying time (administer other medications 1 hour prior) • Sulfonylureas and insulin ↑ risk of hypoglycemia	If patient has not lost ≥4% of baseline body weight by wk 16, discontinue therapy

SMOKING CESSATION

Guidelines Summary

- The model for treatment and intervention of tobacco use and dependence is summarized by the "5 A's":
  - **ASK.** Identify and document tobacco use status for every patient and every visit.
  - **ADVISE.** Urge every tobacco user to quit in a strong and personalized manner.
  - **ASSESS.** Evaluate if your patient is willing to make a quit attempt.
  - **ASSIST.** For patients willing to make a quit attempt, offer treatment options and additional counseling; for those not willing, use motivational strategies to promote quitting.
  - **ARRANGE.** Schedule follow-ups with those patients willing to make a quit attempt; for those not willing to make an attempt, address willingness to quit at the next visit.
- Tobacco dependence is a chronic disease that often requires repeated intervention and multiple attempts to quit. Effective treatments exist that can significantly increase rates of long-term abstinence.
- It is essential that healthcare providers consistently identify and document tobacco use status and treat every tobacco user seen in a healthcare setting.
- Tobacco dependence treatments are effective across a broad range of populations. Clinicians should encourage every patient willing to make a quit attempt to use the counseling treatments and medications recommended.
- Brief tobacco dependence treatment is effective. Clinicians should offer every patient who uses tobacco at least the brief treatments shown to be effective.

Medications for Smoking Cessation

Generic • Brand • Dose/Dosage Forms	Contraindications	Primary Side Effects	Key Monitoring	Pertinent Drug Interactions	Med Pearls
Mechanism of action – partial $\alpha_4\beta_2$ nicotinic receptor agonist; prevents nicotine stimulation of the mesolimbic dopamine system					
Varenicline ☆ • Chantix • 0.5 mg daily × 3 days, then 0.5 mg BID × 4 days, then 1 mg BID × 11 wk • Tabs	Hypersensitivity	• Somnolence • Abnormal dreams • N/V • Constipation • Suicidal/homicidal ideation • Irritability • Depression • Mania • Hostility • Agitation • Anxiety • Panic • Psychotic symptoms • Hallucinations • Paranoia • Delusions • Seizures • Hypersensitivity • Rash (including Stevens-Johnson syndrome)	• Nicotine consumption • Mood changes • Psychotic symptoms • Suicidal/homicidal ideation	• Concurrent use with nicotine replacement products may ↑ risk of N/V • ↑ effects of alcohol	• Start 1 wk prior to target stop day • Take after meal and with full glass of water
Mechanism of action – inhibits neuronal uptake of norepinephrine and dopamine					
Bupropion ☆ • Zyban • 150 mg daily × 3 days, then 150 mg BID × 7–12 wk • ER tabs	• Seizure disorders • Anorexia or bulimia • Abrupt discontinuation of alcohol, benzodiazepines, barbiturates, or antiepileptic drugs • Use of MAOI within 2 wk • Use of MAOI within 14 days • Hypersensitivity • Concurrent use of linezolid or methylene blue	• Insomnia • Xerostomia • Dizziness • Nausea • Constipation • Suicidal/homicidal ideation • Irritability • Depression • Mania • Hostility • Agitation • Anxiety • Panic • Psychotic symptoms • Hallucinations • Paranoia • Delusions • Seizures • Hypertension • Anaphylaxis	• Nicotine consumption • Mood changes • Psychotic symptoms • Suicidal/homicidal ideation • Seizure activity	• CYP2B6 substrate • CYP2D6 inhibitor • CYP2B6 inhibitors may ↑ effects/toxicity • CYP2B6 inducers may ↓ effects • May ↑ effects/ toxicity of CYP2D6 substrates • ↑ risk of hypertensive crises with MAOIs	• Start 1 wk prior to target stop day • Can be coadministered with nicotine replacement patches

Medications for Smoking Cessation *(cont'd)*

Generic • Brand • Dose/Dosage Forms	Contraindications	Primary Side Effects	Key Monitoring	Pertinent Drug Interactions	Med Pearls
Mechanism of action — supplements nicotine, which exhibits primary effects via autonomic ganglia stimulation					
Nicotine • Nicoderm CQ, Nicorelief, Nicorette, Nicotrol, Thrive • Gum: 1 piece every 1–2 hr PRN during wk 1–6, then 1 piece every 2–4 hr PRN during wk 7–9, then 1 piece every 4–8 hr PRN during wk 10–12 as needed; max = 24 pieces/day) • Inhaler: 6–16 cartridges/day; duration of treatment = 3 mo • Transdermal patch: >10 cigarettes/day: 21 mg/day × 6 wk, then 14 mg/day × 2 wk, then 7 mg/day × 2 wk; ≤10 cigarettes/day: 14 mg/day × 6 wk, then 7 mg/day × 2 wk • Lozenge: 1 lozenge every 1–2 hr PRN during wk 1–6, then 1 lozenge every 2–4 hr PRN during wk 7–9, then 1 lozenge every 4–8 hr PRN during wk 10–12 as needed; max = 20 lozenges/day) • Nasal spray: 1 spray in each nostril 1–2 ×/hr (max = 80 sprays/day); duration of treatment = 3 mo	• Smoking or chewing tobacco • Post-myocardial infarction • Life-threatening arrhythmias • Worsening angina	• Headache • Mouth or throat irritation • Dyspepsia • Cough	• Nicotine consumption • Nicotine toxicity (severe headache, dizziness, confusion)	None	• Can be coadministered with bupropion • Gum or lozenge: use 4-mg dose if smoke first cigarette within 30 min of waking; otherwise, use 2-mg dose • Do not eat or drink within 15 min of using gum or lozenge • Oral inhalation: patient should continuously puff for ~20 min

Over-the-Counter Medications

22

This chapter covers the following drug classes:

- **Vitamins**
- **Common herbals and supplements**
- **Decongestants**
- **Antihistamines**
- **Cough suppressants and expectorants**
- **Antidiarrheals**
- **Laxatives**
- **Antifungals**
- **Pediculocides**
- **Atopic dermatitis medications**
- **Poison ivy medications**
- **Sunscreens**

This chapter provides an overview of basic treatment for common ailments treatable by pharmacists. It also makes recommendations as to when self-treatment is not appropriate.

VITAMINS

Water-Soluble Vitamins

Vitamin	Function	Deficiency Manifestation	Recommended Daily Allowance (RDA)
B$_1$ (thiamine)	• Energy metabolism and production • Maintenance of nerve function	• Beriberi • Wernicke-Korsakoff syndrome	• Males: 1.2 mg • Females: 1.1 mg
B$_2$ (riboflavin)	• Energy metabolism and production • Maintenance of vision and skin	• Sore throat • Lesions of the lips and mucosa of the mouth • Glossitis • Normochromic, normocytic anemia	• Males: 1.3 mg • Females: 1.1 mg
B$_3$ (niacin)	• Energy metabolism and production • Maintenance of nervous and digestive systems and skin	Pellagra	• Males: 16 mg • Females: 14 mg
B$_5$ (pantothenic acid)	Energy metabolism and production	Paresthesia	5 mg
B$_6$ (pyridoxine)	• Production of red blood cells • Balance of sodium and potassium	Neuropathy	• Age 19–50 yr: 1.3 mg • Males >50 yr: 1.7 mg • Females >50 yr: 1.5 mg
B$_7$ (biotin)	• Fatty acid synthesis • Metabolism of amino acids	• Dermatitis • Enteritis • Hair loss	30 mcg
B$_9$ (folic acid)	• DNA synthesis • Production of red blood cells	• Neural tube defects • Megaloblastic anemia	400 mcg
B$_{12}$ (cobalamins)	• Nerve function • Production of red blood cells • DNA synthesis	Megaloblastic anemia	2.4 mcg
C (ascorbic acid)	• Antioxidant • Enhances immune system	Scurvy	• Males: 90 mg • Females: 75 mg

Fat-Soluble Vitamins

Vitamin	Function	Deficiency Manifestation	RDA
A	Vision	• Night blindness • Xerophthalmia • Hyperkeratosis	• Males: 900 mcg (3,000 units) • Females: 700 mcg (2,330 units)
D	• Calcium and phosphorus regulation • Bone health	Rickets	• Age 19–70 yr: 15 mcg (600 units) • Age >70 yr: 20 mcg (800 units)
E	• Antioxidant • Smooth muscle and nerve function	Hemolytic anemia	15 mg
K	Blood clotting	Bleeding	• Males: 120 mcg • Females: 90 mcg

COMMON HERBALS AND SUPPLEMENTS

Common Usage

- Saw palmetto
  - Used in men to improve symptoms of benign prostatic hyperplasia (BPH)
- Glucosamine and chondroitin
  - Used widely for treating osteoarthritis and joint structure support
  - Glucosamine: Important for maintaining elasticity, strength, and resiliency of the cartilage in articular (movable) joints
  - Chondroitin: Promotes flexibility of cartilage
- Fish oils or omega-3 fatty acids
  - Used primarily for hypertriglyceridemia
  - Contain eicosapentaenoic acid (EPA) and docosahexaenoic acid (DHA), and are believed to be efficacious in many people
- St. John's wort
  - Used for mild to moderate depression
  - Used in Europe for centuries for mild to moderate depression and its efficacy is comparable with tricyclic antidepressants; one study suggests it is no more effective than a placebo or sertraline in moderate to severe depression; it should not be used with other selective serotonin reuptake inhibitors (SSRIs) or serotonin norepinephrine reuptake inhibitors (SNRIs)

- Coenzyme Q10
  - Used for cardiovascular diseases, including angina, heart failure, and hypertension, and may help with myalgias due to statin therapy
- Melatonin
  - Used for insomnia, particularly when adjusting to shift-work cycles or jet lag
  - Naturally secreted from the pineal gland and appears to be the sleep-regulating hormone of the body; adults experience about a 37% decrease in daily melatonin output between 20 and 70 years of age
- Echinacea
  - Used as an immune stimulant
  - Has been studied extensively in the area of flu and cold prevention/treatment
- Black cohosh
  - Used for women's health problems, especially postmenopausal symptom relief and painful menses
  - Should be avoided in pregnancy and lactation
- Ginger
  - Used primarily for motion sickness, dyspepsia, and nausea
  - Lacks sedative effects of other antinausea treatments
  - Has been studied in pregnant women at less than 17 weeks' gestation
- Ginkgo biloba
  - Used for vascular dementia, Alzheimer's, and ischemic stroke
  - The ginkgolides are potent platelet-activating factor antagonists
- Ginseng
  - Used to treat diabetes mellitus
  - May also help reduce mental and physical stress

Over-the-Counter Medications

Name • Alternate Name • Dose	Contraindications	Primary Side Effects	Key Monitoring Parameters	Pertinent Drug Interactions	Med Pearls
Mechanism of action – inhibits production of dihydrotestosterone (DHT), inhibits receptor binding, and accelerates the metabolism of DHT					
Serenoa repens • Saw palmetto • BPH: 160 mg BID	• Pregnancy or lactation • Age <12 yr	Nausea/vomiting (N/V)	BPH symptoms	• May ↑ toxicity of estrogens or estrogen-containing contraceptives • May ↑ risk of bleeding with warfarin	Data from meta-analysis do not support use
Mechanism of action – glucosamine is an amino-sugar that is naturally produced and is a key substrate in the synthesis of macromolecules for connective tissues; chondroitin absorbs water, adding to cartilage thickness, and is found in natural physiologic connective tissue; inhibits synovial enzymes that may contribute to cartilage destruction					
Glucosamine/ chondroitin • Glucosamine: 500 mg TID • Chondroitin: 400 mg TID	• Glucosamine: active bleeding • Chondroitin: none	• Flatulence • Abdominal cramps • ↑ blood glucose	Osteoarthritis pain	May ↑ risk of bleeding with antiplatelets or anticoagulants	
Mechanism of action – inhibit diacylglycerol transferase which leads to a ↓ in hepatic synthesis of triglycerides					
Omega-3 fatty acids • Fish oils • Hypertriglyceride-mia: 2–4 g/day	Active bleeding	Gastrointestinal upset	Lipid panel	May ↑ risk of bleeding with antiplatelets or anticoagulants	
Mechanism of action – ↑ concentrations of serotonin in the central nervous system (CNS) and may have some monoamine oxidase inhibitor (MAOI) effects					
Hypericum perforatum • St. John's wort • 300 mg TID	• Pregnancy or lactation • Concurrent use with CYP2C19, CYP3A4, or P-glycoprotein substrates	• Nausea • Xerostomia • Itching • Photosensitivity • Fatigue • Dizziness • Insomnia • Jitteriness • Headache	Depression symptoms	• CYP2C19 and CYP3A4 inducer • May ↓ effects of CYP2C19 or CYP3A4 substrates • ↑ risk of serotonin syndrome with MAOIs, SSRIs, SNRIs, triptans, tricyclic antidepressants (TCAs), fentanyl, lithium, dextromethorphan, meperidine, buspirone, linezolid, methylene blue, and tramadol	Minimum of 4–6 wk of therapy is recommended before results seen
Mechanism of action – involved in adenosine triphosphate generation and serves as a lipid-soluble antioxidant providing protection against free-radical damage within the mitochondria					
Ubiquinone • Coenzyme Q10 • 20–300 mg/day in 2–3 divided doses	None	• Abdominal discomfort • Headache • N/V	Heart failure symptoms	• May ↓ anticoagulant effects of warfarin • May ↑ risk of cardiotoxicity with anthracyclines	None

Over-the-Counter Medications *(cont'd)*

Name • Alternate Name • Dose	Contraindications	Primary Side Effects	Key Monitoring Parameters	Pertinent Drug Interactions	Med Pearls
Mechanism of action — supplements the naturally deficient concentrations of melatonin					
N-acetyl-5-methoxytryp-tamine • Melatonin • 1–5 mg at bedtime	Autoimmune disease	• Morning sedation or drowsiness • Headache • Dizziness • Nausea	Sleep quality/ quantity	• CYP1A2 inhibitor • May ↑ effects/toxicity of CYP1A2 substrates	Drugs that deplete vitamin B$_6$ may inhibit the ability of the body to synthesize melatonin
Mechanism of action — may stimulate white blood cell function, including cell-mediated immunity					
Echinacea purpurea/ angustifolia/ pallida • Echinacea • 50–1,000 mg TID on day 1, then 250 mg 4 × /day	• Hypersensitivty to plants in Asteraceae/ Compositae family (including ragweed, chrysanthemums, marigolds, daisies) • Immunosup-pressed patients • Rheumatoid arthritis • Systemic lupus erythematosus • Multiple sclerosis • Tuberculosis	• Itching • Rash • N/V	Cold symptoms	• CYP1A2 inhibitor • CYP3A4 inducer • May ↑ effects/toxicity of CYP1A2 substrates • May ↓ effects of CYP3A4 substrates • May ↓ effects of immunosuppressants	Should not use for >10 days in acute infection
Mechanism of action — contains phytoestrogens, which mimic estrogen					
Actaea racemosa or *Cimicifuga racemosa* • Black cohosh • 20–40 mg BID	• History of or at risk for breast cancer • Pregnancy or lactation • Aspirin sensitivity	• N/V • Rash • Hepatotoxicity	Menopausal symptoms	• CYP2D6 inhibitor • May ↑ effects/toxicity of CYP2D6 substrates	Contains salicylates
Mechanism of action — has local affects in the gastrointestinal (GI) tract and in the CNS					
Zingiber officinale • Ginger • 500–2500 mg/ day in 2–4 divided doses	Active bleeding	Generally well tolerated	Degree of nausea	May ↑ risk of bleeding with antiplatelets or anticoagulants	Use during pregnancy for morning sickness remains controversial
Mechanism of action — the flavonoid component protects neurons and retinal tissue from oxidative stress and injury					
Ginkgo biloba • Ginkgo • 120–240 mg/day in 2–3 divided doses	• Pregnancy or lactation • Active bleeding	• Nausea • Constipation • Headache • Dizziness • Palpitations • Allergic skin reactions	Mini mental state exam	May ↑ risk of bleeding with antiplatelets or anticoagulants	None

Over-the-Counter Medications   *(cont'd)*

Name • Alternate Name • Dose	Contraindications	Primary Side Effects	Key Monitoring Parameters	Pertinent Drug Interactions	Med Pearls
Mechanism of action – ↓ postprandial glucose levels and stimulates the release of insulin					
Panax quinquefolius • Ginseng (American) • Usual: 100–400 mg daily • Diabetes: up to 3 g/day, 2 hr before a meal	Active bleeding	• Insomnia • Headache • Anorexia	Blood glucose	• May ↑ risk of bleeding with antiplatelets or anticoagulants • May ↑ effects of glucose-lowering drugs	Should not use for >3 mo

DECONGESTANTS

Guidelines Summary

- A pharmacist may appropriately recommend a decongestant once it is determined that the patient does not have any of the following:
  - Fever (temperature >101.5°F)
  - Chest pain
  - Shortness of breath
  - Uncontrolled hypertension
  - Cardiac arrhythmias
  - Insomnia
  - Anxiety
  - Worsening of symptoms or development of additional symptoms during self-treatment
  - Concurrent underlying chronic cardiopulmonary disease
  - Acquired immune deficiency syndrome or chronic immunosuppressant therapy
  - Frail patients of advanced age
  - Children <2 years of age
  - Current use of MAOIs
- Topical decongestants should not be recommended for longer than 3 days due to the risk of rhinitis medicamentosa, a condition of rebound nasal congestion brought on by overuse of intranasal vasoconstrictive medications.

Decongestants

Generic • Brand • Dose	Contraindications	Primary Side Effects	Key Monitoring Parameters	Pertinent Drug Interactions	Med Pearls
Oral Decongestants					
Mechanism of action – alpha-1 adrenergic stimulant					
Phenylephrine • Sudafed PE Maximum Strength • 10 mg every 4 hr PRN	• Uncontrolled hypertension • Ventricular tachycardia • Use of MAOI within 2 wk	• Restlessness • Hypertension • Tremor • Tachycardia • Insomnia	• Blood pressure • Heart rate • Anxiety	↑ risk of hypertensive crisis with MAOIs	Available OTC without restrictions
Pseudoephedrine • Sudafed • IR: 60 mg every 4–6 hr PRN • ER: 120 mg every 12 hr or 240 mg daily					• Available behind the counter • Must provide photo identification and sign log book to purchase • Amount purchased limited to ≤3.6 g/day or 9 g/mo
Topical Decongestants					
Oxymetazoline • Afrin • Intranasal: 2–3 sprays in each nostril BID	Hypersensitivity	• Dryness of nasal mucosa • Stinging • Rebound congestion	Rebound congestion	↑ risk of hypertensive crisis with MAOIs	Not recommended for longer than 3 days
Naphazoline • Clear Eyes • Ophthalmic: 1–2 drops every 6 hr PRN					
Phenylephrine • Neo-Synephrine • 1–2 sprays in each nostril every 4 hr					

ANTIHISTAMINES

Guidelines Summary

- Contact dermatitis
  - Identify the cause: Chemicals, acids, solvent, fragrances, metals, poison ivy, etc.
  - Clean the area with mild soap and water.
  - Refer patient to physician if the rash causes edema or invades the eyelids, external genitalia, anus, or massive areas of the body.
  - Treatment includes topical treatment with hydrocortisone, bicarbonate pastes, and antihistamines.
- Allergic rhinitis and common cold
  - A pharmacist may appropriately recommend an antihistamine once it is determined that the patient does not have any of the following:
    » Symptoms of otitis media or sinusitis
    » Symptoms of lower respiratory tract infection
    » History of nonallergic rhinitis
- Insomnia
  - Transient or short-term insomnia with no underlying problems are appropriate for self-treatment.
  - Discuss good sleep hygiene practices—no caffeine after 5 P.M., no exercise in the evening.
  - If diphenhydramine is recommended, it should be taken at bedtime only as needed.
  - Patients who complain of continuing insomnia after 14 days of treatment should be referred to a physician.

Antihistamines

Generic • Brand • Dose/Dosage Forms	Contraindications	Primary Side Effects	Key Monitoring Parameters	Pertinent Drug Interactions	Med Pearls
First-Generation Histamine H₁ Antagonists					
Mechanism of action – competes with histamine for H_1 receptor sites on effector cells in the GI tract, blood vessels, and respiratory tract					
Clemastine • Tavist Allergy • 1.34 mg BID-TID (max = 8.04 mg/day) • Tabs	• Hypersensitivity • Concurrent use with MAOIs • Lactation • Asthma	• Sedation • Dry mouth • Constipation • Blurred vision • Urinary retention	Mental alertness	• Concurrent use with MAOIs may ↑ risk of anticholinergic effects • Additive effects with other anticholinergic medications	• Paradoxic reactions (including stimulatory effects) may be seen • Have more anticholinergic effects than second-generation H₁ antagonists • Diphenhydramine also available as injection • NOT for OTC use in children <2 yr
Chlorpheniramine • Chlor-Trimeton • IR: 4 mg every 4–6 hr PRN (max = 24 mg/day) • ER: 12 mg every 12 hr (max = 24 mg/day) • ER tabs, solution, tabs	• Hypersensitivity • Narrow angle glaucoma • BPH • Asthma			• CYP2D6 substrate • CYP2D6 inhibitors may ↑ effects/toxicity • Additive effects with other anticholinergic medications	
Brompheniramine • J-Tan PD • 1–2 mg every 4–6 hr PRN (max = 6 mg/day [2–5 yr]; 12 mg/day [6–11 yr]) • Solution, tabs	None			Additive effects with other anticholinergic medications	
Diphenhydramine • Benadryl, Sominex, Unisom, ZzzQuil • Allergy: 25–50 mg every 4–8 hr PRN (max = 300 mg/day) • Insomnia: 50 mg at bedtime PRN • Caps, chewable tabs, solution, strips, suspension, tabs	• Hypersensitivity • Lactation			Additive effects with other anticholinergic medications	
Doxylamine • Sleep Aid • 25 mg at bedtime PRN • Solution, tabs					

Antihistamines *(cont'd)*

Generic • Brand • Dose/Dosage Forms	Contraindications	Primary Side Effects	Key Monitoring Parameters	Pertinent Drug Interactions	Med Pearls
Second-Generation Histamine H$_1$ Antagonists					
Mechanism of action – long-acting tricyclic antihistamines with selective peripheral H$_1$-receptor antagonistic properties; less blood-brain barrier penetration					
Loratadine • Alavert, Claritin • 10 mg daily • Caps, chewable tabs, ODTs, solution, tabs	Hypersensitivity	• Some sedation • Headache • Dizziness • Xerostomia	Relief of symptoms	Additive effects with other anticholinergic medications	• Available in combination with pseudoephedrine • Desloratadine (Clarinex) only available Rx • NOT for OTC use in children <2 yr
Cetirizine • Zyrtec • 5–10 mg daily • Caps, chewable tabs, ODTs, solution, tabs					• Available in combination with pseudoephedrine • Most sedating of the second-generation antihistamines • NOT for OTC use in children <2 yr
Fexofenadine • Allegra, Mucinex Allergy • 60 mg BID or 180 mg daily • ODTs, suspension, tabs		Headache			• Avoid taking with fruit juices • Available in combination with pseudoephedrine • Least sedating of the second-generation antihistamines • NOT for OTC use in children <2 yr

COUGH SUPPRESSANTS AND EXPECTORANTS

Guidelines Summary

- The primary goal of treating a cough is to reduce the number and severity of cough episodes.
- Cough suppressants (antitussives) should only be used to treat nonproductive coughs; should not be used for productive coughs.
- Codeine and dextromethorphan are the cough suppressants of choice for nonproductive cough.

- Antihistamines also have antitussive properties.
  - Diphenhydramine is a better choice for a cough associated with allergies but is highly sedating.
  - A second-generation antihistamine can also be considered since they are associated with less sedation.
- Expectorants include guaifenesin and water. Expectorants can be used to thin out the mucus or phlegm associated with a productive cough; they do NOT act as a cough suppressant.
- Patients should be excluded from self-treatment if they have any of the following:

Cough with thick yellow sputum or green phlegm	Unintended weight loss
Drenching nighttime sweats	History of asthma, COPD, or heart failure
Foreign-object aspiration	Cough duration >7 days
Fever (temperature >101.5°F)	Children <2 yr of age
Hemoptysis	Cough worsens during self-treatment

Cough Suppressants

Generic • Brand • Dose/Dosage Forms	Contraindications	Primary Side Effects	Key Monitoring Parameters	Pertinent Drug Interactions	Med Pearls
Mechanism of action – depresses the medullary cough center					
Dextromethorphan • Robitussin, Delsym • IR: 10–20 mg every 4 hr or 30 mg every 6–8 hr • ER: 60 mg BID • Max = 120 mg/day • Caps, ER suspension, gel, lozenges, solution, strips	Use of MAOI within 2 wk	• Confusion • Irritability	Relief of symptoms	• CYP2D6 substrate • CYP2D6 inhibitors may ↑ effects/toxicity • ↑ risk of serotonin syndrome with MAOIs, SSRIs, SNRIs, triptans, TCAs, fentanyl, lithium, meperidine, buspirone, linezolid, methylene blue, St. John's wort, and tramadol	• Not for OTC use in children <2 yr • Chemically related to morphine; lacks narcotic properties except in overdose • May require Rx for use in children and adolescents in some states
Codeine • 7.5–15 mg every 4–6 hr (max = 120 mg/day)	• Hypersensitivity • Respiratory depression • Paralytic ileus • Severe or acute asthma • Gastrointestinal obstruction	• N/V • Constipation • Sedation	• CNS depression • Relief of symptoms	• CYP2D6 substrate • CYP2D6 inhibitors may ↑ effects/toxicity • Other CNS depressants, including alcohol, may ↑ CNS depressant effects	10% of a codeine dose is demethylated in the liver to form morphine

Expectorant

Generic • Brand • Dose/Dosage Forms	Contraindications	Primary Side Effects	Key Monitoring Parameters	Pertinent Drug Interactions	Med Pearls
Mechanism of action – expectorant; irritates the gastric mucosa and stimulates respiratory tract secretions, thereby ↑ fluid volumes and ↓ mucous viscosity					
Guaifenesin • Mucinex • IR: 200–400 mg every 4 hr PRN • ER: 600–1,200 mg BID PRN • Max = 2,400 mg/day • ER tabs, oral packets, solution, tabs	Hypersensitivity	• Dizziness • Kidney stone formation	Relief of symptoms	None	More effective with water intake

ANTIDIARRHEALS

Guidelines Summary

- Acute diarrhea can be managed with fluids, electrolyte replacement, dietary interventions, and nonprescription drug treatment.
- Persistent and chronic diarrhea requires medical care, and patients are not candidates for self-treatment if either forms of diarrhea is present.
- Patients should be excluded from self-treatment if any of the following apply:
  - <6 months of age
  - Severe dehydration
  - >6 months of age with persistent high fevers greater than 102.2°F
  - Blood, mucus, or pus in the stool
  - Protracted vomiting or severe abdominal pain
  - Pregnancy
  - Chronic or persistent diarrhea

Antidiarrheals

Generic • Brand • Dose/Dosage Forms	Contraindications	Primary Side Effects	Key Monitoring Parameters	Pertinent Drug Interactions	Med Pearls
Mechanism of action – acts directly on opioid receptors on intestinal muscles to inhibit peristalsis and prolong transit time					
Loperamide • Imodium A–D • 4 mg, followed by 2 mg after each loose stool, (max = 16 mg/day) • Caps, chewable tabs, solution, suspension, tabs	• Hypersensitivity • Abdominal pain without diarrhea • Children <2 yr • Primary tx for acute dysentery, acute ulcerative colitis, bacterial enterocolitis, and pseudomembra-nous colitis (*C. difficile*)	• Constipation • Abdominal cramping • Abdominal distention	• Bowel movement frequency • CNS depression • Paralytic ileus • S/S of dehydration	None	None
Mechanism of action – possesses both antisecretory and antimicrobial effects; may also provides some anti-inflammatory effects					
Bismuth subsalicylate • Pepto-Bismol • 524 mg every 30–60 min PRN for up to 2 days (max = 4,200 mg/day) • Chewable tabs, suspension	• Children or adolescents with influenza or chickenpox (due to risk of Reye's syndrome) • Hx of GI bleed • Pregnancy • Hypersensitivity to salicylates	• Discoloration of tongue and feces (grayish-black) • Hearing loss • Tinnitus	Bowel movement frequency	May ↓ absorption of tetracyclines and fluoroquino-lones (separate by 2 hr)	None
Mechanism of action – helps reestablish normal intestinal flora; suppresses the growth of potentially pathogenic microorganisms by producing lactic acid, which favors the establishment of an aciduric flora					
Lactobacillus • Culturelle, Lactinex • Culturelle: 1 caplet daily or BID • Lactinex: 4 tabs 3–4 × /day • Caps. chewable tabs, granules, powder, tabs, wafers	Hypersensitivity to milk protein	• Flatulence • Bloating	Bowel movement frequency	None	Lactinex must be stored in refrigerator
Lactase enzyme • Lactaid • 1–2 capsules taken with milk or meal	None	None	Bowel movement frequency	None	• Used in the treatment of lactose intolerance • Prevents osmotic diarrhea

LAXATIVES

Guidelines Summary

- Lifestyle modifications
  - Educate patient about high fiber and increased hydration in diet.
  - Encourage patients to avoid postponing defecation.
  - Monitor bowel habits with a daily diary.
  - Encourage patients to maintain moderate exercise.
- Patients should be excluded from self-treatment if they have any of the following:
  - Marked abdominal pain or significant distention or cramping
  - Marked or unexplained flatulence
  - Fever
  - N/V
  - Paraplegia or quadriplegia
  - Daily laxative use
  - Unexplained changes in bowel habits and/or weight loss
  - Bowel symptoms that persist for 2 weeks
  - History of irritable bowel disease
- Pharmacologic therapy begins with bulk-forming agents and proceeds to osmotic laxatives.
- If these options are not helpful, stimulant laxatives should be considered.
- Enemas, suppositories, and lubricants are also available as options.

Medications for Constipation

Generic • Brand • Dose/Dosage Forms	Contraindications	Primary Side Effects	Key Monitoring Parameters	Pertinent Drug Interactions	Med Pearls
Mechanism of action – bulk-forming laxatives that work by absorbing water in the intestine to form a viscous liquid that promotes peristalsis					
Psyllium • Metamucil, Konsyl • 2.5–30 g/day in divided doses • Caps, packets, powder	• Fecal impaction • GI obstruction	• Abdominal cramps • Diarrhea	Bowel movement frequency	May ↓ absorption of other medications (space apart by 2 hr)	Take with full glass of water
Calcium polycarbophil • FiberCon • 2 tabs 1–4 × /day • Tabs					
Methylcellulose • Citrucel • 2 caps up to 6 × /day • 1 tbsp up to 3 × /day • Powder, tabs					

Medications for Constipation   (cont'd)

Generic • Brand • Dose/Dosage Forms	Contraindications	Primary Side Effects	Key Monitoring Parameters	Pertinent Drug Interactions	Med Pearls
Mechanism of action – osmotic laxative that causes water retention in the stool					
Polyethylene glycol 3350 • GlycoLax, MiraLax • 17 g daily • Packets, powder	• GI obstruction • Hypersensitivity	• Abdominal cramps • Diarrhea • Bloating	Bowel movement frequency	None	Can reconstitute with 8 oz of water, juice, cola, or tea
Mechanism of action – stimulant laxatives that stimulates peristalsis by directly irritating the smooth muscle of the intestine					
Senna • Ex-Lax Maximum Strength, Senokot • 17.2 mg daily up to 34.4 mg BID • Chewable tabs, solution, tabs	• Fecal impaction • GI obstruction	• Abdominal cramps • Diarrhea	Bowel movement frequency	None	None
Bisacodyl • Dulcolax, Fleet Laxative • 5–15 mg PO daily • Rectal: 10 mg daily • Enema, suppository, tabs				Effect may be ↓ by milk, dairy products, or antacids (separate by 1 hr)	
Mechanism of action – stool softeners that ↓ surface tension of the oil-water interface of the stool, resulting in enhanced incorporation of water and fat which facilitates stool softening					
Docusate sodium • Colace • 100 mg PO BID • Rectal: 1 enema 1–3 × /day • Caps, enema, solution, tabs Docusate calcium • Kao-Tin • 240 mg daily	• Fecal impaction • GI obstruction	• Diarrhea • Cramping	Bowel movement frequency	None	Take with full glass of water
Mechanism of action – osmotic laxative that promotes bowel evacuation by causing osmotic retention of fluid which distends the colon with ↑ peristaltic activity					
Magnesium hydroxide • Phillips Milk of Magnesia • 1–2 tbsp daily or BID • Chewable tabs, suspension	Hypersensitivity	Diarrhea	Bowel movement frequency	May ↓ absorption of tetra-cyclines and fluoroquinolones (separate by 2 hr)	• Take with full glass of water • Use with caution in patients with renal impairment
Mechanism of action – lubricant laxative that eases passage of stool by ↓ water absorption and lubricating the intestines					
Mineral oil • Fleet Oil • 1–2 tbsp at bedtime • 1 enema × 1 • Enema, oil	• Children <6 yr • Pregnancy • Elderly • Difficulty swallowing	• Abdominal cramps • Diarrhea • Aspiration pneumonia	Bowel movement frequency	May ↓ absorption of fat-soluble vitamins (A, D, K, E)	Aspiration is possible, especially in elderly population

ANTIFUNGALS

Guidelines Summary

- Patients should be excluded from self-treatment if they have any of the following:
  - Causative factor unclear
  - Nails or scalp involved
  - Face, mucous membranes, or genitalia involved
  - Signs and symptoms of possible secondary bacterial infection
  - Excessive and continuous exudation, fever, malaise
- Apply a thin layer of medication to affected area for 2–4 weeks (product dependent), even after the signs and symptoms disappear.

Topical Antifungal Medications to Treat Tinea

Generic • Brand • Dose/Dosage Forms	Contraindications	Primary Side Effects	Key Monitoring Parameters	Pertinent Drug Interactions	Med Pearls
Mechanism of action – squalene epoxidase inhibitor results in deficiency of ergosterol within the fungal cell					
Butenafine • Lotrimin Ultra, Mentax • Apply daily × 2 wk (corporis/cruris) or 4 wk (pedis) • Cream	Hypersensitivity	• Burning • Contact dermatitis • Erythema • Irritation • Stinging	Clinical signs of improvement	None	Used to treat tinea pedis, tinea cruris, and tinea corporis
Terbinafine • Lamisil, Lamisil AT • Apply 1–2 × /day × ≥1 wk • Cream, gel					
Mechanism of action – binds to phospholipids in the fungal cell membrane, altering cell wall permeability and resulting in loss of intracellular elements					
Clotrimazole • Lotrimin AF • Apply BID	Hypersensitivity	• Burning • Contact dermatitis • Erythema • Itching	Clinical signs of improvement	None	Used to treat tinea pedis, tinea cruris, and tinea corporis
Miconazole • Desenex, Micatin • Apply BID × 2 wk (cruris) or 4 wk (corporis/pedis) • Cream, lotion, ointment, powder, powder spray, solution, spray					

Topical Antifungal Medications to Treat Tinea   *(cont'd)*

Generic • Brand • Dose/Dosage Forms	Contraindications	Primary Side Effects	Key Monitoring Parameters	Pertinent Drug Interactions	Med Pearls
Mechanism of action – distorts the hyphae and stunts mycelial growth in susceptible fungi					
Tolnaftate • Tinactin • Apply BID × 2 wk (cruris) or 4 wk (corporis/pedis) • Cream, powder, powder spray, solution, spray	Hypersensitivity	• Burning • Contact dermatitis • Erythema • Itching	Clinical signs of improvement	None	Used to treat tinea pedis, tinea cruris, and tinea corporis
Mechanism of action – inhibits conversion of yeast to the hyphal form (active form) and interferes with fatty-acid biosynthesis					
Undecylenic acid • Fungi-Nail • Apply BID × 4 wk • Solution	Hypersensitivity	High alcohol concentrations may cause burning	Clinical signs of improvement	None	Used to treat tinea pedis and toe fungus

PEDICULOCIDES

Guidelines Summary

- All members of a household that contain a person with a lice infestation should be screened for lice and treated if they are infected.

- Treatment includes ovicidal agents. Retreatment is only needed for ovicidal agents if lice continue to be seen. Weakly ovicidal agents will require retreatment to make sure all nits have hatched and will be exposed to medication.

- Nonpharmacologic treatment includes washing all items such at hats, towels, and bedding that came into contact with the infected person within 48 hr of treatment in hot water and dried with hot air. If something cannot be washed in a washing machine, other options include dry cleaning or placing the items within a plastic bag for a two-week period.

- Patients should be excluded from self-treatment if they have any of the following:
  - Children <2 yr
  - Hypersensitivity to chrysanthemums
  - Secondary skin infection in lice-infested areas
  - Pregnancy
  - Lactation

Medications to Treat Pediculosis

Generic • Brand • Dose/Dosage Forms	Contraindications	Primary Side Effects	Key Monitoring Parameters	Med Pearls
Mechanism of action – inhibits respiration of lice by respiratory spiracle obstruction				
Benzyl alcohol • Ulesfia • 4–48 ounces based on length of hair • Lotion	None	• Pruritus • Erythema • Local irritation • Eye irritation	Eradication of lice and nits	• Rx only • Apply to *dry* hair, saturate scalp, leave on for 10 min, rinse, then repeat in 7 days
Mechanism of action – inhibits sodium influx into nerve cell membranes, causing repolarization and paralysis of the lice				
Permethrin • Elimite, Nix • Cream, lotion	Hypersensitivity	• Pruritus • Erythema • Scalp rash • Burning • Stinging • Scalp discomfort	Eradication of lice and nits	• Elimite is Rx only • Wash hair with conditioner-free shampooo, towel dry, apply sufficient amount of lotion or cream to saturate scalp and hair, leave on for no longer than 10 minutes, rinse with warm water, comb hair with nit comb; may repeat in 7 days, if needed • Do not use near eyes or inside the nose, ear, mouth, or vagina • Elimite can also be used for scabies
Mechanism of action – neurotoxicity caused by stimulation of nerve cells to produce repeated discharges and subsequent paralysis				
Pyrethrins and piperonyl butoxide • A–200, Licide, Pronto Plus, RID • Gel, oil, shampoo, solution	None	• Pruritus • Burning • Stinging • Skin irritation	Eradication of lice and nits	• Apply to *dry* hair, leave on for 10 minutes, wash and rinse, comb hair with nit comb, then repeat in 7–10 days • Do not use near eyes, in eyebrows or eyelashes, or inside nose, mouth, vagina • Solution should only be applied to bedding (not for human use)
Mechanism of action – ↑ permeabilty of cell membranes to chloride, resulting in hyperpolarization and death of lice				
Ivermectin • Sklice • Lotion	None	• Burning • Skin irritation	Eradication of lice and nits	• Rx only • Apply to *dry* scalp and hair, leave on for 10 minutes, rinse with warm water, comb hair with nit comb; do not repeat • Also available as cream (Soolantra) for rosacea
Mechanism of action – inhibits cholinesterase in lice, causing death				
Malathion • Ovide • Lotion	• Hypersensitivity • Neonates or infants	• Chemical burns • Local irritation • Stinging • Conjunctivitis	Eradication of lice and nits	• Rx only • Apply to *dry* hair and scalp, dry hair naturally (do not cover), shampoo off after 8–12 hr, comb hair with nit comb; may repeat in 7–9 days if needed

Medications to Treat Pediculosis *(cont'd)*

Generic • Brand • Dose/Dosage Forms	Contraindications	Primary Side Effects	Key Monitoring Parameters	Med Pearls
Mechanism of action – CNS excitation and involuntary muscle contractions produce paralysis and death of lice				
Spinosad • Natroba • Suspension	None	• Erythema • Local irritation • Dry skin	Eradication of lice and nits	• Rx only • Apply to *dry* scalp and hair, leave on for 10 minutes, rinse with warm water, may then shampoo, comb hair with nit comb; may repeat in 7 days if needed
Mechanism of action – stimulates the nervous system of lice, causing seizures and death				
Lindane • Only available generically • Shampoo	• Hypersensitivity • Premature infants • Uncontrolled seizure disorders • Crusted skin conditions	• Ataxia • Dizziness • Burning • Neurotoxicity • Seizures • Dermatitis	• Eradication of lice and nits • Mental status • Seizures	• Rx only • Apply to *dry* hair and massage in for 4 min, add in water to form a lather, rinse hair thoroughly, comb hair with nit comb; do not repeat • Can also be used for pubic lice or scabies

ATOPIC DERMATITIS MEDICATIONS

Guidelines Summary

- Treatment of atopic dermatitis includes skin hydration, removal of known irritants, and topical steroid creams.
- Patients should be excluded from self-treatment any of the following apply:
  - Age <2 years
  - Severe dermatitis or pruritus
  - Large body area involvement
  - Skin infection

Medications for Atopic Dermatitis

Generic • Brand • Dose/Dosage Forms	Contraindications	Primary Side Effects	Key Monitoring Parameters	Med Pearls
Mechanism of action – ↓ inflammatory mediators through the induction of phospholipase A2 inhibitory proteins and release of arachidonic acid				
Hydrocortisone • Cortaid • Applied up to 3–4 × /day • Cream	• Hypersensitivity • Diaper dermatitis	• Acneiform eruptions • Skin irritation • Dry skin • Hypopigmentation	Response to therapy	Avoid use on weeping lesions

POISON IVY MEDICATIONS

Guidelines Summary

- Remove clothing worn during exposure to urushiol. Wash exposed clothing separately to avoid contaminating other items.
- Wash skin with soap and water to remove urushiol.
- Treatment focuses on the relief of itching and may include the use of topical calamine or hydrocortisone.
- Avoid topical anesthetics, antihistamines, and antibiotics for mild symptoms to prevent sensitization of the skin and a drug-induced dermatitis.
- Nonpharmacologic treatment can include the use of colloidal oatmeal baths, tepid showers, and baking soda compressed.
- Patients should be excluded from self-treatment if they have any of the following:
  - Involvement of rash on the face, eyes, or genitalia
  - Difficulty breathing
  - Exposure to smoke from a burning poison ivy, poison oak, or poison sumac plant
  - Age <2 years
  - Widespread rash involving >25% of body surface area
  - Presence of infection
  - Presence of rash >2 weeks
  - Presence of numerous bullae

Medications for Poison Ivy

Generic • Dose/Dosage Forms	Contraindications	Primary Side Effects	Key Monitoring Parameters	Med Pearls
Mechanism of action – possesses astringent properties to dry weeping lesions; works as a skin protectant				
Calamine • Apply as often as necessary • Lotion	Hypersensitivity	Local irritation	Response to therapy	Do not use on open lesions

SUNSCREENS

Sunscreen

- The American Academy of Dermatology recommends that everyone wear sunscreen any day they will be outside and exposed to sunlight.
- Application of sunscreen should include agents that are:
  - Broad spectrum to cover exposure to both ultraviolet (UV) A and UVB rays
  - Water-resistant
  - Sun Protection Factor (SPF) of 30 or higher, which will block 97% of UVB rays
- Sunscreen terms
  - SPF is measure of a suncreen's ability to block UVB rays. SPF is a factor that can estimate how much time one can spend in the sun without getting burned. If a burn would normally start in 10 minutes, using a product with an SPF of 30 will allow an exposure of approximately 300 minutes without a burn (30 times longer).
  - Water-resistant sunscreen is effective for up to 40 minutes in water.
  - Very water-resistant sunscreen is effective for up to 80 minutes in water.
- Guidelines for the application of sunscreen
  - Sunscreen should not be applied to infants ≤6 mo.
  - Use enough sunscreen to coat the skin; may need ≥1 ounce to cover the body.
  - To protect lips, use a lip balm with at least an SPF of 30.
  - Apply 15 minutes before exposure to sun.
  - Reapply every 2 hours or after swimming.
  - Creams are best for application on dry skin and the face.
  - Sprays may be used, but ensure all areas have been covered.
  - Gels may be used for areas covered in hair.
  - Stick formulations are good for administration around the eyes.

Part Three

Pharmaceutical Sciences, Calculations, Biostatistics, and Clinical Trial Design

Pharmaceutics

23

This chapter covers the following:

- **Physical pharmacy**
- **Pharmaceutical dosage forms**

Pharmaceutics encompasses a number of disciplines, including dosage form design, biopharmaceutics, and pharmacokinetics. This chapter focuses on dosage form design (drug dosage forms and the physical and chemical properties that allow these products to be manufactured).

PHYSICAL PHARMACY

Physical pharmacy is a branch of pharmaceutics that deals principally with the physical and chemical properties of drugs. It is a highly mathematical subject, but the NAPLEX is not concerned with these aspects except as they relate to chemical kinetics.

Preformulation

Preformulation is an important stage of drug development where the pharmaceutical company characterizes the following physicochemical properties of the drug.

Solubility and Lipophilicity

Every drug must be solubilized before it can be absorbed by the body. A drug must possess at least some aqueous solubility in order to be effective; poorly soluble compounds show incomplete and unpredictable absorption. However, at least some lipophilicity must also be present, as drugs must be able to pass through biological membranes in order to reach their sites of action, which are often intracellular.

Dissolution rate is improved by ↓ particle size, which ↑ the surface area of the drug that comes into contact with the body fluids.

Ionization Behavior

Most drugs are administered as salts and therefore carry a positive or negative charge in solution. That is, when such a drug goes into solution, a fraction of the molecules dissociate into ions (i.e., charged compounds). The proportion of ionized to unionized drug is very important because the two behave differently in the body:

- Ionized drug: More soluble, but cannot cross body membranes
- Unionized drug: Less soluble, but can cross body membranes

Remember: Until the drug is absorbed across the body membranes, it cannot get to the site of action, but it needs to go into solution before that can happen. The equilibrium between the more soluble ionized form and the more absorbable unionized form of the drug is crucial.

The Henderson-Hasselbalch equation (see formula that follows) can be used to calculate exact ratios of ionized to unionized drug; however, the "Ionization Behavior of Weak Acids and Bases" table below will give you a rough estimate of the ionization behavior of weak acids and bases when comparing the pH of the absorption site to the pK_a. In most cases, you will be able to obtain a sufficiently accurate answer by using the table instead of the actual equation, saving valuable exam time.

$$pH = pK_a + \log \frac{[\text{Salt}]}{[\text{Acid}]} \text{ or } pH = pK_a + \log \frac{[\text{ionized}]}{[\text{unionized}]} \text{ if the drug is an acid}$$

$$pH = pK_a + \log \frac{[\text{Base}]}{[\text{Salt}]} \text{ or } pH = pK_a + \log \frac{[\text{unionized}]}{[\text{ionized}]} \text{ if the drug is a base}$$

Ionization Behavior of Weak Acids and Bases

	Acidic Drug	Basic Drug
$pH > pK_a$	More ionized	More unionized
$pH = pK_a$	Equal	Equal
$pH < pK_a$	More unionized	More ionized
Note that for pH more than 2 units away from pK_a, expect almost complete ionization/unionization.		

The acid or base form is the unionized form and the salt form is the ionized form of the corresponding acid or base. Accordingly, ionized and unionized can be substituted in the above equations in order to calculate the amount of ionization or unionization at a particular pH value. To identify which equation to use, you must first know if the drug in question is an acid or a base.

It is impossible to tell if a drug is an acid or a base by looking only at the pK_a. Some acids have a higher pK_a (phenytoin = 8.3) than do some bases (morphine = 8.0). You can tell if a drug is an acid or base, however, by what type of salt is used in its formulation. Weak acids form sodium, calcium, potassium, or other cationic salts; weak bases form hydrochloride or other anionic salts.

For example, warfarin is formulated as the sodium salt. Therefore, warfarin is an acid. The positively charged sodium ion is used to displace the proton (i.e., hydronium ion or positively charged hydrogen) from the proton-donating acid in its formulation. In solution, warfarin disassociates from sodium into a negatively charged molecule (i.e., ionized form). If the solution is acidic (e.g., gastric fluid), a proton is likely to be donated back to the negatively charged warfarin to produce the uncharged drug (unionized form). Of course, this is a dynamic state in which the drug is going back and forth between the ionized and unionized form based on the pH of the environment. Determining this ratio provides information about the drug's solubility and its ability to cross biological membranes in any given environment. This is the power of the Henderson-Hasselbalch equation and of the table presented.

Stability

Physical, chemical, and microbiological stability are all very important in preformulation studies. While physical instability does not generally result in ↓ drug concentrations, it can lead to problems with dose uniformity and pharmaceutical elegance (e.g., the mottled appearance that can develop in tablets over time or the formation of a nonsuspendable sediment in a liquid dosage form).

Most drugs degrade by either zero- or first-order kinetics (see "Rate and Half-Life Equations" table). Drugs following zero-order degradation have a constant degradation rate that is independent of the drug concentration. First-order degradation, however, is concentration-dependent; therefore, the amount of drug degrading per unit of time is not constant.

Rate and Half-Life Equations

Order	Rate Equation		Half-Life Equation
Zero	$C = C_0 - k_0 t$		$t_{1/2} = 0.5 \dfrac{C_0}{k_0}$
First	$\log C = \log C_0 - \dfrac{k_0 t}{2.303}$	$C = C_0 e^{-kt}$	$t_{1/2} = \dfrac{\ln 2}{k_1} = \dfrac{0.693}{k_1}$

Where C is equal to concentration, C_0 is the initial concentration, K_0 is the zero-order degradation constant, t is time, $t_{1/2}$ is half-life, and K_1 is the first-order degradation constant.

With equations, it is possible to calculate the concentration (or amount) of drug at any given time if its degradation rate constant is known. It is not, however, useful to memorize the first-order equation for the NAPLEX because the calculator provided does not include the exponential function (e). Therefore, the only way to calculate the concentration (or amount) of drug at any given time is to estimate the amount by understanding what the degradation constants represent.

The first thing to do is identify if the question is related to a zero-order or first-order process. If a graphical representation is presented for any problem, a zero-order process will be linear with a constant degradation over time. Therefore, the units for zero-order degradation constants are in terms of amount per unit time (e.g., mg/hr). First-order degradation will be a nonlinear decline that is asymptotic to the x-axis on a graph similar to a drug concentration-time curve seen in pharmacokinetics. The units of the first-order degradation constant are in terms of $time^{-1}$ (e.g., yr^{-1}).

After identifying whether the degradation process is zero-order or first-order, the second step is to estimate how much drug is remaining (or degraded) over some amount of time. This is simple for zero-order processes because a constant amount is being lost over time. For example, if the starting amount of drug is 1,000 mg and 10 mg per year is degraded (i.e., $K_0 = 10$ mg/yr), after 10 years it will have lost 100 mg of drug and have 900 mg remaining. Many zero-order degradation problems can be rationalized without memorizing the equations in the table.

The estimation of amount of drug remaining following first-order degradation is not as straightforward and requires an in-depth understanding of the first-order degradation constant. The degradation constant is in terms of $time^{-1}$, as mentioned. This represents a percentage of drug lost per unit of time that is being presented. For example, a K_1 of 0.2 yr^{-1} indicates that 20% of the drug is lost every year. Thus, if the starting amount of drug is 1,000 mg of drug, 20% will be lost of that in the first year, or 200 mg, leaving 800 mg. The key in these estimations is to remember that in year 2, the starting amount is 800 mg because 200 mg was lost in year 1. To calculate the amount of drug lost after 2 years, subtract 20% of 800 mg (i.e., 160 mg) from 800 mg. Therefore, the amount of drug remaining after 2 years will be 800 mg minus 160 mg, for a total of 640 mg. This process must be repeated for year 3 and so on.

Solid-State Properties

Crystallization

Solids are present in crystalline or amorphous forms, or as a combination of the two. Crystalline forms show fixed geometric patterns, whereas the atoms in amorphous solids are randomly placed (as they would be in a liquid).

- Crystalline solids have definite melting points, whereas amorphous solids melt over a range of temperatures.
- Amorphous solids are more soluble than the corresponding crystalline forms.
- Solids tend to revert to the more stable crystalline form on storage.

Polymorphism

Polymorphs are one of several crystalline structures that have the same chemical formula but show different physical properties. The properties they exhibit can vary substantially, however, and this leads to pharmaceutical companies patenting different polymorphic forms based on variations in solubility, bioavailability, solid-state stability, or processing behavior (such as improved powder flow or tablet compaction).

A pharmacy-related example of polymorphism is ritonavir, a protease inhibitor used to treat human immunodeficiency virus. Initially, it was thought to exist in only one polymorphic form, with relatively poor aqueous solubility. It was marketed in a soft gelatin capsule, which contained an ethanol/water cosolvent system. After drug approval, several batches failed quality control tests. It was discovered that a second polymorphic form with even lower solubility had formed, causing the drug to precipitate out of the cosolvent system. The product had to be reformulated to include Kolliphor (polyethoxylated castor oil) as a solubilizing agent.

Rheology

Rheology is the science of flow properties, which is especially important when discussing liquid and semisolid dosage forms.

Viscosity and fluidity are two common terms associated with rheology. Viscosity refers to the resistance offered when part of the liquid flows past another part; fluidity is essentially the opposite. Viscous liquids are thick and slow-moving; fluid liquids are thin and flow more readily.

Testing

Numerous quality assurance tests exist for dosage forms. The four tests used for tablets and sometimes capsules are as follows: friability, hardness, disintegration, and dissolution testing.

Friability and hardness testing evaluate the ability of tablets to withstand manufacturing, packaging, and shipping. Hardness testing measures the force required to cause a tablet to break, and friability testing measures what percentage weight of a tablet is lost after it is tumbled for a specified amount of time in a friabilator.

Disintegration testing is performed by placing tablets into mesh-bottomed cylinders that are immersed in a solution and agitated at a specified rate.

PHARMACEUTICAL DOSAGE FORMS

Oral Delivery: Solids

Traditional/Immediate Release

The different types of immediate-release tablets are described in the following table.

Types of Immediate-Release Tablets

Type of Tablet	Key Features	Example
Compressed	All ingredients contained in a single layer; designed to be swallowed whole; may or may not be coated	Various
Multi-compressed	Contain separate layers of drug, for various reasons (incompatibility of drugs, immediate- plus extended-release in the same tablet, etc.)	Mucinex (guaifenesin)
Chewable	Disintegrate rapidly when chewed; usually mannitol-based (pleasant mouth feel, sweet taste)	Children's vitamins Dilantin Infatabs (phenytoin)
Buccal	Dissolve in cheek cavity; may be designed to erode slowly or quickly	Fentora (fentanyl)
Sublingual	Dissolve under the tongue; erode quickly and are absorbed rapidly	Nitrostat (nitroglycerin)
Effervescent	Contain drug that dissolves rapidly after adding to water; results in carbonated liquid that masks taste	Alka-Seltzer

Many immediate-release tablets are coated. This process can help mask unpleasant tastes and odors, as well as improve the appearance of the tablet, protect the drug from the atmosphere, and allow it to be swallowed more easily. The two types of coating used for immediate-release products are sugar and film coatings.

Extended Release

The different types of extended-release tablets are described in the following table.

Types of Extended-Release Tablets

Type of Tablet	Key Features	Example
Enteric coating	Coating remains intact until drug reaches small intestine; can protect drug from stomach acid and enzymes, or can protect stomach from irritating drugs	Enteric-coated aspirin
Diffusion-controlled reservoir system	Beads or pellets are coated with polymer that releases drug at varying speeds; may involve several release rates	Drug-eluting stents
Diffusion-controlled matrix system	Drug is mixed into an inert plastic matrix; drug dissolves and leaves matrix	Glucotrol XL (glipizide)
Wax	Remains intact in GI tract and is eliminated in feces (inform patient that this is normal)	Desoxyn (methamphetamine)
Hydrophilic	Water causes matrix to swell; drug diffuses through gel layer, and may also be released as matrix erodes	Slo-Niacin (niacin)
Dissolution-controlled system	Rate of release affected by dissolution and tablet or bead erosion (some hydrophilic matrices fall into this category as well as diffusion-controlled)	Cardizem CD (diltiazem)
Ion-exchange resin	pH conditions of GI tract cause drug to be released from resin	Inderal (propanolol)
Osmotically controlled system	Tablet pulls water into system, then releases drug at controlled rate by osmotic pressure; tablet shell eliminated in feces (inform patient that this is normal)	Glucotrol XL (glipizide)
Complex formation	Drug is combined with other agents, forming a slowly soluble chemical complex	Rynatan allergy products

Rapid Release

The various types of rapid-release solid dosage forms are described in the following table.

Types of Rapid-Release Solid Dosage Forms

Type of Product	Key Features	Example
Tablets	Product can contain large doses of drug	Claritin RediTabs (loratidine)
Strips	Dissolves before children can spit it out; cannot put large doses of drug into product	Zuplenz (ondansetron)
Lollipops	Absorbed through buccal mucosa	Actiq (fentanyl)

Oral Delivery: Liquids

Oral liquid dosage forms have the same advantages as other oral products, with the additional advantage of being easy to swallow for small children and others who cannot easily swallow solid dosage forms. Several disadvantages exist as well. Liquids are less portable and convenient than solids. Incorrect doses are much more likely, as patients or caregivers could measure using an inappropriate measuring device (i.e., not all spoons are standard size), and product may be spilled before being consumed. Also, taste can be a large issue, as more of the drug will reach a patient's taste buds than with the same drug in a tablet or capsule.

Solvents

Water is the most common solvent for pharmaceutical products; purified water prepared by distillation, reverse osmosis, or ion-exchange treatment is acceptable for oral use. Other commonly used solvents include ethyl alcohol, glycerin, sorbitol, propylene glycol, and some edible oils. Typically, solvents other than water are included to improve solubility and, in some cases, add sweetness to the final product (e.g., glycerin, sorbitol, and propylene glycol). Only small amounts of sorbitol and glycerin should be present in a given dose of liquid, as they may act as osmotic laxatives in higher quantities.

Types of Liquids

Single-phase liquid dosage forms are all variants of the solution. One or more soluble substances are dissolved in one or more solvents, including water. Therefore, the drug(s) must be water-soluble and stable in aqueous solution. The presence of other excipients in varying amounts results in the following designations:

Types of Single-Phase Liquid Dosage Forms

Type of Product	Key Features	Examples
Syrups	• Contain sugar or sugar substitutes • Contain little or no alcohol • Thickeners improve mouth feel and physically conceal the drug from taste buds • Taste pleasant; often used with children	Various cough/cold preparations
Elixirs	• By definition alcoholic, but some nonalcoholic commercial products are mislabeled as elixirs • Slightly sweet; artificial sweetener usually used since sucrose is not very soluble in alcohol • Less viscous than syrups	• Diphenhydramine • Phenobarbital • Digoxin
Tinctures	• 15–80% alcohol • Usually consist of drug extracted from plant material • Unpleasant taste; not commonly used today	• Opium tincture (1,000 mg morphine/100 mL) • Paregoric (camphorated opium tincture; 40 mg morphine/100 mL)

Types of Single-Phase Liquid Dosage Forms   *(cont'd)*

Spirits	• Alcoholic solutions of aromatic or volatile substances • High concentration of alcohol • Active ingredient may precipitate out when added to aqueous preparations	Flavoring agents
Aromatic waters	• Aqueous solutions of volatile oils • Very dilute	Flavoring and perfuming agents
Fluid extracts	• Similar to, but more potent than, tinctures • Used as drug source, not as dosage form	Herbal medications

Suspensions are multiphase products that contain finely divided solid particles distributed through the liquid phase. Some advantages exist over single-phase liquids. Drugs that have an unpleasant flavor are preferred as suspensions, since the drug does not interact with the taste buds as much when it is not dissolved. Also, drugs that have poor stability in water do not degrade as readily in suspension as they do in solution.

The primary concern with making suspensions is to have a particle size that is small enough to remain suspended in the dispersion medium of choice while not being so small that the particles start to attract each other and form clumps that will not resuspend. This can be achieved by two techniques, used separately or in combination: (1) use of structured vehicles and (2) controlled flocculation.

- Structured vehicles: ↑ viscosity and slow the sedimentation of suspended particles. These natural and synthetic polymer solutions are often used (cellulose gels, acacia, bentonite).
- Controlled flocculation: Add materials that promote loose aggregation of suspended particles, but keep their surfaces apart by charge or interaction of polymer chains. These particles will settle, but loosely, and resuspend easily.

Emulsions are dispersions that consist of nonmiscible liquids. These products are thermodynamically unstable and require an emulsifying agent to keep them combined properly.

Only oil-in-water (O/W) emulsions are used for oral dosage forms, as water needs to be in the external phase to be palatable to the patient; otherwise, all the patient would taste would be the oil in the outer portion of the product. Topical products can be either O/W or water in oil (W/O). Three types of emulsifiers are used, depending on the product being made:

- Surfactants: Contain hydrophilic and hydrophobic portions, which remain at the interface of the oil, and water phases to stabilize the product. Often used in combination.
- Hydrophilic colloids: Water-soluble polymers that form a film around oil droplets in O/W emulsions. Tend to ↑ viscosity of the product.
- Finely divided solids: Form a film of particles around the droplets of the dispersed phase, but allow interaction with the dispersion medium as well.

Topical Delivery

Topical products are used for three primary reasons: (1) to protect injured areas of the skin from the environment; (2) to hydrate the skin; and (3) to apply medication to the skin for local effect.

Powders and liquids are used as topical delivery systems, though not as frequently as semisolid preparations. Of the types of liquids mentioned in the oral delivery section, solutions, suspensions, and emulsions may all be used topically. Two external-use–only liquid products are:

- Liniments: Alcoholic solutions used to irritate the skin and relieve more deep-seated pain or discomfort (Heet, Absorbine Jr), or oleaginous emulsions used as emollients or protective agents. Liniments are applied by rubbing and are not suitable for application to bruised or broken skin.

- Collodions: Contain pyroxylin in an alcohol/ether base that evaporates, leaving an occlusive film on the skin; used to hold edges of incised wounds together.

Ointment Bases

Five types of ointment bases exist:

- Hydrocarbon/oleaginous: Greasy, petroleum-based products used for emollient effect (Vaseline, petrolatum)

- Anhydrous absorption: Greasy products that form W/O emulsions when aqueous solutions are added; can be used to incorporate solutions into an otherwise lipophilic base (hydrophilic petrolatum, anhydrous lanolin)

- W/O emulsion: Similar to anhydrous absorption bases, but already contain some water (hydrous lanolin, cold cream)

- O/W emulsion (water-removable): Creamy emulsions that are easily washed from the skin; may be diluted with water to form lotions (hydrophilic ointment, Lubriderm)

- Water-soluble: Greaseless, water-washable bases containing no oleaginous compounds; cannot add large amounts of water or will soften too much (PEG ointment)

Other topical product definitions are:

- **Creams:** Terminology often used to describe emulsion bases; soft, cosmetically acceptable topical products
- **Pastes:** Very thick semisolids containing at least 20% solids by weight
- **Gels:** Jelly-like dispersions that are water-soluble, water-washable, and greaseless

Rectal, Vaginal, and Urethral Delivery

Rectal, vaginal, and urethral dosage forms such as suppositories and enemas are less frequently prescribed than many other types of dosage form, but they do have an important place in certain types of therapy. They can be useful for local therapy in rectal or vaginal conditions, or when protecting susceptible drugs from GI tract degradation or first-pass metabolism.

Pulmonary Delivery

Metered-Dose Inhalers

Metered-dose inhalers (MDIs) are primarily used to deliver medications, including bronchodilators and corticosteroids, for the treatment of asthma and chronic obstructive pulmonary disease. While MDIs are portable and able to deliver precise quantities of potent drugs, many patients have difficulty using them properly.

Dry-Powder Inhalers

Dry-powder inhalers (DPIs) avoid some of the difficulties with MDIs. They are generally easier for patients to use correctly, since the device can be primed before use and the patient does not have to coordinate their breaths with device actuation. Ease of use, however, depends significantly on the particular type of device.

The Diskus device is a classic example of the discrete-dose style of DPI. Individual doses are contained in foil packets, protecting them from humidity and allowing for dose consistency if the device is dropped. Some discrete-dose devices are single-dose units, and the drug is added when the device is ready to be actuated (Rotahaler, Aerosilizer, Handihaler); this is often a necessity if a drug is heat-sensitive and must be kept refrigerated until use, such as Spiriva (tiotropium bromide). The Twisthaler, on the other hand, is an example of a reservoir device. All of the doses are contained in a central compartment; and if the device is dropped or exposed to humidity, all doses are affected. Of currently marketed products, only the Twisthaler and Flexhaler are reservoir devices.

Nebulizers

Nebulizers allow the drug to be delivered directly to the lung in high concentration and without the use of propellant. Two types exist: (1) jet and (2) ultrasonic. Jet nebulizers can be used with either solutions or suspensions, and operate by the Bernoulli principle, whereby compressed air from the machine flows at high speed over the medicated liquid, atomizing it and carrying it to the patient. Ultrasonic nebulizers can only be used with solutions. Ultrasonic nebulizers use the vibrations of high-frequency sound waves to move liquid from the machine through the face mask. Vibrations are timed to coincide with inhalation; therefore, less medication is lost with the ultrasonic than with the jet nebulizers.

Nasal Delivery

Nasal delivery shares many of the advantages of pulmonary delivery. Drugs that are inactivated by the GI tract or that undergo first-pass metabolism are protected, and large-molecule drugs can be absorbed across the nasal mucosa. The nose has a dense vasculature, which aids in absorption. Viscosity enhancers and mucoadhesives are often included in the formulations to ↑ residence time, as nasal drainage can be a problem. In addition to the many drugs available via nasal delivery (e.g., desmopressin, calcitonin, butorphanol, corticosteroids), the route shows promise for vaccine delivery, with FluMist being the first approved example.

The most commonly used nasal products are saline solutions for dry nasal mucosa, nasal decongestants, and intranasal corticosteroids.

Parenteral Delivery

Injectable products have many advantages over other dosage forms but also have more potential complications. No drug is lost to first-pass metabolism or acid- or enzyme-mediated degradation in the GI tract, which makes injection a particularly useful route for protein drug delivery. Additionally, the products must be sterile (see following table for various sterilization methods used), free from undesired particulate matter, and pyrogen-free.

Sterilization Methods Used in Industry

Method	How Does It Work?	Advantages	Disadvantages	Products Sterilized by This Method
Steam sterilization	Heat coagulates and kills microorganisms	• Method of choice when applicable • Lower heat than dry heat sterilization	• Cannot use with heat- or moisture-sensitive drugs • Autoclave can have cools spots	• Aqueous solutions in closed containers • Surgical instruments • Glassware
Dry heat sterilization	Heat coagulates and kills microorganisms	Useful for moisture-sensitive material	• Cannot use with heat-sensitive drugs • Autoclave can have cool spots	• Glassware • Surgical equipment • Oleaginous materials • Powders • Moisture-sensitive material
Filtration	Bacteria and particulate matter are physically removed by membrane filters	Inexpensive	• Technique failure • Membrane defects • Drug can absorb to membrane	• Small volumes of thin liquid • Heat-sensitive liquid formulations
Ionizing radiation	Gamma radiation mutates and kills bacteria	Effective for most microorgranisms	Expensive setup	Sterilizing plastic medical devices
Gas sterilization	Ethylene and propylene oxide gases alkylate microbial protein	Good for heat- and moisture-sensitive materials	• Possibility of toxic residue • Explosion hazard • Expensive setup • Cannot penetrate glass to sterilize material in sealed containers	• Heat-sensitive material • Moisture-sensitive material • Medical and surgical equipment wrapped in plastic

Multiple-dose injectable products must contain a preservative in order to ensure that the product remains sterile after the initial use.

Ocular and Otic Delivery

Drug delivery to the eye is complicated by two factors: (1) drug loss due to blinking and lacrimal drainage and (2) poor drug penetration through the corneal membrane. Polymers are typically used as viscosity enhancers to prolong the retention time and ↓ lacrimal drainage; some polymers, such as hyaluronic acid, have mild adhesive properties that prolong the retention time even further.

Most ocular products are solutions; however, suspensions, ointments, and gels may also be used. These dosage forms prolong drug contact with the eye and may be preferable in some situations.

Ocular products must be sterile when dispensed, and all multidose products must contain preservative. This helps prevent serious ocular infections, which can lead to corneal ulcers and blindness.

Otic products are generally solutions or suspensions, which frequently contain glycerin or propylene glycol to ↑ the viscosity and maximize contact between the product and the ear canal. The hygroscopic nature of these solvents also helps them draw moisture out of the tissues, which can ↓ inflammation and the amount of moisture available for any microorganisms to grow. Most otic products fall into one of the following categories:

- Anti-infective and anti-inflammatory products: May contain analgesics and local anesthetics to ↓ pain associated with otitis externa or otitis media
- Ear-wax removal agents: Contain surfactants (which emulsify ear wax) or peroxides (which release oxygen and disrupt the integrity of the ear wax), which facilitate removal of the ear wax

Transdermal Delivery

Transdermal delivery differs from topical delivery in that the drug is intended for systemic use. The drug molecules must therefore be small enough to penetrate the stratum corneum and reach the general circulation. Some transdermal ointments (nitroglycerin ointment) exist, but most products are available as transdermal delivery systems (patches).

Patches

Transdermal patches attach to the skin with adhesive and contain the drug either in a polymer matrix or in a drug reservoir covered by a rate-controlling membrane. An excess amount of drug is typically present to ensure that a concentration gradient exists, causing the drug to exit the patch and enter the skin passively. Patches provide more uniform blood concentrations than conventional release products and can improve patient compliance since, depending on the drug, they can be worn for 1 to 7 days. GI absorption problems and first-pass metabolism also are avoided with transdermal delivery.

Biopharmaceutics and Drug Disposition

24

This chapter covers the following:

- **Drug liberation and absorption**
- **Drug distribution**
- **Drug metabolism**
- **Drug excretion**

Biopharmaceutics deals with the relationship between the physicochemical properties of a drug; the dosage form in which the drug is available; and its route of administration, with the rate and extent of its absorption and elimination from the body. It is the science that links together traditional pharmaceutics (physical pharmacy and dosage form design) with pharmacokinetics. The acronym LADME (liberation, absorption, distribution, metabolism, and excretion) is often used to describe the main processes addressed by biopharmaceutics.

DRUG LIBERATION AND ABSORPTION

A key concept to remember is that drugs are administered as dosage forms, not individual chemicals. Once taken, they must first be liberated from the dosage form in question and absorbed into the bloodstream before they become available in the systemic circulation. The exception is IV administered drugs, as they are delivered directly into the systemic circulation.

Liberation from a dosage form can be as simple as powder from a capsule being released from the capsule shell after ingestion, or as complicated as the slow release of drug from a tablet or transdermal patch matrix. Oral compressed tablets are the most commonly dispensed dosage form; in this case, liberation of the drug requires disintegration of the tablet into smaller drug particles that then undergo dissolution.

If a drug is not already in solution within the dosage form (as in an oral syrup or elixir), it must first undergo dissolution. Undissolved drug particles cannot cross biological membranes and are therefore trapped at their site of administration. For oral dosage forms, this means that any drug that is not absorbed will continue down the gastrointestinal (GI) tract and will be lost in the feces. In the case of an eye drop given in suspension form, the drug particles remain on the corneal surface until the drug either dissolves and passes through the corneal membrane or is lost via lacrimal drainage. Similarly, topical products remain on the skin surface, and IM and subcut injections remain in the tissues until the drug is dissolved in the body fluids.

The rate and extent to which the drug contained in the dosage forms described above is absorbed into the systemic circulation is the **bioavailability**. This property plays a very important role in the biopharmaceutics and pharmacokinetics of drugs. The liberation and dissolution of a drug can be affected by processing factors and excipients, which can in turn affect bioavailability. Other factors affecting bioavailability are addressed later in this chapter.

One physicochemical property that can affect bioavailability is particle size. A ↓ in the particle size of a drug formulation will ↑ the drug's surface area, which leads to more rapid dissolution. This is an important factor for drugs with low water solubility; finely milling or micronizing drugs such as griseofulvin and nitrofurantoin can dramatically improve their oral bioavailability.

Many excipients can affect product bioavailability. Some examples are listed in the following table.

Excipients That Affect Product Bioavailability

Excipient Category	Examples	Effect on Drug Particles	Effect on Bioavailability
Disintegrants	Starch, microcrystalline cellulose	Breaks tablet into smaller particles, ↑ dissolution	Possible ↑
Surfactants	Tweens, Spans	Low concentration: ↓ surface tension and ↑ dissolution rate	Possible ↑
		High concentration: Form micelles with drug inside, ↓ dissolution	Possible ↓
Lubricants	Magnesium stearate	Has tendency to waterproof particles in large concentration, making them less soluble	Possible ↓

Drug Transport Across Membranes

There are several ways for drugs to cross body membranes that you should be aware of: (1) passive diffusion, (2) carrier-mediated transport, (3) endocytosis, and (4) drug efflux. In passive diffusion, the drug crosses cell membranes based on a concentration gradient, moving from regions of higher concentration to areas of (relatively) lower concentration. For this mechanism to be practical, the drug must be small enough to be absorbed across cells and lipid-soluble enough to interact with the cell membranes. The rate of transport is described by Fick's first law of diffusion:

$$\frac{dC}{dt} = \frac{DA(C_s - C)}{h}$$

While it is unlikely that the NAPLEX will require you to perform calculations based on this equation, you should be familiar with the items that affect it: The concentration gradient ($C_S - C$), the thickness of the membrane being crossed (h), the surface area of the membrane (A), and the diffusion coefficient of the drug (D).

As would be expected, drugs diffuse more slowly through thicker membranes. Body locations with larger surface area tend to promote faster diffusion, as there is more available membrane through which the drug molecule can diffuse. The small intestine is thus a prime location for drug absorption, as the surface area is very large due to the presence of villi and microvilli.

Another key factor to remember is that the GI membranes are more permeable to the drug in the unionized form. The unionized form of the drugs does not carry a net positive or negative charge. In an acidic environment, a weakly acidic drug would be primarily in its unionized form. It would therefore be expected that weakly acidic drugs would be better absorbed in the highly acidic environment of the stomach. However, the absorption of weakly acidic drugs generally increases as the drug moves from the stomach to the intestines. The aforementioned factors in Fick's first law play a large role in absorption, such as a ↓ membrane thickness and ↑ surface area of the small intestine. Furthermore, even though the unionized form of a drug is more permeable to cell membranes, the ionized form of the drug is more soluble. Therefore, basic drugs will be more soluble in the highly acidic environment of the stomach. Because of this, poorly soluble, weakly basic drugs may be poorly absorbed if taken with drugs that ↓ gastric acid secretion. For example, ketoconazole and atazanavir both exhibit ↓ rate and extent of absorption when taken with antacids, H_2 blockers or proton pump inhibitors. The extent of drug ionization at any given pH can be estimated by the Henderson-Hasselbalch equation, as detailed in the Ionization Behavior section of the Pharmaceutics chapter.

Not all drugs are absorbed by passive diffusion; many undergo carrier-mediated transport processes. Active transport, which requires input of energy and occurs against a concentration gradient, is the most common type of carrier-mediated transport process.

Unlike passive diffusion, the process can be saturated or competitively inhibited by chemically similar substrates. Many drugs are transported via transport systems designed to move amino acids and vitamins across cell membranes. Some drugs undergo simultaneous passive diffusion and active transport.

The final method of drug transport with which you should be concerned is drug efflux. In this case, transporters pump drugs and other substances out of cells rather than into them. P-glycoprotein (P-gp) is the key efflux protein, and it is linked to multidrug resistance in tumor cells. In this case, resistance occurs because the transporter pumps drug out of the tumor tissue before it can accumulate to an effective concentration. P-gp is also expressed on the intraluminal surface of the GI tract. In this location, it pumps substrates out of the plasma and back into the intestinal lumen, resulting in a $\downarrow$ net absorption (and bioavailability) of some drugs. Digoxin, corticosteroids, and immunosuppressants are just a few of the drugs that can be affected in this way. There is significant overlap between drugs that are inhibitors of the cytochrome P450 3A (CYP3A) isoenzyme and inhibitors of P-gp. Therefore, many drugs that are known inhibitors of the CYP3A4/5 can enhance absorption and $\uparrow$ the plasma concentrations of digoxin even though that digoxin is not a CYP3A4/5 substrate. The amiodarone–digoxin interaction is a clinically relevant example of an interaction involving P-gp that results in $\uparrow$ plasma digoxin concentrations since amiodarone is an inhibitor of P-gp.

Barriers to Drug Absorption

Several factors can affect drug absorption (see following table). Food intake can affect absorption and bioavailability in a variety of ways, including $\uparrow$ the pH in the stomach, which can in turn affect drug dissolution and absorption ($\uparrow$ dissolution and absorption for weak acids and $\downarrow$ dissolution and absorption for weak bases). Chemical stability may be affected as well, which can in turn $\downarrow$ the amount of drug available for absorption.

Food-Related Absorption and Bioavailability Variations

Process	Explanation	Examples
Food-drug complexation	Can bind and make drug insoluble; prevent absorption	Tetracycline or fluoroquinolone complexes with calcium and iron in food and supplements ($\downarrow$ bioavailability)
Alteration of pH	Food acts as buffer in stomach; $\uparrow$ pH	• $\uparrow$ dissolution (and subsequent absorption) of weak acids • $\downarrow$ dissolution (and subsequent absorption) of weak bases
Gastric emptying	Foods and some drugs can slow gastric emptying and delay drug onset or speed-up gastric emptying and $\downarrow$ drug effect	Metoclopramide and erythromycin can $\uparrow$ gastric emptying

Food-Related Absorption and Bioavailability Variations *(cont'd)*

Process	Explanation	Examples
Gastric acid secretions	• Pepsin may ↑ drug metabolism • Bile salts ↑ dissolution of poorly soluble drugs, but can form complexes with other drugs	Bile acid-drug complexes: neomycin, nystatin
Competition for specialized absorption mechanisms	Competitive inhibition of drugs by nutrients with similar chemical structures	Amino acids can compete with drugs (e.g., cephalexin) transported by the peptide transporter (PEPT1)
↑ volume and viscosity of GI contents	Presence of food can lead to: • Slower drug dissolution • Slower diffusion of dissolved drug from GI tract	This can affect several drugs
Food-induced changes in first-pass metabolism	↑ bioavailability due to inhibition of CYP450 isoenzymes (primarily CYP3A)	Grapefruit juice may ↑ bioavailability of numerous 3A substrates (e.g., cyclosporine, verapamil, saquinavir)
Food-induced changes in blood flow	• Giving some drugs with food ↑ bioavailability due to ↑ blood flow to the GI tract and liver following a meal • A larger fraction of drug escapes first-pass metabolism because the enzyme system becomes overwhelmed	Drugs with metabolism sensitive to rate of presentation to liver: • Propranolol • Hydralazine

DRUG DISTRIBUTION

Once in the bloodstream, some proportion of the drug may be bound to the plasma proteins while the remainder remains unbound. A key point to remember is that only drug that is unbound can pass out of the plasma to reach the site of action. The amount of drug that is bound to plasma protein is in dynamic equilibrium with the amount that is not.

Volume of Distribution

In the average 70-kg (~155-lb) patient, blood volume is approximately 5 L and total body water is about 40 L. After absorption, a drug will distribute into the body fluids; since the total amount of drug placed into the body is known and the concentration of drug in the plasma can be measured, the volume of fluid through which the drug seems to have distributed throughout the body can be determined. This volume is referred to as the *apparent* volume of distribution (V_d), because it is not a physical volume. Rather, it is a calculated number, dependent on physicochemical properties of the drug, which helps compare the behavior of different drugs. Thus, the apparent V_d may be a much larger value than what is physiologically possible (i.e., $\geq 1,000$ L). This indicates that the drug either is primarily distributed into extravascular tissue or is highly protein bound. This phenomenon can be visualized by the following equation to determine a drug's apparent V_d:

$V_d = \dfrac{dose}{C_p}$ when dose = IV bolus and C_p is unbound plasma drug concentration measured immediately after injection for a one-compartment drug.

Plasma Protein Binding

Most drugs exhibit plasma protein binding, and this affects their V_d. Proteins are large molecules that cannot leave the capillaries; therefore, the drug-protein complex remains in the plasma. However, the concentration of protein-bound drug is not usually measured. Therefore, protein binding that results in lower free plasma concentrations of the drug will ↑ the apparent V_d. Because protein binding is reversible, equilibrium exists between bound and free drug. As free drug distributes out of the bloodstream, bound drug is released from plasma proteins to maintain equilibrium.

Certain disease states can alter the concentrations of plasma proteins significantly enough to require drug dose adjustments. Additionally, if a patient is receiving several drugs that all bind to the same plasma protein, one drug may displace another, leading to higher-than-expected drug concentrations and possible toxicity. This is most important in drugs that are more than 95% protein bound, particularly if they have a narrow therapeutic index. Warfarin (99% protein bound) is an excellent example of this potential drug interaction. Even a minor displacement of protein-bound warfarin (e.g., 99% to 98% bound) would double the unbound concentration, thereby increasing the effective concentration from 1% to 2%.

DRUG METABOLISM

Drugs are eliminated from the body by two processes: metabolism and excretion. Metabolism, also referred to as biotransformation, leads to the chemical conversion of drug to active or inactive compounds called metabolites. These metabolites are generally more polar (and hence more water-soluble) than the parent drugs which allows the metabolites to be more efficiently cleared in the urine. Not all drugs undergo metabolism.

Metabolism is most likely to occur in organs that contain high levels of enzymes. Many drug-metabolizing enzymes, including the CYP450 mixed-function oxidases, are found in the liver, which is the primary site of biotransformation.

One concern with oral delivery of certain drugs is presystemic, or first-pass, metabolism. Because the venous outflow of the GI tract travels directly to the liver via the portal vein, drugs administered via the GI tract are susceptible to hepatic metabolism before they reach the systemic circulation.

Metabolism is classified into Phase I and Phase II reactions.

Phase I Reactions

The primary types of Phase I reactions are oxidation, reduction, and hydrolysis. Oxidation is the most common type of metabolism, and many of these reactions are catalyzed by enzymes in the CYP superfamily.

Phase II Reactions

Phase II reactions are synthetic reactions. They are often called conjugation reactions, as a reactive group on the drug is attached to a polar molecule or group originating inside the body.

Examples of Phase II reactions are listed in the following table, with glucuronidation being the most common example.

Phase II Reactions

Type of Phase II Reaction	Drugs Metabolized by This Route
Glucuronidation	• Chloramphenicol • Meprobamate • Morphine
Sulfation	• Acetaminophen • Estradiol • Methyldopa • Minoxidil
Amino acid conjugation	• Salicylic acid
Acetylation	• Isoniazid • Procainamide • Sulfonamides • Hydralazine
Methylation	• Catecholamines • Niacinamide
Glutathione conjugation	• Chlorambucil

Factors Affecting Biotransformation

Several factors can affect metabolizing enzyme activity in the body. Disease states, age, gender, or chemical and nutritional exposure to a variety of substances can lead to enzyme inhibition or enzyme induction. Genetic variability also plays a role. Drug–drug interactions are a common result of the metabolic process, as most marketed drugs are metabolized by multiple pathways, and drugs that inhibit or induce enzyme activity can affect the metabolism of many other drugs.

Enzyme Inhibition

Enzyme inhibition describes the situation when an enzyme is prevented from binding with its substrate. The substrate is therefore unable to be properly metabolized, and plasma concentrations ↑, possibly to toxic levels. In cases where a prodrug must be activated by metabolism, enzyme inhibition may limit, delay, or prevent drug activity. Enzyme inhibitors can act by competitive or noncompetitive means.

The following table contains a partial list of common enzyme inhibitors.

Drugs Involved in Inhibition of Metabolic Enzymes

CYP1A2	CYP2C9	CYP2C19	CYP2D6	CYP3A
fluvoxamine	fluconazole	cimetidine	bupropion	indinavir
ciprofloxacin	amiodarone	esomeprazole	fluoxetine	nelfinavir
		lansoprazole	paroxetine	ritonavir
		omeprazole	quinidine	clarithromycin
		pantoprazole	duloxetine	itraconazole
		fluoxetine	sertraline	ketoconazole
		fluvoxamine	terbinafine	nefazodone
		indomethacin	amiodarone	saquinavir
		isoniazid	cimetidine	erythromycin
		ketoconazole	chlorpromazine	fluconazole
		oxcarbazepine	clomipramine	grapefruit juice
		probenecid	doxepin	verapamil
		topiramate	haloperidol	diltiazem
		voriconazole	methadone	cimetidine
				amiodarone

Enzyme Induction

Enzyme inducers stimulate enzyme activity, which leads to ↓ plasma concentrations of the enzyme's targets. In most cases, this means a ↓ in both activity and adverse effects of the drug. If active or toxic metabolites are produced, however, drug activity and toxic effects may be ↑. Although there are exceptions, the inducers commonly affect all of the inducible CYP enzymes including CYP1A2, CYP2B6, CYP2C9, CYP2C19, and CYP3A. The CYP2D6 isoenzyme is not inducible.

Some drugs undergo a phenomenon called auto-induction, wherein they stimulate their own metabolism. Carbamazepine is a key example of a drug of this type. Due to auto-induction, administration of carbamazepine especially during the initial 3–5 weeks of therapy can lead to ↓ blood concentrations and therapeutic activity.

Drugs Involved in Induction of Metabolic Enzymes

Seizure medications	• Carbamazepine • Phenytoin • Phenobarbital
Tuberculosis medications	• Rifampin

DRUG EXCRETION

Unlike metabolism, excretion eliminates the substances without further chemical change. The kidney is the primary organ involved, and most substances are excreted in the urine. Polar, water-soluble drugs are usually excreted unchanged; lipophilic drugs are generally excreted as metabolites. There are three components to renal excretion:

1. Glomerular filtration
   - Blood passes through the capillary network (glomerulus) inside Bowman's capsule.
   - Fenestrated endothelium allows paracellular transport of most solutes (other than macromolecules) into Bowman's capsule.
   - Filtrate (including drug) moves from Bowman's capsule into renal tubules.
   - All nonprotein-bound, small-molecule drugs undergo glomerular filtration; the concentration of drug or metabolite in the filtrate will be equal to the concentration of unbound drug in the plasma.

2. Tubular reabsorption
   - Many nutrients and ions are actively reabsorbed into the bloodstream.
   - Water is reabsorbed, and filtrate becomes more concentrated as it moves along the tubule.
   - No transporters exist for reabsorption of drug; passive diffusion process is dependent on filtrate pH. Acidic (citrus fruits, cranberry juice, aspirin) and basic (milk products, sodium bicarbonate) foods and drugs can alter urine pH enough to affect reabsorption.
     » In alkaline urine: Acidic drugs are ionized → less reabsorbed → more readily excreted in urine
     » In acidic urine: Basic drugs are ionized → less reabsorbed → more readily excreted in urine

  » Phentobarbital (weak acid) overdose: Treated by alkalinizing urine with sodium bicarbonate injection

3. Tubular secretion

- This occurs simultaneously with tubular reabsorption.
- This removes certain substances from the blood and secretes them back into the filtrate.
- This occurs against the concentration gradient and is an energy-requiring process that uses protein transporters.
- Only ionized drugs are bound to and secreted by the transporter proteins; drugs that are highly ionized at pH 7.4 will be secreted to a greater extent.
- Plasma protein binding has little effect on this process; transporters can strip drug off of protein.
  - » Competitive process; can lead to drug interactions
    - – Saturable process; at high dose, process plateaus → less drug excreted → higher plasma concentration than expected

The rate of renal excretion of drugs is the net result of the above processes. It depends on blood flow in addition to the physicochemical properties of the drugs in question. More rapid blood flow through the nephron generally leads to an ↑ in all three processes, with an overall higher drug excretion rate. Glomerular filtration rate (GFR) is normally about 120 mL/min, but may vary widely with the patient's age, body weight, and concomitant disease states. The GFR for an individual is determined by calculating the clearance of creatinine, an endogenous substance that is not reabsorbed or secreted. This value gives an indication of kidney function. A common way to estimate a patient's creatinine clearance (CrCl) is using the Cockroft-Gault equation listed here and should be memorized for the NAPLEX.

$$\text{CrCl (mL/min)} = \frac{(140 - \text{age}) \times \text{wt (kg)}}{\text{Serum Creatinine (mg/dL)} \times 72} (\times 0.85 \text{ if female})$$

Nonrenal Excretion

Drugs may also be excreted by the liver into the bile; at this point, one of two things can happen:

- Biliary excretion: Bile (including drug) is emptied into the small intestine, where it is eventually excreted from the body in the feces.
- Enterohepatic recycling: The drug is partially reabsorbed from the intestines (based on pK_a and partition coefficient) and re-enters the bloodstream. Drugs undergoing this process may show a secondary peak in plasma concentration; with multiple dosing regimens, the blood-concentration curve can be altered significantly.

Pharmacogenomics

This chapter covers the following:

- **Definitions**
- **Phase I metabolism**
- **Phase II metabolism**
- **Drug targets**

Variants (i.e., mutations) in the human genome account for a portion of the clinical variability observed between patients receiving the same drug therapy. *Pharmacogenomics* describes the impact of genetics on the pharmacokinetics and pharmacodynamics of drugs. The most clinically relevant variants that alter drug pharmacokinetics and pharmacodynamics are located in genes that encode drug-metabolizing enzymes, target receptors, or the human leukocyte antigen (HLA). These genes and the effects of genetics on drug therapy are the focus of this chapter.

DEFINITIONS

Proteins (including enzymes) that have different expression profiles are considered to be polymorphically expressed. The expression profile is commonly determined by the presence of functional versus nonfunctional alleles. Alleles are a specific form of a gene. Humans have two alleles for each gene, one inherited from each parent. Therefore, patients may have:

- Two functional alleles known as the wild-type (i.e., extensive or normal metabolizer)
- One functional and one nonfunctional allele (i.e., intermediate metabolizer)
- Two nonfunctional alleles (i.e., poor metabolizer)

Genetic polymorphisms result in allele expression that can lead to a number of metabolism-related issues. For the NAPLEX, it is important to understand how the functional classification of enzymes can alter dosage requirements. For example, you will likely be told if a patient fits into one of the three categories listed. It is unlikely that you will be expected to memorize the nomenclature for functional and nonfunctional alleles for even the most common cytochrome P450 (CYP) enzymes. However, it is useful to know that alleles follow a star nomenclature system, with *1 considered the wild-type for most enzymes. Therefore, if a patient is said to express the *1/*1, it is highly likely that she would be considered an extensive or normal metabolizer. If only one *1 is present, he may be an intermediate metabolizer, and if no *1 is present she may be a poor metabolizer.

Of course, patients cannot always be simply categorized into one of the three groups listed, and individuals can have polymorphisms that may increase or reduce function to varying extents. For example, polymorphisms of the CYP2D6 enzyme can produce an allele with supraenzymatic activity. These patients would be classified as ultrarapid metabolizers. For the NAPLEX, once you identify the expression profile of a patient, you will likely need to make dosage adjustments to avoid subtherapeutic consequences or toxic effects, depending on the category into which a patient falls and whether the metabolite of the drug is active or inactive.

PHASE I METABOLISM

Cytochrome P450

CYP enzymes, in particular, are highly polymorphic and follow the nomenclature outlined. As mentioned, CYP2D6 can be problematic, with individuals classified as poor, intermediate, extensive, and ultrarapid metabolizers. The percentage of poor metabolizers varies somewhat by ancestry. Approximately 5–10% of Caucasians, 1–2% of Asians, and up to 20% in African Americans are poor metabolizers. When making dosage adjustments, it is important to consider whether (1) the parent drug is active and/or (2) the major metabolite via the CYP pathway in question is active. For example, codeine is metabolized by CYP2D6. Poor metabolizers of CYP2D6 receive less benefit from codeine, because it must be metabolized into morphine to exert its full analgesic effect. Pharmacists should be aware of this variability, since poor metabolizers may be falsely labeled as drug-seekers when in fact codeine is an ineffective analgesic for them. These patients should instead be placed on analgesics not activated by CYP2D6, such as morphine itself.

The importance of the field of pharmacogenomics has dramatically increased the ability to determine a patient's genotype. In addition to CYP2D6, the enzymes CYP1A, CYP2C9, and CYP2C19 are polymorphically expressed. Understanding the drugs metabolized by these pathways and their active metabolites is important for the NAPLEX. The following table lists selected drugs metabolized by the most common CYP enzymes.

Common Drugs Metabolized by Pathway

CYP1A2	CYP2C9	CYP2C19	CYP2D6	CYP3A
caffeine	warfarin	omeprazole	codeine	clarithromycin
theophylline	phenytoin	esomeprazole	dextromethorphan	erythromycin
	glipizide	lansoprazole	hydrocodone	quinidine
	glyburide	pantoprazole	oxycodone	midazolam
		citalopram	fluoxetine	alprazolam
		voriconazole	haloperidol	diazepam
		clopidogrel	venlafaxine	cyclosporine
			paroxetine	tacrolimus
			duloxetine	amlodipine
			risperidone	diltiazem
			propranolol	nifedipine
			metoprolol	verapamil
			tamoxifen	atorvastatin
				lovastatin
				simvastatin
				estrogens
				carbamazepine

PHASE II METABOLISM

Glucuronidation

Phase II reactions are synthetic reactions. They are often called conjugation reactions, because a reactive group on the drug is attached to a polar molecule or group originating inside the body. Like Phase I enzymes, Phase II enzymes can be polymorphically expressed with altered function.

Irinotecan is a cytotoxic agent used in colorectal cancer that has an important pharmacogenomic profile related to its drug toxicity. The active metabolite of irinotecan is SN-38. SN-38 is primarily eliminated by glucuronidation through the UGT1A1 enzyme. The presence of UGT1A polymorphisms can predict severe drug toxicities before ironotecan is administered. Homozygotes for the UGT1A1*28 allele have Gilbert's syndrome, which affects bilirubin elimination. Homozygotes for the UGT1A1*28 allele also demonstrate significantly reduced elimination of SN-38, predisposing patients to life-threatening myelosuppression.

DRUG TARGETS

Somatic Mutations

Currently, the greatest clinical application of pharmacogenomics involves identifying somatic mutations within the field of oncology. *Somatic mutations* refer to genetic variants that occur within the tumor itself and are not a part of the patient's germline. Therefore, screening for somatic mutations requires a biopsy of the tumor; saliva will only reveal the germline DNA. For example, somatic mutations within the epidermal growth factor receptor tyrosine kinase family can help guide the treatment of various cancers, such as non–small cell lung carcinoma.

Vitamin K Epoxide Reductase Complex Subunit 1 (VKORC1)

The VKORC1 gene encodes for the vitamin K epoxide reductase complex subunit 1, which converts inactive vitamin K epoxide to active vitamin K. Active vitamin K is required for several coagulation factors. Patients with mutations at position 1639 (1639G>A) in the VKORC1 gene demonstrate diminished VKORC1 expression. Since VKORC1 is the target for warfarin, patients with diminished VKORC1 expression require lower maintenance doses of warfarin. These patients have a correspondingly higher risk of warfarin-related adverse events at normal doses.

Human Leukocyte Antigen

The strongest evidence for adverse effects that have been associated with HLA polymorphisms are serious skin hypersensitivity reactions resulting in Stevens-Johnson syndrome (SJS) or toxic epidermal necrolysis (TEN). Carbamazepine and phenytoin have a strong association with the development of SJS/TEN in patients carrying the HLA-B*1502 allele. The highest allele frequency for this mutation is found in Asian populations, so patients of Asian descent are commonly tested for this mutation before receiving carbamazepine or phenytoin therapy. Additionally, abacavir has a strong association with the development of hypersensitivity reactions in patients carrying the HLA-B*5701 allele. Patients should be tested for this mutation before receiving abacavir therapy, and abacavir should be avoided in patients who test positive for this mutation.

Pharmacokinetics

26

This chapter covers the following:

- **Plasma drug concentration profiles**
- **Theoretical compartments**
- **Basic pharmacokinetic parameters**
- **Oral dosing**
- **Multiple dosing factor and accumulation factor**
- **Nonlinear pharmacokinetics**

PLASMA DRUG CONCENTRATION PROFILES

Plasma drug concentration versus time curve graphs are used extensively in pharmacokinetics. A known dose of drug is given to a patient, and blood samples are taken at various time intervals following drug administration. The concentration of drug in plasma following IV and oral administration is measured and plotted in the following figure. The shape of the curve depends on the relative rates of absorption (oral drug), distribution, and elimination of the drug.

Plasma Concentration versus Time Curves for Intravenous and Oral Drug Administration

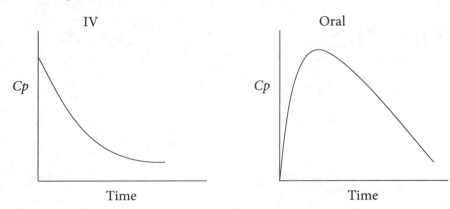

The preceding graphs represent drug plasma concentration (Cp) versus time profiles following an IV bolus and oral administration of a mock drug. Following IV administration, the drug will reach its maximum plasma concentration (C_{max}) at time 0 (leftmost point on the X-axis). Therefore, the time to maximum plasma concentration (T_{max}) is at time 0 following an IV bolus.

Following the lag time for absorption, a rise in drug plasma concentration is seen until it reaches a plateau, which represents the C_{max} on the oral curve. The time of this plateau (i.e., C_{max}) is the T_{max}. At T_{max}, there is a brief time period where this is no net change in drug plasma concentration. This represents the time when the rate of drug absorption is equal to that of elimination. Beyond the C_{max}, elimination will be greater than absorption and is represented by a decline in the drug plasma concentration.

THEORETICAL COMPARTMENTS

From a pharmacokinetic perspective, the body is considered to consist of compartments, inside each of which the drug can be considered evenly distributed.

- One-compartment model
  - Central compartment includes plasma and well-perfused tissue with rapid distribution (e.g., liver, kidneys).
  - Drug distributes rapidly and uniformly to this compartment.
- Two-compartment model
  - Central compartment is still present, and includes plasma and well-perfused organs (e.g., liver, kidneys).
  - There is a slow distribution of drug into a peripheral compartment that consists of poorly perfused tissue (e.g., muscles, connective tissue).

One-Compartment Model

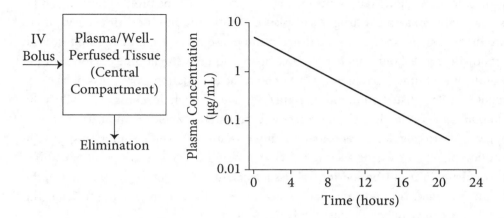

The basic structure of a one-compartment drug is displayed on the left, with a corresponding plasma concentration-time curve on the right. Note that the Y-axis is on a logarithmic scale, which linearizes the relationship. At time 0, the drug is administered into the central compartment. This can be observed on the concentration-time curve by the C_{max} at time 0. The central compartment represents plasma and tissue to which the drug rapidly distributes. The slope of the concentration time curve on a log or natural log scale is directly proportional to the first-order elimination rate constant and therefore the drug half-life. The elimination rate constant can be calculated by taking the difference of the natural log of two concentrations and dividing by the difference of the two corresponding times.

Two-Compartment Model

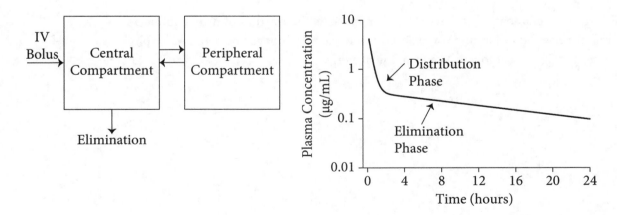

The general structure of a two-compartment model is displayed on the left of the figure. The right side of the figure represents the log concentration-time profile following an IV bolus of a two-compartment drug. As displayed on the concentration-time curve, there are two distinct slopes labeled as the distribution phase and the elimination phase. The C_{max} following an IV bolus in a two-compartment model is still at time 0. However, the slope of the line at time 0 is representative of both the elimination from the central compartment and slow distribution into peripheral tissue. This phase, commonly called the *distribution phase* of the drug, is not directly representative of elimination. Therefore, it is inappropriate to calculate an elimination rate constant or half-life while a drug is in the distribution phase. Once drug accumulates in the peripheral tissue to a point of equilibrium (i.e., drug diffuses from peripheral tissue back into the central compartment), the change in the concentration-time curve is solely due to the elimination of the drug. The half-life of the drug can be calculated only in the elimination phase.

BASIC PHARMACOKINETIC PARAMETERS

Bioavailable Fraction

The bioavailable fraction (F) is the portion of dose administered that reaches the systemic circulation. For IV administration, $F = 1$. A drug given by any other route can have an F ranging from 0 to 1; the F will never be >1. Two factors can $\downarrow$ the F of a drug:

- Incomplete absorption
- First-pass metabolism

Elimination Rate Constant

The first-order elimination rate constant, k, represents the fraction of drug eliminated per unit time, and thus has units of reciprocal time (i.e., hr^{-1}). It can be obtained graphically (see the figure that follows) or from the drug $t_{1/2}$:

$$k = \frac{\ln 2}{t_{1/2}} = \frac{0.693}{t_{1/2}}$$

Graphical Calculation of Elimination Rate Constant

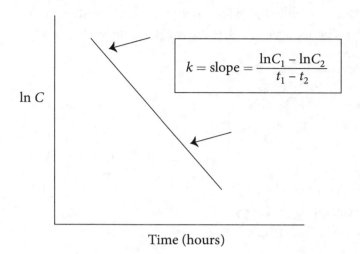

$$k = \text{slope} = \frac{\ln C_1 - \ln C_2}{t_1 - t_2}$$

ln C

Time (hours)

Half-Life

The elimination $t_{1/2}$ of a drug is the time required for its serum concentration to ↓ by half. It can be obtained mathematically or graphically:

$$t_{1/2} = \frac{\ln 2}{k} = \frac{0.693}{k}$$

The $t_{1/2}$ can also be calculated from clearance (CL) and volume of distribution (V_d). While these parameters do not influence or depend on one another, half-life depends on both of them:

$$t_{1/2} = 0.693 \times \left(\frac{Vd}{CL}\right)$$

Clearance

CL refers to the efficiency of the body in removing drug from the blood. The liver and kidney are the primary organs involved, and body CL refers to the sum of the hepatic (CL_h) and renal clearances (CL_r), plus any CL from other organs, usually negligible:

$$CL = CL_h + CL_r$$

Knowledge of drug CL can help determine when dosage adjustments are needed in patients with hepatic or renal impairment.

Volume of Distribution

Apparent V_d describes the volume of body fluids required to account for all drugs in the body. Several equations can be used to calculate apparent V_d, depending on the information you have available:

$$V_d = \frac{\text{Dose}}{C_{peak}} = \frac{F \times \text{Dose}}{\text{AUC} \times k} = \frac{CL \times t_{1/2}}{0.693}$$

V_d has the following effect on $t_{1/2}$:

- Small V_d
  - Drug mostly located in blood
  - Liver and kidneys only clear drug in blood
  - Fewer passes needed to rid body of drug
  - Shorter $t_{1/2}$
- Large V_d
  - Drug is extensively distributed into extravascular tissues
  - Liver and kidneys only clear drug in blood
  - More passes are required to clear drug from body
  - Longer $t_{1/2}$

Area under the Curve

Area under the curve (AUC) is a measure of the extent of drug exposure. It is defined as the area under the drug plasma level – time curve from $t = 0$ to infinity. It can be calculated by the trapezoidal rule, or by the other listed equations, and has units of concentration/time. S is the salt factor for a given drug formulation and refers to the percentage of administered product that is the active moiety (the acid or base, not the salt).

Trapezoidal rule:

$$\text{AUC} = \frac{C_{n-1} + C_n}{2} (tn - t_{n-1})$$

where n refers to the concentration and time associated with it and $n-1$ is the previous concentration and associated times.

Other equations:

$$\text{AUC} = \frac{F \times S \times D_0}{CL} = \frac{F \times D_0}{k \times V_d}$$

AUC is often directly proportional to dose, such that ↑ the dose of a drug from 500 mg to 1,000 mg will lead to a twofold ↑ in AUC.

MULTIPLE DOSING

Two things affect how much drug accumulates between the first dose and a dose at steady state:

- Elimination constant or half-life
- Dosing interval

We cannot control the half-life; it is dependent on the drug in question. However, the dosing interval can be adjusted to increase or decrease the drug accumulation factor. A simple estimation of this can be described by:

- Dosing interval < drug half-life → C_{SS} will be much higher than the concentration after the first dose.
- Dosing interval = drug half-life → C_{SS} will be twice as high as the concentration after the first dose.
- Dosing interval > drug half-life → C_{SS} will be similar to the concentration after the first dose (because the drug is almost completely washing out before the next dose is given).

Peak-to-Trough Ratio

Multiple intermittent dosing results in peak and trough drug concentrations. As will be discussed, a dose and dosing interval (τ) are calculated to achieve a desired steady-state plasma concentration average ($C_{SS, avg}$). The $C_{SS, avg}$ represents the average concentration between the peak and trough. Shorter dosing intervals for a particular dose will lead to a decreased $P{:}T$ ratio, meaning that less fluctuation in peak-to-trough is occurring.

Loading Doses

Loading doses are often used to achieve target plasma drug concentrations as quickly as possible. These large initial doses (which may be given as either a single dose or divided doses over a specified period of time) are especially important in life-threatening conditions such as myocardial infarction, status asthmaticus, and status epilepticus. Loading doses should not be used when there is not an urgent need to achieve target blood concentrations immediately or the patient cannot be supervised for possible toxicity. Loading doses for narrow-therapeutic-index drugs should ideally occur within a clinical setting.

$$F \cdot \text{Loading dose} = C_{ss(target)} \times V_d$$

Loading doses are commonly given by the IV route, so the F will be equal to 1 in these cases. If an oral loading dose is being administered, the bioavailability of the drug MUST be taken into consideration.

If the patient already has drug in his or her system, this needs to be taken into consideration. Simply take the desired concentration ($C_{ss(target)}$) and subtract out the concentration already in the system. Just be sure the units are identical when performing this calculation.

Constant IV Infusion

Constant-rate infusions do not generate fluctuations in plasma concentrations. Determining the rate for such infusions is relatively simple:

1. Determine the target steady-state plasma concentration (C_{SS}).
2. Find the appropriate population CL.
3. Look up S (if drug is a salt).
4. Calculate infusion rate (R). (The infusion rate is in the units of amount per time [e.g., mg/min].)

$$R = \frac{C_{SS} \times CL}{S}$$

In most instances, S will be equal to 1 and can be ignored. Clearance adjustment factors may be available for some drugs.

Intermittent Oral Dosing

Dose rate in intermittent oral dosing is calculated in a similar fashion to IV infusions. Remember to take F into account with oral dosing, however, since bioavailability may not be equal to IV products. The equation to calculate a dosing rate (dose divided by dosing interval, τ) for an intermittent infusion or oral dosing to a desired steady-state plasma concentration is displayed:

$$\frac{F \times \text{Dose}}{\tau} = C_{SS,\,avg} \times CL$$

where F is the bioavailability (equal to 1 for IV infusion), dose is the amount administered, τ is the dosing interval, Css, avg is the average steady-state plasma concentration, and CL is the clearance. This is an important equation that can be used to calculate maintenance dosing of drugs to desired steady-state concentrations.

NONLINEAR PHARMACOKINETICS

So far, this chapter has referred to general pharmacokinetic principles. These principles are applicable to most drugs without significant modification, and they result in linear mathematical models. Several assumptions are made when different or multiple doses are given:

- Drug clearance remains constant.
- Doubling the dose results in a doubling of the concentration and AUC.

These assumptions are not always accurate. With some drugs, giving a single low dose of the drug leads to the expected linear pharmacokinetics. However, when higher doses are given, or when the medication is taken chronically, the drug no longer fits the linear pharmacokinetic profile.

Pharmacokinetic Relationships: Linear versus Nonlinear

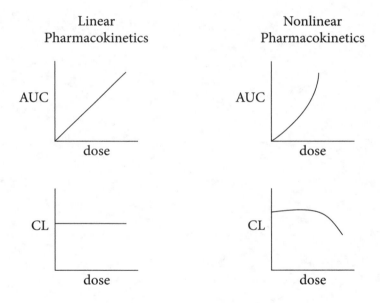

Nonlinear pharmacokinetics generally occur when one or more enzyme- or carrier-mediated systems are saturated. These systems are often referred to as capacity-limited.

Most elimination processes can be saturated if enough drug is given. Certain drugs (phenytoin in particular) show nonlinear behavior even at normal drug doses.

For drugs exhibiting nonlinear behavior, dose increases lead to half-life increases, and AUC is not proportional to the amount of bioavailable drug. The behavior is described by the Michaelis-Menten equation:

$$\frac{dC}{dt} = \frac{V_{max} - C_{SS}}{K_m + C_{SS}}$$

V_{max} (the maximum elimination rate) and K_m (the Michaelis constant, equal to one-half the concentration at V_{max}) are dependent on both the drug and the enzyme system.

Calculations

27

This chapter covers the following:

- **Problem-solving techniques**
- **Fundamentals of units and measurement**
- **Density, specific gravity, and specific volume**
- **Percentage, ratio strengths, and parts per million**
- **Dosage calculations**
- **Dilution, concentration, and alligation**
- **Electrolyte solutions**
- **Compounding calculations**

PROBLEM-SOLVING TECHNIQUES

Ratio-Proportion and Dimensional Analysis

Ratio-proportion is a one-step calculation technique that is probably the easiest to use for simple (one- or two-step) calculations. In this process, you set up a likeness between a fraction involving known quantities and one that includes your unknown, and solve the equation by cross multiplying. An example is given here, illustrating how to convert 3 fluid ounces to milliliters:

$$\frac{30\,\text{mL}}{1\,\text{fl oz}} = \frac{x\,\text{mL}}{3\,\text{fl oz}}$$

$$(30\,\text{mL})(3\,\text{fl oz}) = (x\,\text{mL})(1\,\text{fl oz})$$

$$\frac{(30\,\text{mL})(3\,\text{fl oz})}{(1\,\text{fl oz})} = x\,\text{mL}$$

$$x = 90\ \text{mL}$$

To avoid rounding errors, keep as many decimal points as possible until the last step in the calculation. If the question is fill-in-the-blank style, it will instruct you regarding how many decimals points to include in the final answer.

Dimensional analysis is a technique, often used in chemistry and other sciences, which allows you to set up long calculations in a single step. Using the short example given earlier, the problem would be solved:

$$3 \text{ fl oz} \times \frac{(30 \text{ mL})}{(1 \text{ fl oz})} = 90 \text{ mL}$$

As you can see, the fluid ounces cancel out and leave you with the correct units of milliliters. This serves as an internal error-check and may be helpful in longer, more complex problems.

FUNDAMENTALS OF UNITS AND MEASUREMENT

- Avoirdupois refers to solid measures only (pounds and ounces).
  - 1 pound = 16 ounces
- Common or household liquid measurements start with the teaspoon.
  - 1 teaspoon (tsp) = 5 mL
  - 3 tsp = 1 tablespoon (T) = 15 mL
  - 2 T = 1 fluid ounce (fl oz) = 30 mL = 1/8 cup
  - 1 cup = 8 fl oz
  - 1 pint = 16 fl oz (or 2 cups)
  - 1 quart = 32 fl oz (or 4 cups)
  - 1 gallon = 128 fl oz (or 16 cups)

Avoirdupois System	Metric System
1 lb	454 g
2.2 lb	1 kg
1 oz	28.4 g
1 grain	64.8 mg

Apothecary System	Metric System
1 tsp	5 mL
1 T	15 mL
1 fl oz	29.6 mL (30 mL is an acceptable estimate)
1 cup	240 mL
1 pint	473 mL
1 quart	946 mL
1 gallon	3,785 mL

Prefix	Conversion Factor	Example
Kilo (k)	1,000 or 10^3	1 kilograms (kg) = 1,000 grams (g)
Deci (d)	0.1 or 10^{-1}	1 deciliter (dL) = 0.1 liters (L)
Centi (c)	0.01 or 10^{-2}	1 centimeter (cm) = 0.01 meters (m)
Milli (m)	0.001 or 10^{-3}	1 milligram (mg) = 0.001 grams (g)
Micro (μ)	0.000001 or 10^{-6}	1 microliter (μL) = 0.000001 liters (L)
Nano (n)	0.000000001 or 10^{-9}	1 nanogram (ng) = 0.000000001 grams (g)

DENSITY, SPECIFIC GRAVITY, AND SPECIFIC VOLUME

Density should be treated like a conversion factor, since you are converting between mass and volume.

Example: 450 mL of phenol weighs 482.56 g. What is its density? Express your answer in g/mL.

$$\frac{482.56 \, \text{g phenol}}{450 \, \text{mL}} = 1.07 \, \text{g/mL}$$

Specific gravity (SG) is the density of a substance relative to a reference substance (usually water). It is a unitless number, because it is equal to density divided by density—the units cancel out. Since water has a density of 1 g/mL, the SG will be numerically identical to the density of the substance expressed in g/mL.

Example: 150 mL of formaldehyde weighs 121.82 g. What is its specific gravity?

$$\frac{\dfrac{121.82 \, \text{g formaldehyde}}{150 \, \text{ml}}}{\dfrac{1 \, \text{g water}}{1 \, \text{mL}}} = 0.81$$

Thus, formaldehyde has a SG of 0.81, which is the same as the density if presented in g/mL.

PERCENTAGE, RATIO STRENGTHS, AND PARTS PER MILLION

Since drugs are administered as dosage forms that contain more than just the active ingredient, the amount of the active ingredient needs to be expressed.

Percent describes the number of parts of active drug relative to 100 parts of the total. In pharmacy, simply stating % is incomplete; you must attach the appropriate descriptor from the following list:

- % w/w: g of active drug per 100 g of product
- % w/v: g of active drug per 100 mL of product
- % v/v: mL of active drug per 100 mL of product

Examples:

    (1)   10% w/v = 10 g of drug in every 100 mL of the total

    (2)   10% w/w = 10 g of drug in every 100 g of the total

Ratio strength is another way of expressing concentration, in terms of parts of active drug related to any number of parts of the whole. Ratio strength is usually expressed in terms of 1 part of active drug relative to the total number of parts of the product, as opposed to percent, which is any number of parts of active drug relative to 100 parts of product.

Example: Express 1 g of epinephrine in 1 L of solution as a percent strength and as a ratio strength.

First convert the units to g and mL:

    1 L = 1,000 mL

To convert to **percentage strength**, set the denominator on the right side of the ratio-proportion equation to 100 and calculate for the numerator.

$$\frac{1\,\text{g epinephrine}}{1,000\,\text{mL}} = \frac{\text{g active}}{100\,\text{mL product}} = 0.1\%\,\text{w/v}$$

To convert to **ratio strength**, set the numerator on the right side of the ratio-proportion equation to 1 and calculate for the denominator.

$$\frac{1\,\text{g epinephrine}}{1,000\,\text{mL}} = \frac{1\,\text{active}}{x\,\text{mL product}} = 1{:}1,000\,\text{w/v}$$

Parts per million (ppm) is a special case of ratio strength. Instead of fixing the numerator as 1, in this case you fix the denominator constant as 1,000,000. Parts per billion (ppb) and trillion (ppt) are handled in an analogous fashion.

DILUTION, CONCENTRATION, AND ALLIGATION

In some cases, you may receive a prescription in which you need to either dilute a product you have on hand or make a product more concentrated. These problems can generally be solved by:

1. Using the equation: (initial quantity, Q_1) × (initial concentration, C_1) = (final quantity, Q_2) × (final concentration, C_2)

   $$Q_1 \times C_1 = Q_2 \times C_2$$

2. Determining the quantity of active ingredient needed and then calculating the quantity of the available solution (usually a concentrated stock solution) that will provide the needed amount of active ingredient

Example:

If 250 mL of a 15% v/v solution of methyl salicylate in alcohol are diluted to 1,500 mL, what will be the percentage strength of this diluted solution?

$$250 \text{ mL} \times 15\% = 1,500 \text{ mL} \times x\%$$

$$x = 2.5\% \text{ v/v}$$

Alligation

Alligation is a method of solving problems that involves mixing multiple products that have different percentage strengths.

Alligation Alternate

This method allows calculation of the number of parts of two or more components of a given strength when they are mixed to prepare a mixture of a desired strength. Crosswise subtraction is used to determine the amounts needed of each component. This method can be used regardless of how concentration is expressed (mg/mL, ratio, parts, %).

Example:

In what proportion should a 20% benzocaine ointment be mixed with an ointment base to produce a 2.5% w/w benzocaine ointment?

Since there is no active drug in the ointment base, its strength can be expressed as 0%. To complete this problem, set up a table with the high concentration (i.e., 20%) in the upper left corner and the low concentration (i.e., 0%) in the lower left corner. The desired concentration (i.e., 2.5%) is placed in the center column between the low and high concentrations. Subtract diagonally to calculate the parts of the low and high concentration solutions to be mixed. See the following table for the appropriate setup of this problem.

Strengths to Be Mixed	Desired	Difference in Strength Mixed (crosswise subtraction of absolute values)
20%		2.5 parts (2.5−0) of 20% ointment
	2.5%	
0%		17.5 parts (20 − 2.5) of ointment base

Therefore, 2.5 parts of the 20% w/w ointment should be added to 17.5 parts of the ointment base.

For example, if 12 g were to be dispensed in the preceding problem, you would use the following parts.

Parts of high concentration: 2.5 parts

Parts of low concentration: 17.5 parts

Total parts (i.e., high plus low concentration): 20 parts

To calculate the amount of the *high* concentration to be mixed:

$$\frac{2.5\,\text{parts}}{20\,\text{parts}} = \frac{x\,\text{g}}{12\,\text{g}}$$
$$x = 1.5\,\text{g}$$

To calculate the amount of the *low* concentration to be mixed:

$$\frac{17.5\,\text{parts}}{20\,\text{parts}} = \frac{x\,\text{g}}{12\,\text{g}}$$
$$x = 10.5\,\text{g}$$

ELECTROLYTE SOLUTIONS

Millimoles and Milliequivalents

A review of several chemistry concepts will be useful before beginning milliequivalent calculations.

- Moles (mol): Measurement of the amount of a substance; Avogadro's number of particles (6.023×10^{23})
- Atomic weight: Found on the periodic table; 1 mol of that atom weighs that many grams (also, 1 mmol of that atom weighs that many mg)
- Molecular weight (MW): The sum of all the atomic weights for all of the atoms in the molecule. 1 **mole** of the molecule will weigh the value of the molecular weight in

grams. However, in electrolyte solutions and osmolarity calculations, it is necessary to convert to millimoles. This can be visualized in the following important equations:

$$\text{moles} = \frac{\text{Amount (grams)}}{\text{Molecular weight}}$$

$$\text{millimoles} = \frac{\text{Amount (milligrams)}}{\text{Molecular weight}}$$

- Molar solution: The molarity of a solution is the moles of solute in every 1 L of solution. This is an important concept on the NAPLEX, as questions can ask for the answer in terms of molarity; therefore, on the last step of the problem, you would then need to calculate how many moles there are in 1 L for the solutes in the problem.

The following table displays the valence of the most common ions. This information will likely not be provided on the NAPLEX.

Valence	Ions
+1	Sodium, potassium, lithium
+2	Barium, calcium, magnesium, zinc
+3	Aluminum
+1 or +2	Copper
+2 or +3	Iron, manganese
−1	Acetate, chloride, bicarbonate
−2	Sulfate, carbonate
−1, −2, or −3	Phosphate, citrate

In the magnesium chloride example, Mg^{+2} is divalent; it takes two Cl^- to make as much negative charge as one Mg^{+2}. Therefore, the correct formula is $MgCl_2$, not MgCl. NaCl, however, is made up of two monovalent ions, so the charges are equal.

The concept of equivalents is important in pharmacy when dispensing electrolytes or small drug molecules as salts. For example, a prescription that is written for 40 mg of potassium chloride does not contain the same amount of elemental potassium as a prescription written for 40 mg potassium acetate. The reason is that the 40 mg in each prescription is the total weight of potassium and the salt form (i.e., chloride or acetate).

To overcome this problem for electrolytes, the prescriptions will be written in terms of milliequivalents (mEq). For example, a prescription that calls for 40 mEq of potassium chloride will contain the same amount of elemental potassium as a prescription that calls for 40 mEq of potassium acetate.

Use the following equation to calculate mEq:

$$\text{milliequivalents (mEq)} = \frac{\text{Amount (milligrams)}}{\text{Molecular weight}} \times \text{valence}$$

Example:

How many milligrams of potassium citrate powder (MW = 324.41) should be weighed to compound 1 dose of the following prescription?

Rx   Potassium citrate 20 mEq PO TID

Recall that potassium has a valence of +1 and citrate has a −3, so the formula must have 3 potassium ions for every citrate or $K_3(C_6H_5O_7)$.

$$20\,\text{mEq} = \frac{x\,\text{mg}}{324.1} \times 3$$
$$x = 2{,}160\,\text{mg}$$

Therefore, 20 mEq of potassium citrate provides 20 mEq of potassium and 20 mEq of citrate. This means that a quantity of 2,160 mg of potassium citrate would provide 20 mEq of potassium and 20 mEq of citrate.

Osmolarity and Isotonicity

Osmotic pressure is the pressure that exists across a semipermeable membrane due to the free movement of solvent but not solute. Because cell membranes are semipermeable, this concept is important in patients. When administering parenteral drugs, you must balance the osmolarity of your medication with the osmolarity of the body. If not, tissue damage, pain, and possibly death can result due to cells swelling or shrinking with the movement of solvent.

Solutions are considered isotonic when each one has the same osmotic pressure; in pharmacy and medicine, the reference solution is the plasma (280–300 mOsm/L). Hypertonic solutions have higher osmotic pressure than this; hypotonic solutions have lower osmotic pressure. Some other facts you should remember about osmotic pressure are:

- It is a colligative property, based on the number of particles in solution.
- It can be calculated directly, using dissociation constants.
  - NaCl dissociates into sodium and chloride 80% in aqueous solution.
  - For every 100 particles, 80 will have dissociated (making 160 particles) and 20 will not → 180 particles (20 + 160).

    $$\frac{180\,\text{particles after dissociation}}{100\,\text{particles before dissociation}} = 1.8 = i$$

- To calculate the milliosmoles (mOsm) in a given solution, multiply the millimoles by the theoretical number of particles that the compound would dissociate into in solution.

$$mOsm = \frac{Amount\,(mg)}{Molecular\,weight} \times \begin{array}{c} Theoretical\,number\,of\,particles \\ (or\,disassociation\,constant) \end{array}$$

- The NAPLEX may ask for answers to be written in terms of milliosmolarity. Remember: To calculate milliosmolarity you need to calculate the amount of milliosmoles in the quantity of solution in the problem and convert to 1 L at the end.

Example:

Calculate the osmolarity of NS in mOsm/L. MW NS = 58.5 and $i = 1.8$.

NS = normal saline = 0.9% w/v NaCl in water

$$\frac{0.9\,g}{100\,mL} = \frac{x\,g}{1,000\,mL}$$

$x = 9\,g$ or 9,000 mg of NaCl per liter

$$x\,mOsm = \frac{9,000\,mg}{58.5} \times 1.8$$

$$x = 276.9\,mOsm/L$$

COMPOUNDING CALCULATIONS

Use of Prefabricated Dosage Forms in Compounding

Example:

Rx	Aspirin	300 *mg*
	Lactose	*qs*
	M.ft. cap DTD #60	

Using 325-mg aspirin tablets (weighing 430 mg each) as the source drug, how many tablets are needed to compound this prescription? How many grams of the crushed powder should be weighed out?

$$\frac{300\,mg\,ASA}{capsule} \times 60\,capsules \times \frac{tablet}{325\,mg\,ASA} = 55.38\,tablets \rightarrow 56\,tablets$$

$$55.38\,tablets \times 430\,mg\,total\,tablet\,weight = 23,813\,mg = 23.813\,g$$

Reconstitution Calculations

Example:

Cefadroxil powder for oral suspension comes in a strength of 250 mg/5 mL. The reconstitution instructions are to add 70 mL of purified water to yield a final solution volume of 100 mL. How many grams of cefadroxil powder are in the bottle?

$$\frac{250 \text{ mg cefadroxil}}{5 \text{ mL suspension}} \times 100 \text{ mL} = 5{,}000 \text{ mg} = 5 \text{ g}$$

Drip Rate Calculations

IV medications are regulated by one of the following methods:

- Drip chambers
  - Deliver drops of defined volume.
  - Flow is adjusted by the nurse to a set number of *whole* drops per minute.
  - Standard sets are 10 gtt/mL or 15 gtt/mL.
  - Pediatric and critical care drugs may use microdrop infusion sets: 60 gtt/mL.
- Infusion pumps
  - Deliver a rate of mL/hr.
  - Round to the nearest 0.1 mL.

Example:

17 mL of concentrated vancomycin solution is added to a 100-mL piggyback bag of NS. This solution is to be infused over 1 hour. What is the infusion rate?

$$\frac{17 \text{ mL vancomycin} + 100 \text{ mL NS}}{60 \text{ min}} = 117 \text{ mL/60 min} = 117 \text{ mL/hr}$$

What is the infusion rate in drops/min if the drug is administered using an infusion set that delivers 10 gtt/mL?

$$\frac{117 \text{ mL}}{60 \text{ min}} \times \frac{10 \text{ gtt}}{\text{mL}} = 19.5 \text{ gtt/min} = 20 \text{ gtt/min}$$

Calculations Involving Calories

The usual term is Calorie (with a capital C), which is equal to 1 kilocalorie. Therefore, Calories and kilocalories are synonymous.

To calculate the caloric requirements for a hospitalized patient, first calculate that patient's basal energy requirement. The calculated basal energy expenditure is then multiplied by a stress factor (usually between 1 and 2) to obtain a total energy expenditure (TEE).

The normal adult requires 25–35 Cal/kg/day. The Calories provided by a TPN can be estimated as follows:

Dextrose in the hydrated form (D_5W, $D_{70}W$, etc.)	3.4 Cal/g
Carbohydrates	4 Cal/g
Fats	9 Cal/g
Protein	4 Cal/g

Dextrose in water is the hydrated form and is used in TPN. Although dextrose is a carbohydrate, water molecules are attached to the dextrose to make it more soluble. Therefore, when calculating caloric content of a TPN, 3.4 Cal/g should be used for the dextrose content.

To prevent essential fatty acid deficiency, particularly a deficiency of linoleic acid, fats are incorporated into TPNs usually two to three times weekly. Fats are provided through infusion of oil emulsions. Fatty oil emulsions are approximately isotonic, have a milky appearance, and can be infused into peripheral blood vessels. Every milliliter of 10% fat emulsion has 1.1 Calories, whereas every milliliter of 20% fat emulsion has 2 calories.

Calculations Involving Amino Acids

The average adult requires approximately 1 g/kg/day of amino acids. Amino acids are included in TPN primarily to provide protein and nitrogen supplementation. On average, 16% of an amino acid solution is nitrogen content.

Example:

How many milliliters of an 8.5% amino acid solution are required to provide 20 g of nitrogen?

$$\frac{16\,g\,nitrogen}{100\,g\,amino\,acids} = \frac{20\,g\,nitrogen}{x\,g\,amino\,acids}$$

$$x = 125\,g\,amino\,acids$$

$$\frac{8.5\,g\,amino\,acids}{100\,mL} = \frac{125\,g\,amino\,acids}{x\,mL}$$

$$x = 1{,}470\,mL$$

Of importance is the Cal/g nitrogen ratio. The desired ratio is 125/1 up to 150/1. That is, a formula should provide at least 125 Calories for each gram of nitrogen being infused.

Compounding Considerations for TPNs

Both calcium and phosphate are essential components of TPN formulas. Sources of calcium include the chloride and gluconate salts. Phosphorus is supplied as combinations of mono- and disodium phosphates or mono- and dipotassium phosphates. The exact ratio depends on the pH of the solution.

Depending upon the relative concentrations of the soluble calcium salts and the phosphate salts, a chemical reaction may occur forming the very **insoluble dibasic calcium phosphate** ($CaPO_4$). This fine, white precipitate may form slowly and be difficult to visualize, especially if a milky fatty oil emulsion is also included in the TPN.

Methods for lessening the incompatibility problem:

1. Keep Ca and PO_4 concentrations below certain limits (solubility curves are available for various mixtures).
2. Agitate the mixture after each ingredient addition.
3. Add Na or K phosphates first and calcium salt last.
4. Add the Na or K phosphates to the amino acid solution, and the calcium salt to the dextrose solution; then, mix by shaking.
5. Use a 0.2 micron filter for nonfat emulsion formulas; a 1.2 micron filter is needed for fatty oil emulsions.

Biostatistics

28

This chapter contains the following:

- **Descriptive statistics: Summarizing the data**
- **Inferential statistics: Predicting outcomes**
- **Statistical test selection**

DESCRIPTIVE STATISTICS: SUMMARIZING THE DATA

Central Tendency

Central tendency is a general term used to describe the distribution of a set of values or measurements and the simplification to a single value near a point in the dataset that represents where the largest portion of data are located. The following are the most commonly used central tendency measures.

Median (m): The median is the value directly in the middle of the ranked values in a dataset; that is, 50% of all ranked values are smaller than the median and the other 50% of ranked values are larger. The median is **not** influenced by extreme values (outliers). The median is useful in situations in which there are unusually low or high values that would render the mean unrepresentative of the data.

Mean ($\overline{X}$ or μ): The mean is the average of all observations in a dataset. The mean is the most commonly used measure of central tendency because it has properties that make it useful for statistical analyses. It is influenced by extreme values (outliers) and is most useful when the data are symmetrically distributed without outliers (i.e., normal distribution).

Mode: The mode is the value with the greatest frequency of occurrence. It is not generally used because it is often not representative of the data, particularly when the dataset is small.

Variability

An additional measure that describes the variability in a dataset is, therefore, generally provided with a central tendency measure to better describe the dataset. The following are the most commonly used measures of variability.

Standard deviation (SD or σ): The standard deviation is the most common measure of the variability around the mean. It is used with a mean because it is most informative when the dataset is normally distributed, as described below. The mean and standard deviation are commonly used together as the most informative measures of central tendency and variability of a dataset, respectively.

Standard error of the mean (SEM): The standard error of the mean is defined as the variability of the sample means. It is calculated as the SD divided by the square root of the sample size. This will always be smaller than the sample SD. It is sometimes reported in the scientific and medical literature and is an intermediary step in calculating confidence intervals.

Absolute range: The absolute range is simply the difference between the largest and smallest observation in a dataset. A disadvantage is that the range is based solely on two observations and is likely not representative of the whole dataset. Absolute range is particularly susceptible to outliers.

Interquartile range (IQR): Quartiles are calculated in a way similar to the median, which splits a dataset into two equally sized groups. Quartiles split the data into four approximately equal sized groups. The interquartile range is the range between the lower and upper quartiles. Like the median, the interquartile range is not influenced by unusually high or low values and is particularly useful when data are not symmetrically distributed.

- The lower quartile (Q_L or Q_1) is the 25th percentile; that is, 25% of the data are below the value of Q_1.
- The upper quartile (Q_U or Q_3) is the 75th percentile; that is, 75% of the data are below the value of Q_3.

Boxplots are one-dimensional graphs that can be drawn from the range, IQR, and median, as displayed here.

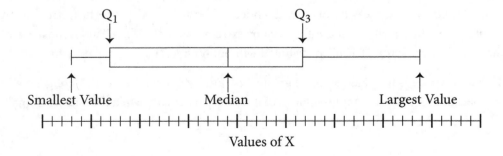

Distributions

Statistical test selection relies heavily on the distribution of data. These distributions can be summarized by a central tendency and variation around that center. The most important distribution is the normal or Gaussian curve. This "bell-shaped" curve is symmetric, with one side the mirror image of the other.

The distribution of any dataset can be assessed visually using a **histogram**. The x-axis represents the actual values in the dataset which, for pharmacy, are usually measures made of patients enrolled in a clinical trial (e.g., systolic blood pressure, creatinine clearance, low-density lipoprotein cholesterol concentrations). The y-axis represents the frequency of the value or the number of patients who had a value within a defined range. An example of a histogram is displayed here.

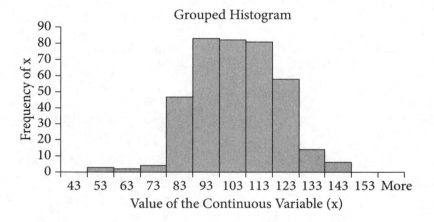

As the sample size (n) displayed in the histogram here approaches the population size (N), the lines on the graph become smooth and look more like following graph for normally distributed data:

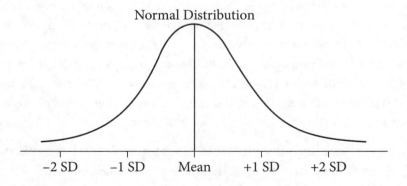

There are important attributes of the Normal Distribution shown in the preceding graph that can be useful in a number of problems on the NAPLEX. Importantly, the data is symmetric about the mean, as shown by the vertical line in the graph. This means that 50% of the values will be greater than the mean and 50% of the values will be less than the mean. Because this is the definition of a median, the mean and median are equal values in a normal distribution. The informative power of the normal distribution comes from the value of the standard deviation:

- The mean ± 1 SD contains 68% of the values in the dataset (or population).
- The mean ± 2 SD contains 95% of the values in the dataset (or population).
- The mean ± 3 SD contains 99.7% of the values in the dataset (or population).

The following graph displays two normal curves with the same means but different standard deviations:

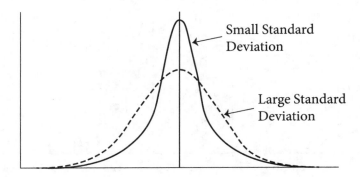

Example:

Patients ($n = 100$) enrolled in a clinical trial have a mean ± SD creatinine clearance of $110 ± 20$ mL/min. Approximately how many patients have creatinine clearance values between 70 and 110 mL/min?

Answer: The value of 70 mL/min is 2 SD away from the mean in the negative direction, and the value of 110 mL/min is the value of the mean. Approximately 95% of the values will be ± 2 SD away from the mean. Because the question is asking for only 2 SD in the negative direction and the normal distribution is symmetrical, it will be half the value of 95%. Half of 95% is 47.5%. Therefore, approximately 47.5% of the sample size of $n = 100$ patients will have values in this range. The answer would be approximately 48 patients have creatinine clearance values in this range.

Not all curves are normally distributed. Sometimes the curve is skewed either positively or negatively. For skewed distributions, the median is a better representation of central tendency than is the mean, and the IQR is a better measure of the variability than is the SD.

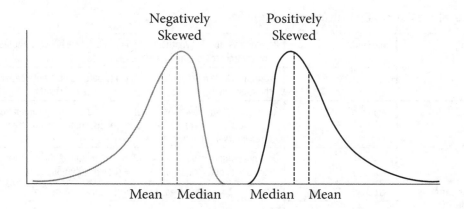

INFERENTIAL STATISTICS: PREDICTING OUTCOMES

The main goal of several studies in the pharmacy literature is to compare measurements from two groups of study patients: a group that receives a standard drug (i.e., control) and a group that receives an investigational drug. Even if both groups are administered placebo, it is highly unlikely that an identical mean and standard deviation of any value will be obtained for both groups. This is due to inherent variability in humans, among other sources, and is termed sampling error. The purpose of inferential statistics is to determine if the observed differences in the measures between the two groups of patients is due to chance (i.e., sampling error) or if one drug is really better than the other.

The following table summarizes important definitions regarding statistical inference.

General Statistical Definitions

Hypotheses	Hypothesis	Theoretical statement that the study is intended to test.
	Null hypothesis	States that there is no difference between the study and control groups.
	Alternative hypothesis	States that the null hypothesis is incorrect; there is a difference between the study and control groups.
Variables	Independent variable	Known variable(s).
	Dependent variable	Variable with a value dependent upon the value of an independent variable.
	Qualitative variable	Variable that yields observations by which individuals can be categorized according to some characteristic or quality.
	Quantitative variable	Variables that yield numerical observations that can be measured through statistical analysis. Qualitative variables can be transformed to quantitative variables by assigning numerical values to the observations.

General Statistical Definitions   *(cont'd)*

Error	Type I error	Rejecting a true null hypothesis: Finding a difference between the study and control groups that does not exist.
	Type II error	Accepting a false null hypothesis: Failing to detect a difference between the study and control groups when a difference truly exists.
Tests	Parametric	Requires prior knowledge of the nature of the data under examination; data must fall under a normal (Gaussian) distribution and be measured on an interval or a ratio scale.
	Nonparametric	Does not require prior knowledge of the distribution of the observations; data need not follow a normal or Gaussian distribution.
Miscellaneous definitions	Accuracy	Measure of how close a measured value is to the expected value.
	Precision	Measure of how close a particular measured value is to the other values in a set of measurements; does not imply proximity between measured values and the expected value.
	Sample	Data set taken under homogeneous conditions; a subset of a population.
	Population	Entire group from which a sample is taken.
	Gaussian (or normal) distribution	A bell-shaped distribution. Given a large enough sample size, the Central Limit Theorem states that the distribution of means will follow this type of distribution even if the population is not Gaussian. • 68% of values fall within $\pm$ 1 SD of the mean • 95% of values fall within $\pm$ 2 SD of the mean • 99.7% of values fall within $\pm$ 3 SD of the mean

Several additional statistical concepts follow, in slightly greater detail. Many of these concepts apply regardless of the statistical test chosen.

Confidence Intervals

Statistical decisions are made based on sampling from a larger population. The true values for the population may be above or below the sample values. For example, the sample mean is unlikely to be the same value as the actual mean of the entire population. Therefore, confidence intervals are calculated from the sample to provide a range of values that is likely to contain the actual population value. The most common confidence interval used is the 95% confidence interval. This interval implies that you are 95% confident that the actual mean value of the population lies within this range of values. The 5% of uncertainty is the same concept as described with the p-value discussed later in this chapter. Therefore, 95% confidence intervals can be used to determine statistical significance with a Type I error rate of 5%, as demonstrated next.

Example:

The following graph displays the 95% confidence intervals for blood pressure measurements following the administration of three drugs. The closed circle represents the sample mean estimate in each group, and the error bars encompass the values of the 95% confidence interval. Which drugs are statistically different from each other?

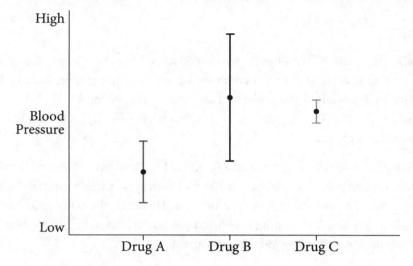

Answer:

When comparing two groups, any overlap of confidence intervals indicates that the groups would have a p-value >0.05 and are not significantly different. Therefore, if the graph represents 95% confidence intervals and each drug is compared with the others, Drugs B and C are no different in their effects, and Drug B is no different from Drug A. Drug A lowers blood pressure to a greater statistically significant extent than Drug C. Of note, comparing these drugs individually to one another as in this example would increase the Type I error rate $>5\%$, as will be discussed (see ANOVA).

Relative Risk and Odds Ratios

A relative risk (RR) is the ratio of the probability of an event occurring in a treatment (i.e., exposed) group to the probability of the event occurring in a control (i.e., nonexposed) group, as displayed in the following equation:

$$RR = \frac{p(\text{exposure group})}{p(\text{nonexposed group})}$$

Example:

In a local hospital over the last year, the frequency of patients with heart failure developing myopathy among those taking statins was 5 out of 100, and among patients not taking statins, it was 2 out of 100 patients. Calculate the relative risk.

Answer:

$$RR = \frac{5/100}{2/100} = 2.5$$

This implies that patients with heart failure who are taking statins were 2.5 times more likely to develop myopathy than patients who were not taking statins. Clearly, there are many variables in a study that could affect the relative risk beyond that of the statin use. Multivariate regression is commonly used in these types of analyses to account for variables beyond the exposure itself.

Similar to the relative risk, an **odds ratio** (OR) is also a measure of association between an exposure and an outcome. An odds ratio will provide a similar estimate to that of a relative risk, but the calculation is not as intuitive. However, the odds ratio has a mathematical advantage and is commonly reported because it is used in logistic regression to account for study variables beyond the exposure.

It is important to be able to make statistical determinations when provided with confidence intervals for relative risks and odds ratios. Simply put, if the 95% confidence interval contains 1, there is no statistically significant effect of the treatment (i.e., exposure). This is demonstrated in the following table for three hypothetical measures:

Relative Risk or Odds Ratio	Confidence Interval	Interpretation
1.98	(1.45–2.53)	Statistically significant (increased risk)
1.25	(0.78–1.53)	No statistical difference (risk the same)
0.45	(0.22–0.68)	Statistically significant (decreased risk)

Number Needed to Treat or Harm

The **number needed to treat (NNT)** is the number of patients receiving a specific treatment or intervention required to prevent one additional outcome (e.g., MI, stroke). The **number needed to harm (NNH)** indicates how many patients must be exposed to a risk factor to cause harm in one patient who otherwise would not have been harmed. To calculate the NNT or NNH, first calculate the **absolute risk reduction (ARR)** or **absolute risk increase (ARI)** of the exposure, respectively. The ARR and ARI are calculated as the difference between the event rates in the control group and the comparative group. The NNT is calculated as the inverse of the ARR, and the NNH is calculated as the inverse of the ARI, as shown in the equations:

$$NNT = \frac{1}{ARR}$$

$$NNH = \frac{1}{ARI}$$

Example:

In a local hospital over the last year, the frequency of patients with heart failure developing myopathy among those taking statins was 5 out of 100, and among patients not taking statins, it was 2 out of 100 patients. Calculate the relative risk.

In the preceding example, the event rate of myopathy in patients taking statins is 5 out of 100, or 5%. The event rate of myopathy in patients not exposed to statins is 2 out of 100, or 2%. In this case, the treatment is increasing the undesirable outcome of myopathy. Taking a statin increases the probability of myopathy from 2% to 5%. Therefore, instead of NNT, we are interested in calculating the NNH. To calculate NNH, first calculate ARI, and then take the inverse.

$$ARI = 5\% - 2\% = 3\%$$

$$NNH = \frac{1}{0.03} = 33$$

This implies that 33 patients exposed to statins would result in one extra case of myopathy that would not have happened under control conditions. These calculations and concepts are very similar for NNT.

p-Value and Statistical Significance

The p-value is the probability that the difference measured between your study group and the control group is the result of random chance rather than a true difference. The p-value is expressed as a value between 0 and 1; therefore, the higher the p-value, the more likely it is that a difference in sample means was due to chance and that a drug had no effect. When the p-value is low (e.g., <5%), it indicates that it was unlikely that the difference was due to chance; therefore, the drug had a statistically significant effect.

The null hypothesis may be rejected if there is a sufficiently small probability that it is true. A significance level (or α) of 0.05 is most commonly chosen, although it should be chosen based on the relative consequences of making a Type I or Type II error in the particular study setting. When a 0.05 significance level is chosen, if $p \leq 0.05$, a statistically significant difference in treatment effect exists between the control and treatment groups. If $p > 0.05$, the results of the study are considered to be not statistically significant, meaning no difference exists between the treatment and control groups. Choosing a larger significance level, like $p = 0.1$, gives a higher probability of rejecting a true null hypothesis (Type I error, or false positive test).

Types of Statistical Error

As defined in the table at the beginning of this chapter, there are two types of error that can be made at the end of a statistical test. The significance level (i.e., alpha, α) is commonly set to 0.05. This means that there is a 5% chance that a **Type I error (α error)** will be made during hypothesis testing. A Type I error is the conclusion that there is a statistical difference when in reality there is not one. Of course, you cannot know from a given experiment if you made a Type I error or not. You can only know the rate at which they occur (i.e., 5%).

The other type of error is **Type II error (β error)**, which is the conclusion that there is not a difference between groups when, in reality, there is a difference. A Type II error can only be made when the p-value is > 0.05 and the conclusion is made that there is no statistical difference between groups. As in a Type I error, one cannot know from a single experiment if a Type II error has been made, but can only calculate the frequency of the error. The Type I error rate is set at 5%, but the Type II error rate varies depending on the variable being measured and the study itself (see "Power and Sample Size"). Type II error rates are commonly designed to be <10% or 20%. The factors that affect Type II error are the same that affect study power.

Power and Sample Size

The power of a study is the ability to detect a difference between study groups if one actually exists. Study power is indirectly related to the likelihood of making a Type II (β) error. Therefore, as study power increases, the likelihood of concluding that there is not a difference when one actually does exist decreases. Therefore, as power increases, Type II error rate decreases. The following factors affect the power of a study:

- **Sample size (*n*):** The closer the sample size is to the actual population size, the easier it is to detect a difference.
- **Difference between the actual population means:** It will be easier to detect a difference between drugs with large effects versus the control or comparator. For example, it is much easier to show that a β-blocker will lower blood pressure compared to a placebo than it would be compared to an angiotensin-converting enzyme (ACE) inhibitor.
- **Variability around the population means (and sample means):** The more variable effect there is, the harder it is to show a difference. For example, if a drug only works in a small percentage of the population, it will be difficult to show statistical significance in a sample from the entire population.
- **Significance level, α:** The Type I error rate directly alters the Type II error rate. This is one reason why the significance level is traditionally set at 5%. If one wanted to decrease the Type I error rate and set it at 1%, it would increase the Type II error rate and, thereby, decrease the power of the study.

Of the factors just listed, the only way to decrease Type II error (increase power) without increasing Type I error is to increase the sample size.

At the conclusion of a study, if the p-value is > 0.05, the actual study power can be calculated. This is done by simply using the actual values of the factors listed about the study (e.g., the sample size, variability, and mean difference). Of course, it would only make sense to calculate the power of a study if the p-value was > 0.05. If the p-value is < 0.05, it is impossible to make a Type II error. Only a Type I error could have been made with a p-value < 0.05, and the power of the study would be irrelevant.

Correlation

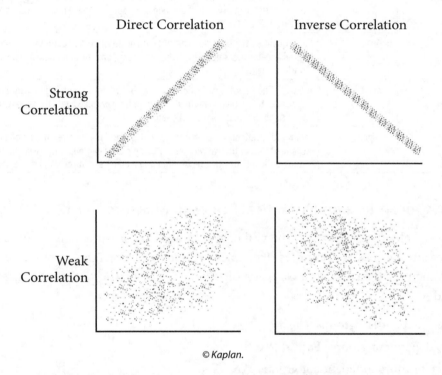

Direct Correlation   Inverse Correlation

Strong Correlation

Weak Correlation

© Kaplan.

A key point to remember is that an observed correlation between two variables does not imply that there is a causal link between the two variables. For example, warm weather causes an increase in both the crime rate and the incidence of sunburn. Crime rate and sunburn incidence will therefore be positively correlated; however, crime does not cause sunburn and sunburn does not cause crime.

STATISTICAL TEST SELECTION

The first thing that must be done when determining what statistical test should be employed is to identify the dependent variable and the scale of measurement that will be used for this variable. These scales are described in the table.

Types of Variables

Qualitative	Nominal	Characteristics that do not have numerical value and do not have order (e.g., gender or race).
	Ordinal	Characteristics that do not have numerical value but have an underlying order to their observations and can be ranked from highest to lowest (e.g., disagree, indifferent, agree, strongly agree).
Quantitative	Interval	Ordered set of categories, similar to an ordinal scale, with the additional requirement that the categories form a series of intervals that are identically spaced. An example is time as read on a clock, 10 A.M., 11 A.M., 12 P.M., 1 P.M., 2 P.M., etc.
	Ratio	Same qualities as an interval scale but with an absolute zero point to indicate a complete absence of the variable being measured. This is the most common type of numerical data in the biomedical and pharmaceutical sciences.
	Ranked	A group of numerical observations that can be arranged according to magnitude, such as in ordinal data. Ordinal data can be transformed into quantitative/ranked data by being assigned values that correspond to each observation's place in the sequence.
	Grouped	Quantitative variables that are categorized, particularly for presentation of data. Nominal variables can be changed to quantitative variables by being placed in groups and assigned numbers. For example, a clinical study could quantify gender by assigning females a value of 1 and males a value of 2.

Tests Appropriate for Numerical Scales of Measurement

Numeric scales (predominantly interval or ratio scales) of measurement are used when the measured values are numbers. Examples include height, weight, or blood pressure level. When the data follows a Gaussian distribution, parametric statistical tests should be used.

- Two independent groups: **_t_-test**
- Two dependent groups: **Paired _t_-test**
- Three or more independent groups: **ANOVA**
- Three or more dependent groups: **Repeated measures ANOVA**

_t_-Test

The _t_-test is one of the most commonly used statistical tests. It compares means obtained from the numeric data of two groups that are independent of each other. This statistical test is commonly used in the pharmacy literature to compare the outcomes of numeric data (e.g., clinical measures, drug concentrations). In a sample of patients who received an experimental drug versus a different (i.e., independent) sample of patients who received a control drug.

Paired *t*-Test

A paired *t*-test is used when the same sample is being used to compare the experimental and the control drug; that is, this test is appropriate when numeric data is being compared between two dependent groups. This is commonly referred to as a crossover design. A paired *t*-test is the appropriate statistical test for numeric or interval data.

ANOVA

When a third group (or more) is added to a study design for comparison, it is not appropriate to perform multiple *t*-tests. For example, an experimental drug to lower blood pressure is being compared to a group of patients taking β-blockers and another group of patients taking ACE inhibitors. In this study design, one cannot perform a *t*-test to compare the experimental drug to the β-blocker group and then perform another *t*-test to compare the ACE inhibitor group. Each time a *t*-test is performed there is a 5% chance of a Type I error; thus, multiple comparisons increase this rate of Type I error greater than 5%. Therefore, if three or more groups are being compared, it is appropriate to use an analysis of variance (ANOVA). An ANOVA will generate one p-value from the three groups. If the p-value is < 0.05, it states that at least one drug was different than another at lowering blood pressure. Importantly, the Type I error rate is maintained at 5% for an ANOVA.

To determine which drug has a statistically significant effect, additional tests are needed. These statistical tests are referred to as *post-hoc tests*. The most commonly used post-hoc test is Tukey's test. The Bonferroni and Scheffe's tests are also post-hoc tests that can be used to determine which groups were statistically different if an overall p-value from the ANOVA was less than 0.05. If a p-value is >0.05 following an ANOVA, no further tests are needed.

Repeated Measures ANOVA

The repeated measures ANOVA is the equivalent of using a paired *t*-test instead of a *t*-test. It, therefore, can be used in crossover studies when there are three or more study periods following appropriate wash-out of the drug between each period. This test is referred to as *repeated measures* because it is commonly used when the same measures are being made in patients throughout a study. For example, in many statin clinical trials, the low-density lipoprotein cholesterol (LDL-C) lowering ability of the statins is not determined at only one point but at several points (e.g., 1, 3, 6, 12, 18, and 24 months). To determine if significant LDL-C lowering occurred in patients during these time intervals, a repeated measures ANOVA must be used. The Dunnett's test is the post-hoc test that should be used if an overall p-value <0.05 is obtained.

When the data does not follow a Gaussian distribution, the same tests used for ordinal data should be employed.

Tests Appropriate for Ordinal Scales of Measurement

Ordinal scales of measurement are used when characteristics have an underlying order to their values but the numbers used are arbitrary (e.g., Likert scales). Various non-parametric tests (e.g., Mann-Whitney U and Wilcoxon Signed-Rank) are used for analyzing such data. Ordinal scales also are used for numeric data that are not distributed normally and that have a small sample size. The following are situations in which a nonparametric test should be considered:

- The outcome is ordinal and the sample is clearly not normally distributed.
- There are values that are too high or too low to obtain accurate measures. It is impossible to analyze such data with a parametric test because the exact value is not determined.
- The sample size is small and the sample is not approximately normally distributed. Data transformation can be done by taking the logarithm of the values. This is common for biological data, which often has outliers in the positive direction (i.e., skewed to the right).

The following table lists parametric tests for normally distributed data and the corresponding nonparametric test for ordinal or non-normally distributed data.

Parametric versus Nonparametric Statistics

Parametric Tests	Nonparametric Equivalent
t-Test $\longrightarrow$	Wilcoxon-Rank Sum (Mann Whitney U)
Paired t-test $\longrightarrow$	Wilcoxon Sign Rank (Sign Test)
ANOVA $\longrightarrow$	Kruskal-Wallis Test
Repeated measures ANOVA $\longrightarrow$	Friedman Test
Note: The Wilcoxon-Rank Sum is the post-hoc test for the Kruskal-Wallis Test	

Tests Appropriate for Nominal Scales of Measurement

Nominal scales are used for characteristics that do not have numerical value (such as gender or race). The Chi-square test and its variants are used to test the null hypothesis that proportions are equal, or that factors or characteristics are not associated with each other.